www.harcourt-international.com

Bringing you products from all Harcourt Health Sciences companies including Baillière Tindall, Churchill Livingstone, Mosby and W.B. Saunders

- ▷ **Browse** for latest information on new books, journals and electronic products

- ▷ **Search** for information on over 20 000 published titles with full product information including tables of contents and sample chapters

- ▷ **Keep up to date** with our extensive publishing programme in your field by registering with eAlert or requesting postal updates

- ▷ **Secure online ordering** with prompt delivery, as well as full contact details to order by phone, fax or post

- ▷ **News** of special features and promotions

If you are based in the following countries, please visit the country-specific site to receive full details of product availability and local ordering information

USA: www.harcourthealth.com

Canada: www.harcourtcanada.com

Australia: www.harcourt.com.au

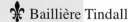 Baillière Tindall   CHURCHILL LIVINGSTONE   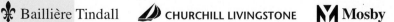 Mosby   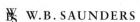 W.B. SAUNDERS

Diseases of the Macula

Photographers

Anne Bolton
Richard Baseler
Robert Fagan
Peter Fontaine
James Gendron
Bogdan Stoj

Artists

T. R. Tarrant
Jenni Miller

Diseases of the Macula

A practical approach

Jack J. Kanski
MD, MS, FRCS, FRCOphth
Honorary Consultant Ophthalmic Surgeon
Prince Charles Eye Unit
King Edward VII Hospital
Windsor, UK

Stanislaw A. Milewski
MD, MA, FACS
Assistant Clinical Professor of Surgery
Department of Ophthalmology
University of Connecticut, USA

With contributions from
Peter H. Judson, MD
Jerry Neuwirth, MD
Michael S. Ruddat, MD
Marion Joseph Stoj, MD
Vaughan Tanner, FRCOphth

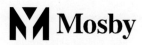

London • Edinburgh • New York • Philadelphia • St Louis • Sydney • Toronto 2002

MOSBY
An imprint of Harcourt Publishers Limited

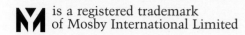
First published 2002

ISBN 0723432414

British Library Cataloguing in Publication Data
A catalogue record for this book is available from the British Library

Library of Congress Cataloging in Publication Data
A catalog record for this book is available from the Library of Congress

Note
Medical knowledge is constantly changing. As new information becomes available, changes in treatment, procedures, equipment and the use of drugs become necessary. The authors and the publishers have taken care to ensure that the information given in this text is accurate and up to date. However, readers are strongly advised to confirm that the information, especially with regard to drug usage, complies with the latest legislation and standards of practice.

Existing UK nomenclature is changing to the system of Recommended International Nonproprietary Names (rINNs). Until the UK names are no longer in use, these more familiar names are used in this book in preference to rINNs, details of which may be obtained from the British National Formulary.

Commissioning Editor: Sue Hodgson
Project Development Manager: Louise Cook
Project Manager: Cheryl Brant
Designer: Andy Chapman
Illustrations Manager: Mick Ruddy

Typeset by IMH(Cartrif), Loanhead, Scotland
Printed in China by the RDC Group

Contents

Preface

Despite great advances in medicine, macular disease remains a very common cause of severe visual impairment, particularly in the elderly. The purpose of this book is to provide a practical and somewhat didactic approach to the diagnosis and management of macular disorders. We have used the term 'macula' liberally and have included diseases that primarily affect the macula such as age-related macular degeneration, as well as those that may have an indirect but nevertheless significant effect on macular function such as vascular and inflammatory diseases. We have not, however, described diseases that primarily affect the peripheral retina such as rhegmatogenous retinal detachment and retinopathy of prematurity. We also felt that the effects of tumors on the macula would not be appropriate for this type of book.

Diseases of the Macula is primarily intended for general ophthalmologists, those in training, and optometrists. In order to facilitate reading we have described the important disease at the beginning of each chapter and the less important towards the end. Selected case studies have been included to enhance understanding of disease processes. The further reading section is not meant to be comprehensive. We have included mainly more recent papers and have only included older publications that have special merit.

J.J.K.
S.A.M.
2001

Acknowledgments

We thank the following colleagues and medical photographic departments for supplying us with additional material without which this book could not have been written:

C. Barry, Lions Eye Institute, Perth (Figures 3.92, 3.141, 5.8, , 5.33, 5.35, 5.66); **K. Bibby** (Figure 4.75); **Prof. A. Dick** (Figure 4.28); **S. Ford, Western Eye Hospital, London** (Figures 2.45, 2.58, 2.68, 2.88, 3.63, 3.117, 3.121, 4.9, 4.21, 4.44, 4.56, 4.70, 4.72); **P. Frith** (Figures 4.36, 4.55); **J. Govan** (Figures 5.68, 5.69); **E. Graham** (Figure 4.24); **K. Jordan** (Figures 2.85, 2.86, 5.37, 5.38); **Prof. S. Lightman** (Figures 4.30, 4.66); **A. Mitchell** (Figures 4.29, 4.76); **P. Morse** (Figures 2.15, 2.57, 2.89, 3.110, 3.131, 3.135, 3.144, 5.19, 5.31, 5.53, 5.54, 5.55, 5.56, 5.57); **K. Nischal** (Figures 3.120, 5.15, 5.25, 5.39); **B. Noble** (Figures 4.48, 4.52, 4.54); **Prof. M. Prost** (Figures 4.96, 4.97); **Royal Eye Hospital, Manchester** (Figures 4.69, 5.62); **J. Salmon** (Figures 2.83, 2.87, 3.107, 4.63, 4.64, 5.66); **K. Sehmi, Moorfields Eye Hospital, London** (Figures 2.103, 5.48, 5.58, 5.64); **A. Shun-Shin** (Figure 5.67); **M. Szreter** (Figure 4.6); **J. Talks** (Figure 2.36); **V. Tanner** (Figure 2.36); **D. Thomas** (Figures 3.101, 3.102, 3.103); **Wilmer Institute, Baltimore** (Figures 1.4, 1.10, 1.20, 1.21, 1.22, 1.23, 1.24, 1.25, 1.26, 1.27, 1.28, 1.29, 1.30, 2.1, 2.4, 2.7, 2.8, 2.13, 2.18, 2.21, 2.35, 2.43, 2.60, 2.76, 2.96, 2.101, 3.1, 3.6, 3.7, 3.9, 3.13, 3.17, 3.18, 3.19, 3.20, 3.21, 3.24, 3.26, 3.28, 3.29, 3.30, 3.31, 3.37, 3.38, 3.39, 3.41, 3.43, 3.47, 3.52, 3.53, 3.54, 3.128, 3.129, 3.130, 4.12, 5.30).

Chapter **1**

Introduction

Applied anatomy

Important landmarks (Figures 1.1 and 1.2)

1. The **macula** is a round area at the posterior pole measuring approximately 5.5 mm in diameter (about four discs). Histologically, it is the region of the retina containing xanthophyll pigment and more than one layer of ganglion cells.

2. The **fovea** is a depression in the inner retinal surface at the centre of the macula. Its diameter is the same as that of an average optic disc (1.5 mm). On ophthalmoscopy, it can be recognized by an oval light reflex arising from the increased thickness of the retina and internal limiting membrane in the parafoveal region.

3. The **foveola** forms the central floor of the fovea and has a diameter of 0.35 mm. It is the thinnest part of the retina and is devoid of ganglion cells (Figure 1.3). Its entire thickness consists only of cones and their nuclei.

4. The **foveal avascular zone** (FAZ) is located inside the fovea but outside the foveola. Its exact diameter is variable and its location can be determined with accuracy only by fluorescein angiography (Figure 1.4).

5. The **umbo** is a tiny depression in the very center of the foveola which corresponds to the ophthalmoscopically visible foveolar reflex that is seen in most normal eyes. Loss of this reflex may be an early sign of damage.

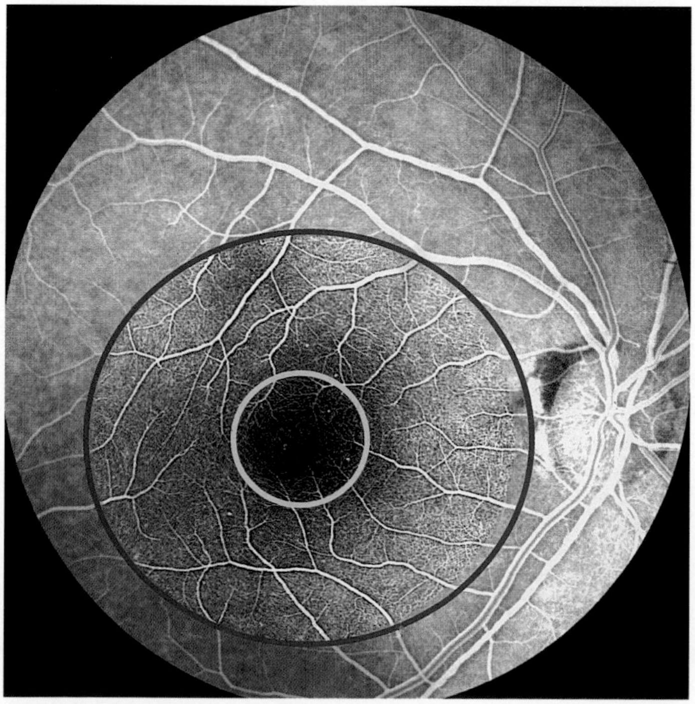

Figure 1.1 Anatomical landmarks: macula (blue circle); fovea (yellow circle)

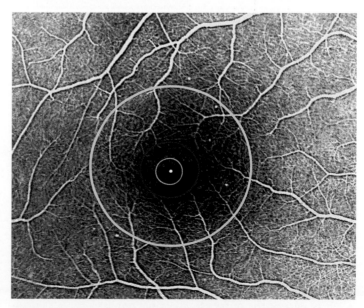

Figure 1.2 Anatomical landmarks: fovea (yellow circle); foveal avascular zone (red circle); foveola (lilac circle); umbo (central white spot)

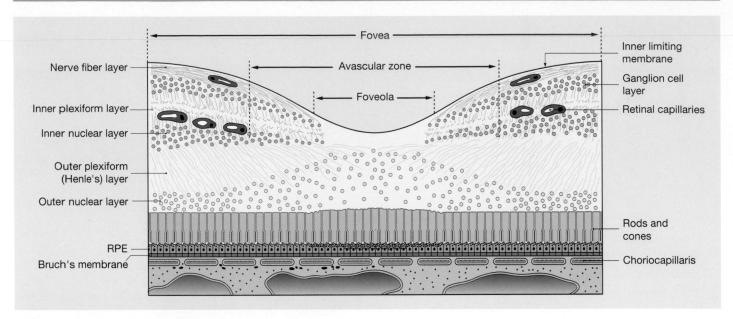

Figure 1.3 Cross-section of the fovea

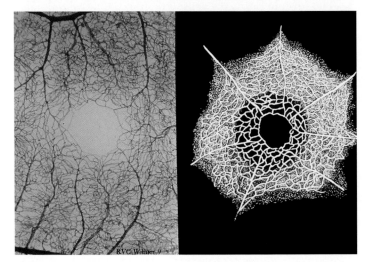

Figure 1.4 Foveal avascular zone

Retinal pigment epithelium

The retinal pigment epithelium (RPE) consists of a single layer of hexagonal cells, the apices of which contain villous processes that envelop the outer segments of the photoreceptors. The RPE cells at the fovea are taller, thinner and contain more and larger melanosomes than elsewhere in the fundus. The adhesion between the RPE and sensory retina is weaker than that between the RPE and Bruch's membrane. The potential space between the sensory retina and RPE is called the subretinal space. A separation between the RPE and sensory retina is called a retinal detachment, and subretinal fluid separates these two layers. The RPE serves two important functions in maintaining the integrity (i.e., dryness) of the subretinal space:

- It is part of the outer blood-retinal barrier.

- It actively pumps ions and water out of the subretinal space.

Bruch's membrane

Bruch's membrane separates the RPE from the choriocapillaris. On electron microscopy it consists of five elements:

- Basal lamina of the RPE.

- Inner collagenous layer.

- Thicker band of elastic fibers.

- Outer collagenous layer.

- Basal lamina of the outer layer of the choriocapillaris.

Changes in Bruch's membrane play a very important part in many macular disorders.

Clinical evaluation of macular disease

Symptoms

1. **Impairment of central vision** is the main symptom of macular disease. Typically, the patient complains that there is something obstructing central vision (positive scotoma) (Figure 1.5a). This is in contrast to the negative scotoma from an optic nerve lesion in which the patient notices a 'hole' in the centre of the visual field (Figure 1.5b).

2. **Metamorphopsia**, is an alteration in image shape which is a common symptom of macular disease (Figure 1.5c) which is not present in patients with optic nerve lesions (Figure 1.5d).

3. **Micropsia**, is a decrease in image size caused by spreading apart of foveal cones, is less common.

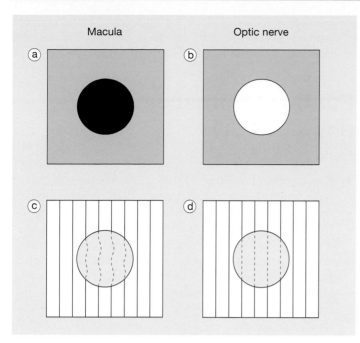

Figure 1.5 Comparison of symptoms between macular and optic nerve disease. (a) Positive scotoma in macular disease; (b) negative scotoma in optic nerve disease; (c) metamorphopsia in macular disease; (d) no metamorphopsia in optic nerve disease

4. **Macropsia**, is an increase in image size caused by crowding of foveal cones, is uncommon. It should be emphasized that colour vision is not significantly impaired in early macular disease, in contrast to lesions of the optic nerve in which loss of colour vision is an early feature.

Methods of examination

1. **Visual acuity** is the easiest and most important test of macular function, particularly for near. In patients with macular disease visual acuity is frequently worse when the patient looks through a pin hole. Hypermetropia, with disparity between the subjective and objective refraction of the eye, is characteristic of a shallow elevation of the sensory retina at the macula.

2. **Indirect slitlamp biomicroscopy** with a contact lens or a strong convex lens is used to examine the macula. Monochromatic light may be useful in detecting subtle macular lesions which may otherwise be overlooked. Green (red-free) light may also enhance detection of superficial retinal lesions such as wrinkling of the internal limiting membrane or cystoid macular edema. It is also useful in delineating the outline of subtle serous elevations of the sensory retina. Lesions involving the RPE and choroid are best detected using light at the red end of the spectrum.

3. **The Amsler grid** test evaluates the 10° of visual field surrounding fixation. It is primarily used for screening of

macular disease and is also useful in the diagnosis of subtle optic nerve lesions. There are seven charts which consists of a 10 cm square divided into smaller 5 mm squares. When it is viewed at one-third of a meter, each small square subtends an angle of 1°. The most useful charts are numbers 1 and 6. The latter has a finer central grid than chart number 1. The test is performed as follows:

- The patient should wear reading spectacles, if appropriate, and cover one eye.

- The patient is asked to look directly at the center dot with the uncovered eye and report any distortion, wavy lines, blurred areas or blank spots anywhere on the grid.

- A patient with an early macular lesion will report that the lines are wavy (Figure 1.6), whereas a patient with an optic nerve lesion will report that some of the lines are missing or faint (see Figure 1.5 d) but not distorted.

4. **Photostress testing** may be useful in demonstrating macular lesions when ophthalmoscopy is equivocal, as in early cystoid macular edema or central serous retinopathy. It may also be used to differentiate visual loss caused by macular disease from that caused by an optic nerve lesion. The test is a gross version of the dark adaptation test in which the visual pigments are bleached by light. This causes a temporary state of retinal insensitivity which is perceived by the patient as a scotoma. The recovery of vision is dependent on the ability of the photoreceptors to re-synthesize visual pigments. The test is performed as follows:

- The best corrected distance visual acuity is determined.

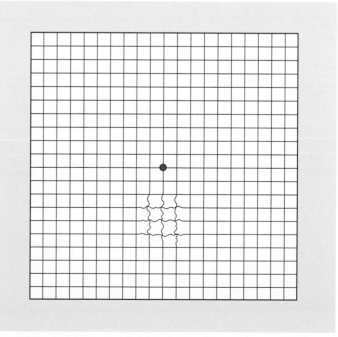

Figure 1.6 Amsler grid chart number 1 showing metamorphopsia just below fixation

- The patient fixates the light of a pen-torch or an indirect ophthalmoscope held about 3 cm away for about 10 seconds (Figure 1.7a).

- The photostress recovery time (PSRT) is measured by the time taken to read any three letters of the pre-test acuity line (Figure 1.7b).

- The test is performed on the other, presumably normal, eye and the results are compared.

In a patient with a macular lesion the PSRT will be longer (sometimes 50 seconds or more) as compared with the normal eye, whereas in a patient with an optic nerve lesion there will be no difference.

5. **Pupillary light reactions** are usually normal in eyes with macular disorders, although extensive retinal disease such as a retinal detachment may be associated with a relative afferent conduction defect (Marcus Gunn pupil). This is in contrast to mild lesions of the optic nerve in which pupillary abnormalities occur early.

6. The **potential visual acuity meter** is used to test macular function in eyes with opaque media. The instrument projects a standard Snellen chart onto the macula through a small area of an immature cataract and the patient is asked to read the letters (Figure 1.8).

Fundus fluorescein angiography

General principles

1. **Fluorescein binding** (Figure 1.9b) is the ability of between 70–85% of fluorescein molecules to bind to serum proteins on entering the circulation (bound fluorescein). The remaining fluorescein molecules remain unbound (free fluorescein). The major choroidal vessels are impermeable to both bound and free fluorescein molecules. However, the walls of the choriocapillaris are extremely thin and contain multiple fenestrations through which free (not bound) fluorescein molecules are able to escape into the extravascular space and also across Bruch's membrane.

2. The **inner blood-retinal barrier** (Figure 1.10a) is composed of the tight junctions of retinal capillary endothelial cells (E) across which neither bound nor free fluorescein molecules can pass. Figure 1.10c shows a normal fluorescein angiogram (FA). The basement membrane (B) and pericytes (P) play only a minor role in confining fluorescein molecules within the lumen of the retinal capillaries. An increase in vascular permeability caused by changes in the intravascular pressure or tissue hydrostatic pressure, or by a change in the capillary walls themselves, will permit leakage of both bound and free fluorescein molecules into the extravascular space (Figure 1.10b). Figure 1.10d shows leakage of fluorescein into the retina due to a breakdown in the inner blood-retinal barrier.

3. The **outer blood-retinal barrier** consists of the RPE and the tight junctional complexes called the zonula occludens (ZO) which are located between adjacent RPE cells. This prevents the passage of free fluorescein molecules across the RPE (Figure 1.11).

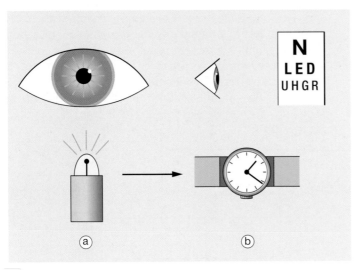

Figure 1.7 The photostress test

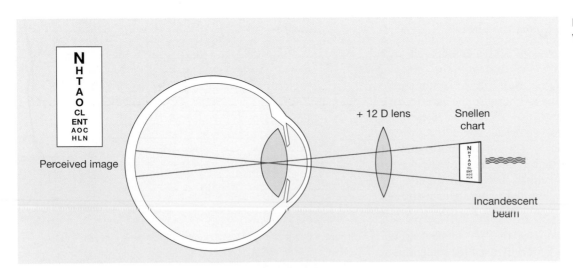

Figure 1.8 The potential visual acuity metre

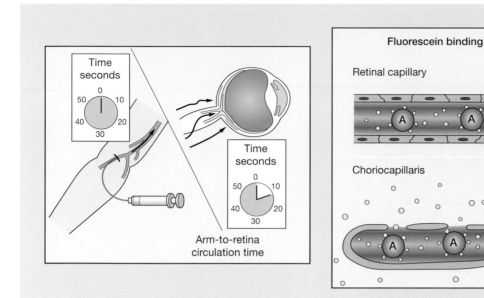

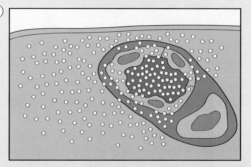

Figure 1.9 (a) Injection of fluorescein into the antecubital vein; (b) principles of fluorescein binding and permeability (A, albumin)

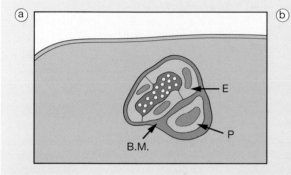

Figure 1.10 The inner blood-retinal barrier (B.M., basement membrane; P, pericyte; E, capillary endothelial cell): Intact barrier (a) & (b); disrupted barrier (c) & (d)

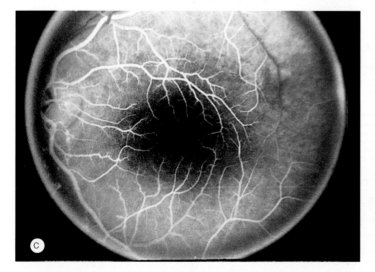

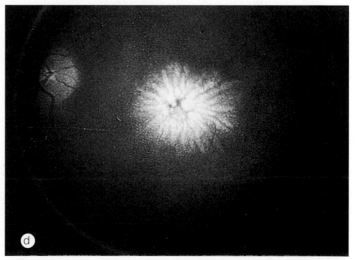

4. **Fluorescence** is the property of certain molecules to emit light energy of a longer wavelength when stimulated by light of a shorter wavelength. The excitation peak for fluorescein molecules is about 490 nm (blue part of the spectrum) and represents the maximal absorption of light energy by fluorescein. Molecules stimulated by this wavelength will be excited to a higher energy level and emit light of a longer wavelength, which will be in the green portion of the spectrum at about 530 nm (Figure 1.12).

5. **Filters** of two types are used to ensure that blue light enters the eye and only yellow-green light enters the camera. White light emitted from the retinal camera passes through a blue excitation filter. The emerging blue light then enters the eye and excites the fluorescein

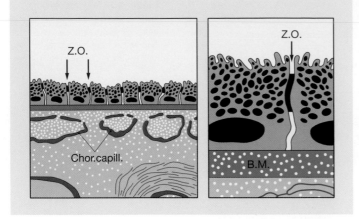

Figure 1.11 The outer blood-retinal barrier (Z.O., zona occludens; B.M., Bruch's membrane)

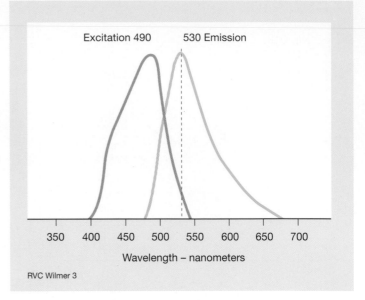

Figure 1.12 Excitation and emission of fluorescence

molecules in the retinal and choroidal circulations to a longer wavelength (yellow-green light). A yellow-green barrier filter then blocks any blue light that may leave the eye allowing only yellow-green light to pass through unimpaired to be recorded on film (Figure 1.13).

Photographic technique

To obtain good quality angiograms, the pupils have to be dilated and the media clear. The technique is as follows:

- The patient is seated in front of the camera with one arm outstretched.

- Fluorescein, usually 5 ml of a 10% solution, is drawn up into a syringe. In eyes with opaque media, 3 ml of a 25% solution may be preferred because it gives better results.

- A 'red-free' photograph is taken.

- Fluorescein is injected rapidly into the antecubital vein (see Figure 1.9a).

- Photographs are taken at approximately one-second intervals, between 5 and 25 seconds after injection.

- After the transit phase has been photographed in one eye, control pictures are taken of the opposite eye. If appropriate, late photographs can also be taken after 10 minutes and, occasionally, after 20 minutes if leakage is anticipated.

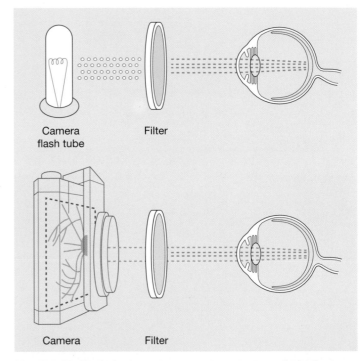

Figure 1.13 Photographic principles of fluorescein angiography

Adverse effects

- Frequent side-effects are discoloration of urine and skin.

- Mild complications are nausea, vomiting, flushing of the skin, itching, hives and excessive sneezing.

- Serious but rare complications are syncope, laryngeal edema, bronchospasm and anaphylactic shock.

It is very important to have a clear plan for managing these eventualities.

Phases of the angiogram

Fluorescein enters the eye through the ophthalmic artery, passing into the choroidal circulation through the short posterior ciliary arteries and into the retinal circulation through the central retinal artery. Because the route to the retinal circulation is slightly longer than that to the choroidal, the latter is filled about 1 second before the former. In the choroidal circulation, often no precise details are discernible, mainly because of the rapid leakage of free fluorescein molecules from the choriocapillaris and also because the melanin in the RPE cells blocks choroidal fluorescence. The angiogram consists of the following overlapping phases.

1. **Choroidal (pre-arterial) phase**, during which the choroidal circulation is filling, but no dye has reached the retinal arteries.

2. **Arterial phase** shows arterial filling and the continuation of choroidal filling (Figure 1.15).

3. **Arteriovenous (capillary) phase** shows complete filling of the arteries and capillaries with early lamellar flow in the veins in which the dye is seen on the lateral wall of the vein (Figure 1.16). Choroidal filling continues and background choroidal fluorescence increases as more free

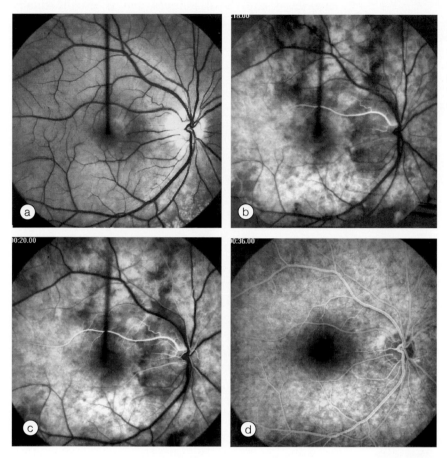

Figure 1.14 Normal choroidal phase in an eye with a cilioretinal artery: (a) Red free; (b) choroidal phase showing patchy filling of the choroid and filling of the cilioretinal artery; (c) arterial phase showing arterial filling and further filling of the choroid; (d) venous phase showing complete choroidal and retinal filling

2. **Arterial phase**, which follows 1 second after the prearterial phase and extends from the first appearance of dye in the arteries until the entire arterial circulation has been filled.

3. **Arteriovenous (capillary) phase**, which is characterized by complete filling of the arteries and capillaries with the appearance of early lamellar flow in the veins.

4. **Venous phase**, which can be subdivided according to the extent of venous filling and arterial emptying into early, mid and late stages.

Interpretation of the angiogram

1. **Choroidal (pre-arterial) phase**, which occurs between 8–12 seconds after dye injection, shows early patchy filling of the choroidal circulation due to the passage of free fluorescein molecules through the fenestrations of the choriocapillaris. A cilioretinal artery, if present, will also become filled at this time because it is derived from the posterior ciliary artery (Figure 1.14).

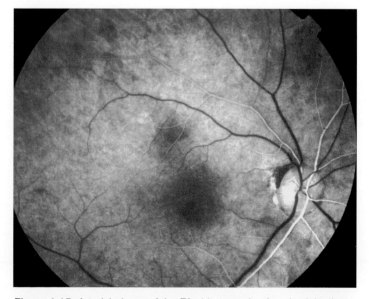

Figure 1.15 Arterial phase of the FA, 11 seconds after dye injection, showing filling of the choroid and retinal arteries

fluorescein molecules leak from the choriocapillaris into the extravascular space. In hypopigmented eyes, this may be so marked that details of the retinal capillaries may be lost. In highly pigmented eyes, background choroidal fluorescence will be less obvious.

4. **Early venous phase** shows complete arterial and capillary filling, and more marked lamellar venous flow (Figure 1.17).

5. **Mid venous phase** shows almost complete venous filling with minimal lamellar flow (Figure 1.18).

6. **Late venous phase** shows complete venous filling with less concentration of dye in the arteries.

5. **Late (elimination) phase** shows the effects of continuous recirculation, dilution and elimination of the dye. With each succeeding wave, the intensity of fluorescence becomes weaker (Figure 1.19). Late staining of the disc is a normal finding. Fluorescein is absent from the angiogram after 5–10 minutes and is usually totally eliminated from the body within several hours of administration.

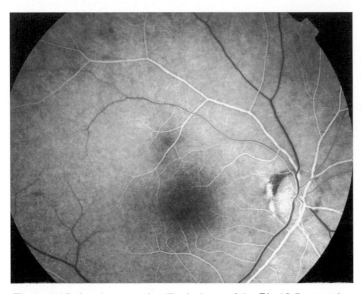

Figure 1.16 Arteriovenous (capillary) phase of the FA, 12.5 seconds after dye injection, showing complete arterial filling and early lamellar venous flow

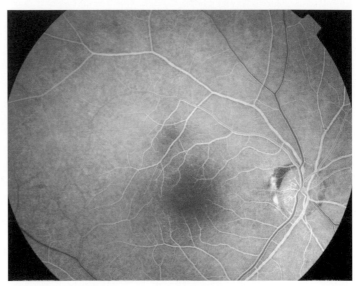

Figure 1.17 Early venous phase of the FA, 13.5 seconds after dye injection, showing marked lamellar venous flow

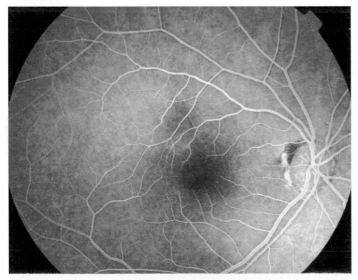

Figure 1.18 Mid venous phase of the FA, 17 seconds after dye injection, showing almost complete venous filling

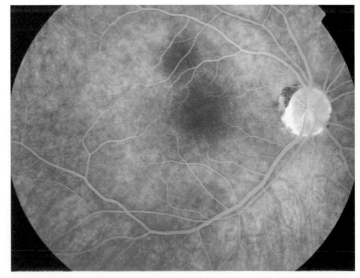

Figure 1.19 Late (elimination) phase of the FA, 5 minutes and 30 seconds after dye injection, showing weaker fluorescence and staining of the optic disc

Dark appearance of the fovea

The normal fovea appears dark (Figure 1.20a) because of the following three phenomena (Figure 1.20b):

- Avascularity of FAZ.

- Blockage of background choroidal fluorescence as a result of increased density of xanthophyll at the fovea.

- Blockage of background choroidal fluorescence because the RPE cells at the fovea are large and contain more melanin than those elsewhere.

Hyperfluorescence

Hyperfluorescence is defined as an abnormal presence of fluorescence or an increase in normal fluorescence. It may be caused by the following phenomena:

1. **Transmission (window) defect** is caused by RPE atrophy or absence which unmasks normal background choroidal fluorescence (Figure 1.21a). It is characterized by early hyperfluorescence which increases in intensity and then fades without changing size or shape (Figure 1.21b).

2. **Pooling of dye** in an anatomical space as a result of breakdown of the outer blood-retinal barrier.

- *In the subretinal space* (Figure 1.22a) as in central serous retinopathy is characterized by early hyperfluorescence (Figure 1.22b) which increases in both intensity and size (Figure 1.22c).

- *In the sub-RPE space* (Figure 1.23a) as in a RPE detachment is characterized by early hyperfluorescence (Figure 1.23b) which increases in intensity but not in size (Figure 1.23c).

3. **Leakage of dye** which may occur from the following vascular structures:

- *Abnormal choroidal vasculature* (as in choroidal neovascularization) is characterized by an early lacy filling pattern of hyperfluorescence (Figure 1.24a) which later increases in size and intensity (Figure 1.24b and 1.24c).

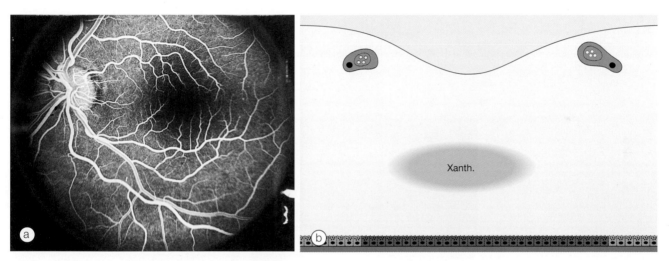

Figure 1.20 Reason for the dark appearance to the fovea on FA (Xanth, xanthophyll) (see the text)

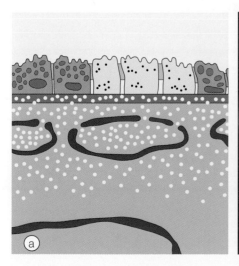
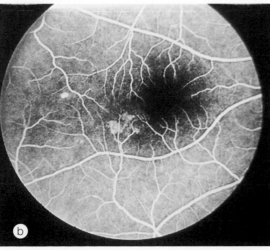

Figure 1.21 Hyperfluorescence due to a RPE window defect (see the text)

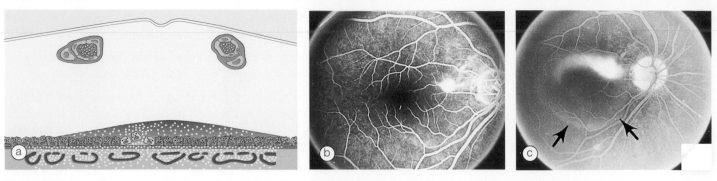

Figure 1.22 Hyperfluorescence due to pooling of dye in the subretinal space in central serous retinopathy

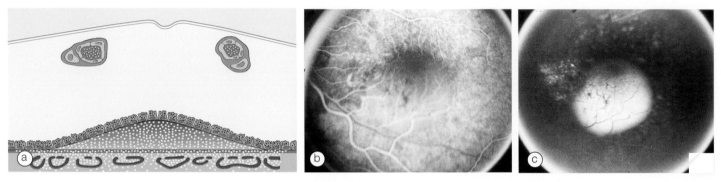

Figure 1.23 Hyperfluorescence due to pooling of dye in the subpigment epithelial space in detachment of the RPE

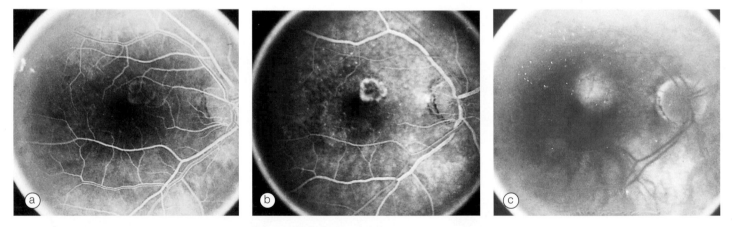

Figure 1.24 Hyperfluorescence due to leakage from a choroidal neovascularization

- *Breakdown of the inner blood-retinal barrier* (as in cystoid macular edema) is characterized by the early hyperfluorescence which increases in size and intensity and gives rise to the characteristic 'flower-petal' pattern seen in the late phase (see Figure 1.10d).

- *Leakage from abnormal retinal or disc vessels* (as in proliferative diabetic retinopathy) (Figure 1.25a) is

characterized by early hyperfluorescence (Figure 1.25b) due to rapid filling of the new vessels followed by increasing intense hyperfluorescence due to leakage (Figure 1.25c).

4. **Staining** of tissues as a result of prolonged retention of dye which is seen in the late phase of the angiogram after the dye has left the choroidal and retinal circulations.

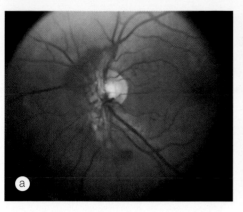
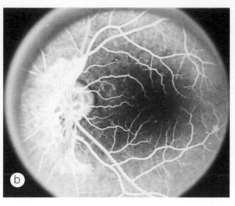
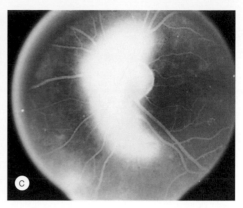

Figure 1.25 Hyperfluorescence due to leakage from disc new vessels in proliferative diabetic retinopathy

Hypofluorescence

Hypofluorescence is a reduction or absence of normal fluorescence. It is caused by either (a) *blockage* (masking) of normal retinal and or background choroidal fluorescence (Figure 1.26) or (b) *filling defects* which prevent normal access of fluorescein dye.

1. **Blockage of retinal fluorescence** is caused by lesions which are located anterior to the retina. The blockage may involve the large superficial vessels, capillary fluorescence, or both according to the location of the lesion as follows:

   • *Vitreous opacities* and *pre-retinal lesions* (such as blood) (Figure 1.27a will block all fluorescence (1.27b and 1.27c).

   • *Deep retinal lesions* (such intraretinal hemorrhages and hard exudates) will only block capillary fluorescence, but not that from the larger retinal vessels.

2. **Blockage of background choroidal fluorescence** is caused by all conditions that also block retinal

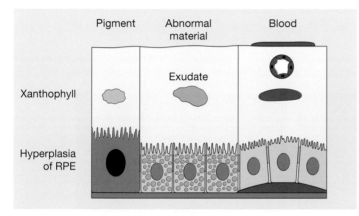

Figure 1.26 Causes of blocked fluorescence

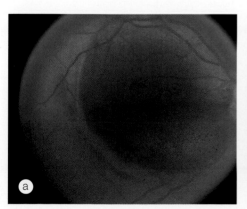
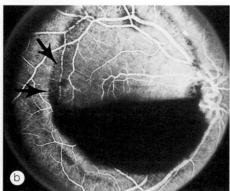
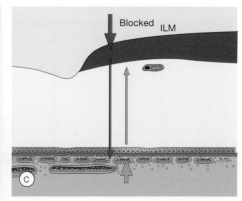

Figure 1.27 Hypofluorescence due to blockage of all fluorescence by a pre-retinal hemorrhage

fluorescence as well as the following which block only choroidal fluorescence:

- *Subretinal or sub RPE lesions* such as blood (Figure 1.28).

- *Increased density of the RPE* such as in congenital hypertrophy of the RPE (Figure 1.29).

- *Choroidal lesions* such as naevi.

The actual cause can be determined only by referring to the clinical findings.

2. Filling defects resulting from one of the following:

- *Vascular occlusion* which prevents access of dye to the tissues. The occlusion may involve the choroidal circulation or the retinal arteries, veins or capillaries (capillary drop-out) (Figure 1.30).

- *Loss of vascular tissue* which may occur in severe myopic degeneration or choroideremia.

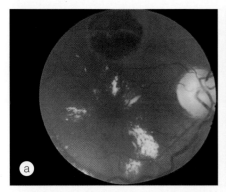
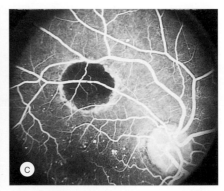

Figure 1.28
Hypofluorescence due to blockage of background choroidal fluorescence by a sub-RPE and subretinal hemorrhages

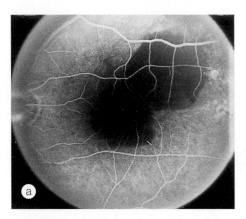
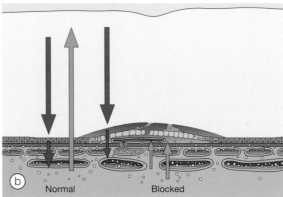

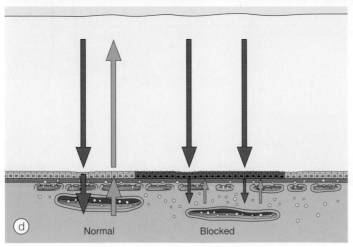

Figure 1.29 Congenital hypertrophy of the RPE and hard exudates (a) causing blockage of background choroidal fluorescence (b)-(d)

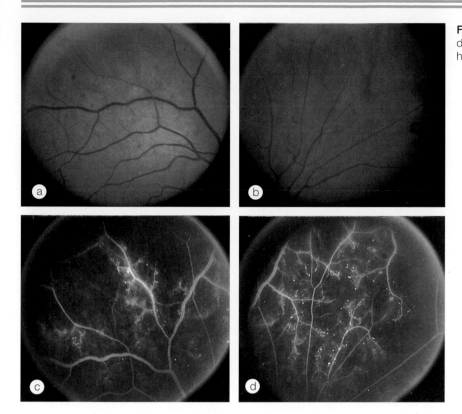

Figure 1.30 Retinal capillary occlusion in diabetic retinopathy (a) & (b) causing hypofluorescence (c) & (d)

Stepwise approach in reporting angiograms

- Comment on the red-free photograph.

- Indicate the phase of the angiogram.

- Indicate whether there is increased or decreased fluorescence as well as any delay in filling.

- Indicate any characteristic features such as smoke-stack or lacy filling pattern.

- State if there is any change in the area or intensity of fluorescence.

It is important to take into consideration the patient's history and ophthalmoscopic findings before drawing conclusions from the angiogram.

Fundus indocyanine green angiography

General principles

Fluorescein angiography is an excellent method of showing the retinal capillaries because the RPE in most eyes provides a uniform dark background. It is therefore a good guide for laser photocoagulation of exudative macular degeneration and retinal vascular disease. It is not, however, helpful in delineating the choroidal circulation. In contrast, indocyanine green (ICG) angiography is of particular value in studying the choroidal circulation. It is also a useful adjunct to FA in angiography in demonstrating disease processes affecting the macula.

1. **ICG binding** is the ability of about 98% of ICG molecules to bind to serum proteins (mainly albumin) on entering the circulation. This phenomenon reduces the passage of ICG through the fenestrations of the choriocapillaris. The dye is not metabolized but is taken up by the parenchymal cells of the liver and then excreted in the bile.

2. **Fluorescence** of ICG is weak and only 1/25 that of fluorescein. The excitation peak is at 805 nm and emission is at 835 nm, which is in the near-infrared spectrum. Infrared light absorbed by the dye readily penetrates normal ocular pigments such as melanin and xanthophyll, as well as exudates or thin layers of subretinal blood. The filters used are infrared barrier and excitation.

Photographic technique

To obtain good quality angiograms, the pupils must be well dilated and the media clear. The technique is as follows:

- The ICG powder is mixed with aqueous solvent to provide 40 mg in 2 ml.

- The patient is seated in front of the camera with one arm outstretched.

- A 'red-free' photograph is taken.

- Between 25 mg and 40 mg of the dye is injected into the antecubital vein.

- Rapid photographs are taken initially and then subsequent photographs are taken at about 3 minutes, 10 minutes and 30 minutes.

- Later phases of the angiogram yield the most information because the dye remains in neovascular tissue after it has left the retinal and choroidal circulations.

If necessary, it is possible to perform ICG angiography simultaneously with or sequentially to fluorescein angiography. ICG videoangiography (ICG-VA) is commonly used as a supplementary test to FA in the diagnosis and treatment of occult choroidal neovascularization (CNV). The two angiographic systems used in performing ICG-VA are the high-resolution digital fundus camera and the scanning laser ophthalmoscope. ICG-guided laser treatment of occult CNV is based on the detection of focal spots or plaques by the digital ICG-VA. The scanning laser ophthalmoscope is better at detecting the vascular net in the very early transit phase of the ICG-VA.

Adverse effects

ICG angiography is associated with a lesser incidence of adverse reactions than fluorescein angiography. Because ICG contains 5% iodine it should not be given to patients allergic to iodine. Its use is also contraindicated in pregnancy.

- The most common mild adverse reactions are staining of stool, nausea, vomiting, sneezing and pruritis.

- Moderate adverse reactions include syncope, skin eruptions, pyrexia, backache, and local skin necrosis.

Phases of the angiogram

Filling of the choroidal circulation can be divided into arterial, capillary and venous phases, similar to the retinal circulation.

1. Early phase

- *First 2 seconds*
  a. Rapid filling of the choroidal arteries and choriocapillaris.
  b. Early filling of choroidal veins.
  c. Major retinal blood vessels are not filled and are seen as dark structures.
  d. A large (watershed) zone of poor perfusion is seen running vertically adjacent to the optic nerve head.

- *2–5 seconds*
  a. Complete filling of larger choroidal veins.
  b. Early filling of retinal arteries.

- *5 seconds – 3 minutes*
  a. Gradual fading of choroidal arterial filling.
  b. Large choroidal veins are visible but less prominent.
  c. Watershed zone is filled.

2. Middle phase (3–15 minutes)

- Fading of choroidal vasculature.

- Fading of retinal vasculature.

3. Late phase (15–60 minutes)

- Hypofluorescence of choroidal vasculature against background hyperfluorescence resulting from staining of extrachoroidal tissue.

- Lack of visibility of retinal vasculature.

Interpretation of the angiogram

1. Early phase, which occurs within 20 seconds of dye injection, shows the following (Figure 1.31a):

- Hypofluorescence of the optic disc associated with poor perfusion of the watershed zone.

- Prominent filling of choroidal arteries and early filling of choroidal veins.

- Retinal arteries are visible but not veins.

2. Early middle phase (3 minutes, 6 seconds) shows the following (Figure 1.31b):

- Filling of the watershed zone.

- Fading of choroidal arterial filling with more prominent filling of choroidal veins.

- Both retinal veins and arteries are visible.

3. Late middle phase (6 minutes, 46 seconds) shows the following (Figure 1.31c):

- Fading of filling of choroidal vessels.

- Diffuse hyperfluorescence as the result of diffusion of dye from the choriocapillaris.

- Retinal vessels are still visible.

4. Late phase (21 minutes, 3 seconds) shows the following (1.31d):

- Hypofluorescence of choroidal vasculature against the background of hyperfluorescence resulting from staining of extrachoroidal tissue.

- Lack of visibility of retinal vasculature.

The dye may remain in neovascular tissue after it has left the choroidal and retinal circulations.

Causes of abnormal fluorescence

1. Hyperfluorescence

- *RPE 'window' defect*.

- *Leakage* of dye from the retinal or choroidal circulations, or the optic nerve head.

- *Abnormal blood vessels*.

2. Hypofluorescence

- *Blockage of fluorescence* by pigment, blood or exudation.

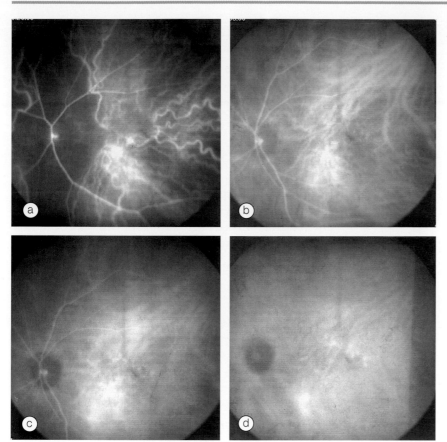

Figure 1.31 Normal ICG angiogram (see the text)

- *Obstruction of the circulation.*
- *Loss of vascular tissue.*
- *RPE detachment* (hyperfluorescent on FA).

Electrophysiological tests

Electrophysiological tests are used mainly in the diagnosis of certain hereditary dystrophies of the fundus, most notably: retinitis pigmentosa, X-linked congenital retinoschisis, rod-cone dystrophies, Stargardt disease and Best disease (see Chapter 5).

Electroretinography

The electroretinogram (ERG) is the record of an action potential produced by the retina when it is stimulated by light of adequate intensity. The recording is made between an active electrode embedded in a contact lens placed on the patient's cornea or a gold foil electrode placed on the eyelid, and a reference electrode on the patient's forehead. The potential between the two electrodes is then amplified and the response displayed (Figure 1.32). The ERG is elicited both in the light-adapted (photopic) and dark-adapted (scotopic) states. The usual ERG response is biphasic as follows (Figure 1.33).

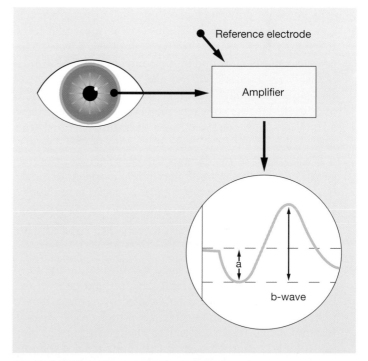

Figure 1.32 Principles of electroretinography

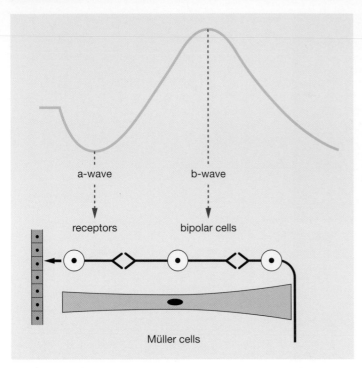

Figure 1.33 Normal electroretinogram. The a-wave is attributed to the photoreceptors and the b-wave to the bipolar cells

1. The **a-wave** is the initial negative deflection which arises from the photoreceptors.

2. The **b-wave** is the positive deflection generated by Müller cells but represents processes occurring in the bipolar cell region. The amplitude of the b-wave is measured from the trough of the a-wave to the peak of the b-wave. The b-wave consists of b1 and b2 subcomponents. The former probably represents both rod and cone activity, whereas the latter is thought to represent cone activity. The amplitude of the b-wave increases with both dark adaptation and increased light stimulus. Because the ERG is a function of the first two neurons of the retina, it is not useful in the diagnosis of disorders affecting the ganglion cells or the optic nerve. It is possible to single out rod and cone responses by using special techniques.

3. **Rod responses** can be isolated by stimulating the fully dark-adapted eye with a flash of very dim light or with blue light.

4. **Cone responses** can be isolated by stimulating the fully light-adapted eye with a bright flash of light or with red light. The cones can also be isolated by using a flicker light stimulus of 30–40 Hz to which rods cannot respond. Cone responses can be elicited in normal eyes up to 50 Hz, after which point the individual responses are no longer recordable (critical flicker fusion).

Electro-oculography

The electro-oculogram (EOG) measures the standing action potential between the electrically positive cornea and the electrically negative back of the eye (Figure 1.34). The EOG is performed as follows:

- The electrodes are attached to the skin near the medial and lateral canthi.

- The patient is then asked to look rhythmically from side to side, making excursions of constant amplitude. Each time the eye moves the cornea makes the nearest electrode positive with respect to the other. The potential difference produced between the two electrodes is amplified and recorded.

- The test is performed in both light-adapted and dark-adapted states.

- As there is much variation in the EOG amplitude in normal subjects, the result is calculated by dividing the level of maximal height of the potential in the light (light peak) by the minimal height of the potential in the dark (dark trough). This ratio is then multiplied by 100 and expressed as a percentage. The normal value is over 185%.

The EOG reflects the activity of the RPE and the photoreceptors. This means that an eye blinded by lesions proximal to the photoreceptors will have a normal EOG. In general, diffuse or widespread disease of the RPE is needed to affect the EOG response significantly.

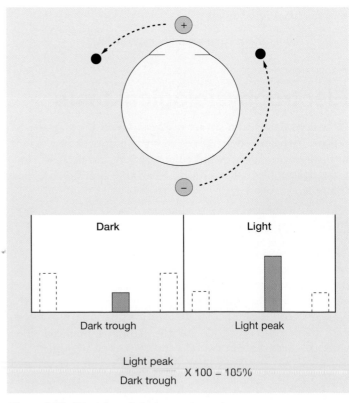

Figure 1.34 Principles of electro-oculography

Principles of laser photocoagulation

Laser is an acronym for **L**ight **A**mplification by **St**imulated **E**mission of **R**adiation. Retinal laser photocoagulation is essentially a destructive form of therapy dependent on the absorption of light energy by ocular pigments (melanin, haemoglobin and xanthophyll) and its conversion into heat. Lasers produce a collimated, coherent monochromatic beam that can deliver a large amount of energy to a small area. The purpose of laser therapy is to produce a therapeutic burn to a pre-selected area while causing minimal damage to surrounding tissue. The main indications for laser photocoagulation are to treat some of the following conditions:

- Retinal vascular diseases.
- Choroidal neovascular membranes.
- High-risk retinal breaks and predisposing peripheral retinal degenerations.
- Selected intraocular tumours.

Ocular pigments

1. **Melanin** is the most important pigment and is present in the cells of the RPE and choroid. The light absorbed by melanin in the RPE is the main source of energy in retinal photocoagulation.

2. **Hemoglobin** best absorbs argon laser energy but is only a significant source of heat when most of the laser energy is concentrated on a blood vessel.

3. **Xanthophyll** is a yellow pigment present in the inner retinal layers of the macula. It becomes a heat source only when blue argon laser photocoagulation is applied close to the fovea.

Wavelengths

An increasing choice of wavelengths is becoming available, each with its own theoretical advantages and disadvantages. The choice of optimum wavelength depends on the absorption spectrum of target tissue. Currently, the main lasers used for retinal photocoagulation are:

1. **Argon**, which emits coherent blue-green light of about 488–515 nm. The beam consists of 70% blue and 30% green light, which can be converted to only green light by the incorporation of a filter. Blue-green wavelengths are well absorbed by all three pigments. However, blue light (488 nm) is undesirable when treating macular disease because it is absorbed by xanthophyll. Green light is absorbed well by melanin and hemoglobin but much less by xanthophyll and is therefore preferred when treatment is required close to the fovea.

2. **Krypton yellow**, which emits light at about 577 nm, is becoming increasingly popular because of its ability to directly coagulate red lesions.

3. **Diode**, which emits infrared light at 780–950 nm.

Practical aspects

1. **Delivery systems**

- *Slitlamp delivery* using a special contact lens is the most common method.

- *Indirect ophthalmoscope* with a condensing lens is most frequently used to treat retinopathy of prematurity.

- *Intraocular* (endolaser) photocoagulation *via* fiberoptic probes can be used during pars plana vitrectomy.

2. **Burn**

- *Spot size* varies between 50–500 μm. It must be remembered that the smaller the spot the greater the energy. Therefore, when changing to a smaller spot size the power level must be reduced. The spot size for focal treatment is usually between 50–100 μm, while panretinal photocoagulation of large areas of the retina requires a larger spot of between 200–500 μm. It is very important to understand the effects on the spot size by different contact lenses. For example, the Goldmann lens does not significantly alter the spot size. However, with other contact lens systems and panfundoscopes the retinal spot size may be larger than the set spot size by 35–50%.

- *Power settings* are from 0–3 W (0–3000 mW). Heavily pigmented fundi will require less energy than hypopigmented fundi to acquire equivalent burns.

- *Exposure time* usually varies from 0.01–5 seconds although treatment of certain intraocular tumours by diode laser photocoagulation (thermotherapy) requires much longer exposure times.

Complications

1. **Foveal damage** may occur as a result of the following mechanisms:

- *Foveal burn*, which usually occurs when treating the temporal retinal periphery with the equatorial mirror. In order to avoid this serious complication it is essential to make constant reference to the fovea.

- *Macular edema* may occur following extensive (panretinal) photocoagulation. Fortunately it usually resolves spontaneously after a few weeks.

- *Macular pucker* is also associated with panretinal photocoagulation, but its effects on visual acuity are permanent.

- *'Spill-over' foveal scarring* may occur months after initial treatment close to the fovea. In this condition the laser scars gradually increase in size to encroach upon the fovea.

2. **Choroidal hemorrhage** may occur when a very small (i.e., 50 μm) but high energy burn ruptures Bruch's

membrane. This may lead to the subsequent formation of choroidal neovascularization.

3. **Contraction of fibrous tissue** is a potentially serious complication which may occur when laser burns are applied too closely. Special care should be taken when treating neovascularization associated with large areas of fibrous tissue, because the energy generated may induce contraction and subsequent tractional retinal detachment.

4. **Effects on visual function** from extensive retinal photocoagulation are night blindness, altered colour and light brightness appreciation, and constriction of visual fields.

5. **Other rare complications** include iris burns, choroidal effusion and vitreous hemorrhage.

Chapter 2

Acquired macular disorders

Age-related macular degeneration

Introduction

1. Prevalence

Age-related macular degeneration (AMD) is the leading cause of irreversible severe visual loss in the Western world in individuals over 60 years old. The prevalence of severe visual loss increases with age. In the USA, at least 10% of individuals between the ages of 65 and 75 years have lost some central vision as a result of AMD. Among those older than 75, 30% are affected to some degree. End-stage (blinding) AMD is found in about 1.7% of all individuals aged over 50 years and in about 18% in those over 85 years.

2. The two types of AMD are:

- *Atrophic* (non-exudative, dry), which is characterized by drusen and geographic atrophy. It is a slowly progressive disease which accounts for 85% of patients with AMD.

- *Exudative* (wet), which is characterized by choroidal neovascularization (CNV), which eventually causes subretinal (disciform) scarring. Although less common, it is frequently devastating and in some cases useful central vision may be lost within a few days. In fact, 88% of legal blindness attributable to AMD is the result of this type. Exudative AMD may occur in isolation or in association with atrophic AMD.

3. Risk factors

- *Systemic*
  a. Age is the most important.
  b. Hypertension.
  c. Smoking.
  d. Positive family history.

- *Ocular*
  a. Presence of soft drusen (see below).
  b. Presence of macular pigmentary changes.
  c. CNV in the fellow eye.

Drusen

Histopathology

Loss of central vision in AMD is the result of changes that occur in response to deposition of abnormal material in Bruch's membrane. This abnormal material is derived from the RPE, and its accumulation is thought to result from failure to clear the debris discharged into this region. Drusen consist of discrete deposits of this abnormal material located between the basal lamina of the RPE and the inner collagenous layer Bruch's membrane (Figure 2.1). The abnormal material also accumulates diffusely throughout Bruch's membrane. Thickening of the inner part of Bruch's membrane is compounded by excessive production of basement membrane-like material by the RPE. It has been postulated that the lipid content of drusen may be a determinant for their subsequent behavior.

Clinical features

Drusen appear as yellow excrescences beneath the RPE which are distributed symmetrically at both posterior poles. They may vary in number, size, shape, degree of elevation and extent of associated changes in the RPE. In some

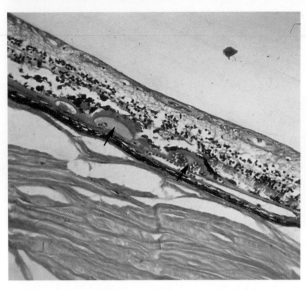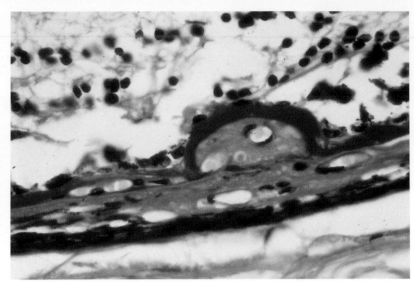

Figure 2.1 Histopathology of drusen (see the text)

patients, drusen may be confined to the region of the fovea, whereas in others the deposits encircle the fovea but spare the fovea itself. Drusen are rarely clinically visible before the age of 45 years; they are not uncommon between the ages of 45 and 60 years and almost universal thereafter. With advancing age they increase in size and number. The following are the three main types:

1. **Hard drusen** are small, round, discrete, yellow-white spots which are associated with focal dysfunction of the RPE (Figure 2.2). In the majority of patients they are innocuous.

2. **Soft drusen** are larger than hard drusen and have indistinct margins (Figure 2.3). With time they may

slowly enlarge and coalesce (Figure 2.4a and 2.4c) to form a solid 'drusenoid' detachment of the RPE best demonstrated on FA (Figure 2.4b and 2.4d). The occurrence of soft and coalescent soft macular drusen is a common precursor to the development of both atrophic and exudative AMD. In some cases drusen may undergo secondary dystrophic calcification and have a glistening appearance (Figure 2.5).

3. **Basal laminar drusen** are innumerable, small, uniform, round, sub-RPE nodules (Figure 2.6). They occur in patients who are younger than those seen with hard or soft drusen and may be associated with pseudovitelliform detachment of the sensory retina, or rarely with CNV.

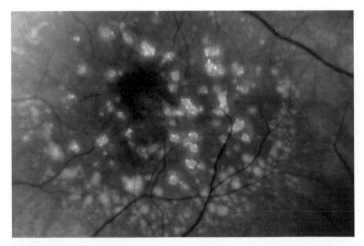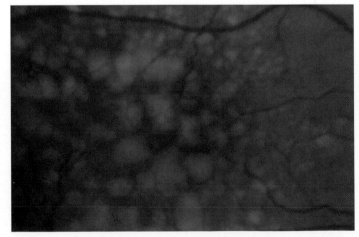

Figure 2.2 Hard drusen

Figure 2.3 Soft drusen

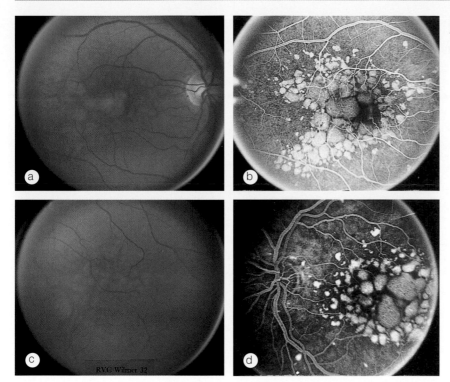

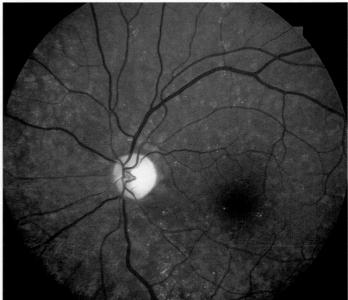

Figure 2.4 Coalescence of soft drusen to form a 'drusenoid' detachment of the RPE (see the text)

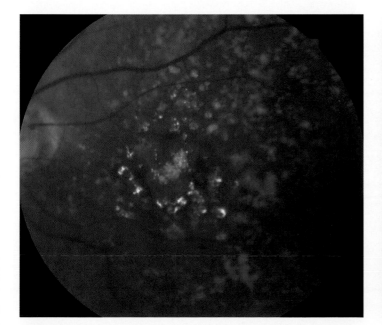

Figure 2.5 Calcified drusen

Figure 2.6 Basal laminar drusen

Fluorescein angiography

Some drusen are brightly fluorescent during angiography, whereas others are not. The degree of fluorescence appears to depend on the quantity of pigment in the overlying RPE, as well as the amount of fluorescein within the drusen themselves.

1. **Hyperfluorescence** of drusen is caused by a window defect resulting from atrophy of the overlying RPE (Figure 2.7b) and late staining (Figure 2.7c). It has also been postulated that hyperfluorescent drusen are hydrophilic (low lipid content) and predispose to the subsequent development of CNV.

2. **Hypofluorescent** drusen are hydrophobic (high lipid content) and, if large and confluent, predispose to the subsequent development of detachment of the RPE. It has also been suggested that a prolonged filling phase of the choroid may indicate the presence of diffuse thickening of Bruch's membrane.

Differential diagnosis

1. **Familial dominant drusen (Doyne honeycomb dystrophy)** is an uncommon condition in which drusen appear during the second and third decades of life. The drusen are symmetrically distributed at the macula and peripapillary region (see Chapter 5).

2. **Hard exudates** in background diabetic retinopathy may, on cursory examination, be confused with drusen. However, unlike drusen they are arranged in rings or clumps and are associated with vascular changes such as microaneurysms and hemorrhages (see Chapter 3).

3. **Type 2 membranoproliferative glomerulonephritis** is a rare disease characterized by hematuria, proteinuria and renal failure. Affected patients show bilateral, symmetrical, diffuse yellow, drusen-like lesions at the posterior pole.

4. **Other causes** of retinal flecks include hereditary conditions such as fundus flavimaculatus, Stargardt

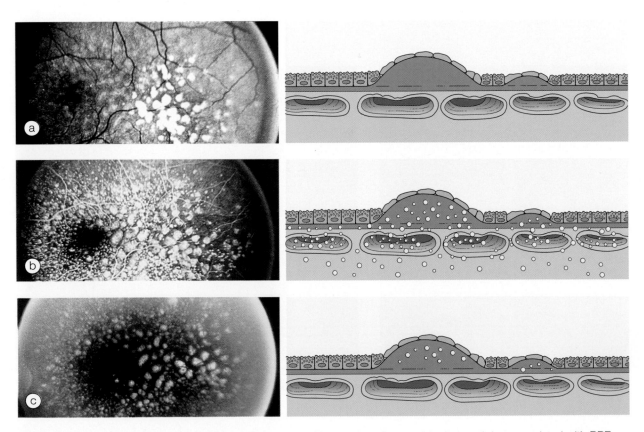

Figure 2.7 Mechanisms of hyperfluorescence of drusen: (a) Prior to dye injection; (b) window defect associated with RPE atrophy; (c) late staining

disease, benign flecked retina, North Carolina macular dystrophy and Alport syndrome (see Chapter 5). In all of these the retinal lesions develop at a much earlier age than drusen.

Drusen and AMD

Although many eyes with drusen maintain normal vision throughout life, a significant number of elderly patients develop impairment of central vision from AMD. The exact role of drusen in the pathogenesis of AMD is still unclear, although it seems probable that their chemical composition may be important. Clinical features associated with an increased risk of subsequent visual loss are large soft and/or confluent drusen, as well as focal hyperpigmentation of the RPE, particularly if one eye has already developed visual loss from AMD.

Prophylactic laser treatment of drusen

A prophylactic treatment for AMD is highly desirable. It has been shown that laser photocoagulation, even with low energies, reduces the number and extent of drusen in eyes with high risk drusen and may also induce a modest improvement of visual function. Although side-effects of treatment are very uncommon, there is a suggestion that such treatment could on rare be occasions be associated with the subsequent development of CNV. For this reason, prophylactic treatment is at present not recommended.

Atrophic age-related macular degeneration

Diagnosis

Atrophic (dry, non-exudative) AMD (Figure 2.8a) is by far the most common type, accounting for about 90% of cases. It is caused by a slowly progressive atrophy of the photoreceptors,

RPE and choriocapillaris (Figure 2.8b), although in some cases it may follow collapse of an RPE detachment (see below). There is no treatment for this type of AMD, although provision of low-vision aids is useful in many patients.

1. **Presentation** is with a gradual mild-to-moderate impairment of vision over several months or years.

2. **Signs** in chronological order are as follows:

- Focal hyperpigmentation or atrophy of the RPE in association with macular drusen (Figure 2.9). At this stage visual acuity may be normal or near-normal.

- Development of sharply circumscribed, circular areas of RPE atrophy associated with variable loss of the choriocapillaris (Figure 2.10). One or both eyes may be affected, and there is variable reduction of visual acuity because the centre of the fovea is usually spared until late in the course of the disease unlike in exudative AMD. When bilateral, the lesions are frequently symmetrical.

- Enlargement of the atrophic areas within which the larger choroidal vessels may become prominent and pre-existing drusen disappear (geographic atrophy) (Figure 2.11). At this stage, visual acuity is usually severely impaired and some patients may benefit from low vision aids.

3. **FA** shows hyperfluorescence due to unmasking of background choroidal fluorescence which may be more extensive than that apparent clinically (see Figure 2.8c).

Differential diagnosis

It should be emphasized that atrophic macular lesions are not pathognomonic for AMD and may be seen in patients with high myopia as well as in the end-stage of the following hereditary dystrophies: Stargardt macular dystrophy, Best disease, central areolar choroidal dystrophy, North Carolina macular dystrophy and Sorsby macular dystrophy (see Chapter 5). Although patients with these conditions develop visual problems earlier than those with AMD, end-stage disease may not develop until much later in life.

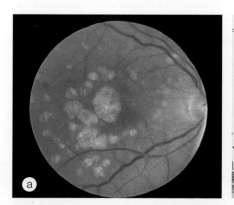 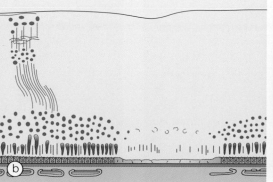 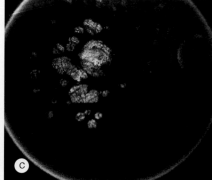

Figure 2.8 (a) Advanced atrophic AMD; (b) focal loss of the photoreceptors, RPE and choriocapillaris; (c) FA showing a window defect

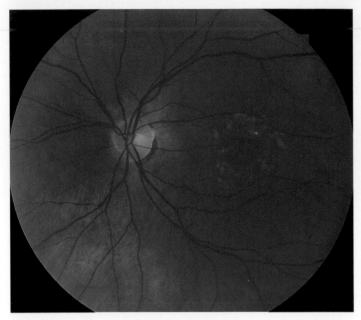

Figure 2.9 Early atrophic AMD showing drusen and mild focal RPE atrophy

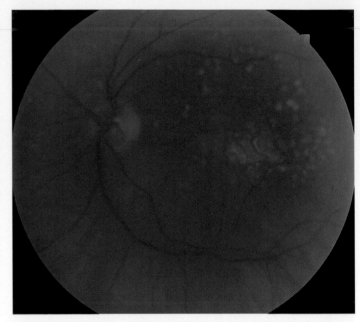

Figure 2.10 Moderate atrophic AMD showing drusen and circular areas of atrophy of the RPE and choriocapillaris

Retinal pigment epithelial detachment

Diagnosis

Detachments of the RPE are thought to be caused by reduction of hydraulic conductivity of a thickened Bruch's membrane, thus impeding the outflow movement of fluid from the RPE towards the choroid.

1. **Presentation** is usually after the fifth decade, with unilateral metamorphosia and a moderate impairment of central vision.

2. **Signs**

   - Sharply circumscribed, dome-shaped elevation at the posterior pole of varying size (Figure 2.12).

   - The sub-RPE fluid is usually clear but may occasionally be turbid.

3. **FA** during the early phase shows hyperfluorescence due to pooling of dye in the sub-RPE space showing the extent of the detachment (Figure 2.13a). During the venous phase there is an increase in the intensity of fluorescence as more dye pools under the detachment (Figure 2.13b).

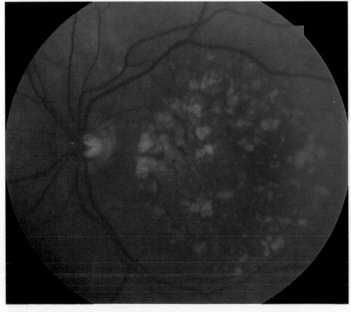

Figure 2.11 Advanced atrophic AMD (geographic atrophy)

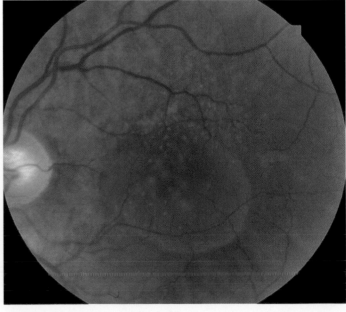

Figure 2.12 Detachment of the RPE

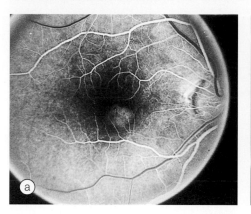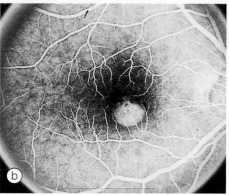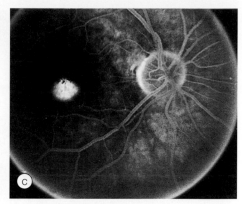

Figure 2.13 FA of RPE detachment: (a) Early hyperfluorescence; (c) & (d) increase in intensity but not in size of hyperfluorescence

The late phase shows that the margins of the detachment are well circumscribed, but there is no increase in the area of hyperfluorescence (Figure 2.13c).

Prognosis

The course and prognosis of an RPE detachment is variable and may follow one of the following patterns:

1. **Spontaneous resolution** without residua may occur, particularly in younger patients.

2. **Geographic atrophy** of the RPE may develop following spontaneous resolution in a minority of patients (see Figure 2.11).

3. **Detachment of the sensory retina** may occur as a result of a breakdown in the outer blood-retinal barrier, allowing passage of fluid into the subretinal space. Because of the relatively loose adhesion between the RPE and sensory retina, the subretinal fluid spreads more widely and is less well defined than in a pure RPE detachment.

4. **Occult CNV** develops in 30–60% of cases (see below).

5. **Tear formation** (see below).

Retinal pigment epithelial tear

Diagnosis

A tear of the RPE may occur at the edge of the attached and detached RPE detachment when tangential stress becomes great enough to rupture the detached tissue. Tears may occur spontaneously in eyes with AMD or following laser photocoagulation of choroidal neovascular membranes in eyes with detachments of the RPE.

1. **Presentation** is with a sudden impairment of central vision.

2. **Signs**

   • Crescent shaped dehiscence in the RPE, located at the edge of a prior serous detachment of the RPE (Figure 2.14a).

   • The flap is retracted and folded.

3. **FA** shows hypofluorescence over the flap with adjacent hyperfluorescence (Figure 2.14b, 2.14c and 2.14d).

Prognosis

Eyes with subfoveal tears usually carry a poor prognosis. Those with detachments of the RPE leading to tears have an especially poor prognosis and are at particular risk of developing visual loss in the fellow eye. However, a minority of eyes maintain good visual acuity in spite of RPE tears, particularly if the fovea is spared.

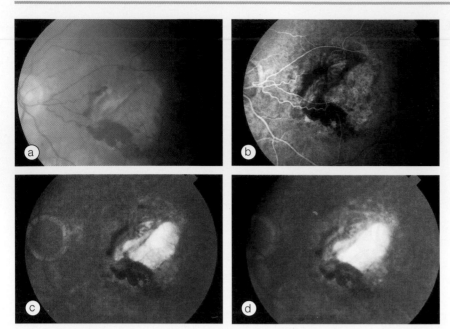

Figure 2.14 FA of a RPE tear (see the text)

Exudative age-related macular degeneration

Pathogenesis

Exudative AMD is caused by CNV consisting of fibrovascular tissue which grows from the choriocapillaris, through defects in Bruch's membrane, into the sub-RPE space and later into the subretinal space. CNV may precede or follow the development of RPE detachment, although these two events are probably not directly related.

Diagnosis

1. **Presentation** is with metamorphopsia and blurring of central vision due to leakage of fluid from CNV. It is at this stage that argon laser treatment may be beneficial.

2. **Signs**

• Many membranes cannot be identified ophthalmoscopically.

• Occasionally, CNV may be detected clinically as a grey-green or pinkish-yellow, slightly elevated, sub-RPE lesion of variable size. If the membrane has broken into the subretinal space, it usually assumes a translucent pale-pink or yellow-white appearance (Figure 2.15).

• Signs associated with leakage from CNV are serous retinal elevation, subretinal blood or sub-RPE blood, and subretinal hard exudates (Figure 2.16).

3. **FA** plays a very important role in the detection and precise localization of CNV in relation to the centre of the FAZ. The following characteristics may be seen.

• *Classic CNV* is characterized by a well-defined membrane which fills with dye in a 'lacy' pattern during the very early phase of dye transit (Figure 2.17b), fluoresces brightly during peak dye transit (Figure 2.17c), and then leaks into the subretinal space and around the CNV within 1–2 minutes (Figure 2.17d). The fibrous tissue within the CNV then stains with dye and leads to late hyperfluorescence. Classic CNV is classified according to its relation to the centre of FAZ as follows:

a. Extrafoveal in which the CNV is more than 200 μm from the center of FAZ.

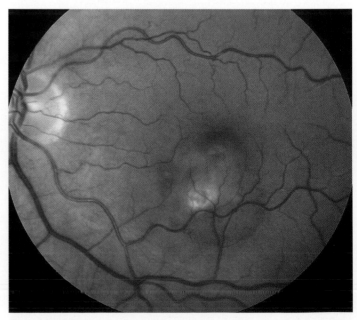

Figure 2.15 Clinical appearance of CNV just below the fovea

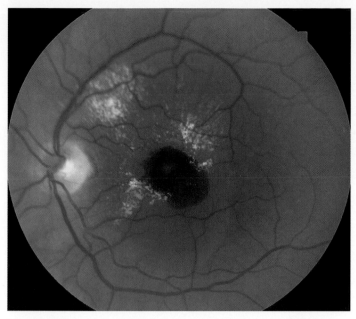

Figure 2.16 Hard exudates and subretinal hemorrhage associated with CNV

- *Fibrovascular RPE detachment* is a combination of CNV and RPE detachment. The CNV fluoresces brighter (hot spot) than the detachment. In other cases, the CNV may be obscured by blood or turbid fluid.

4. **ICG** in certain circumstances may be superior to FA. The longer, near-infrared wavelengths used for excitation (805 nm) and emission (835 nm) can penetrate the RPE and choroid, and the near-infrared light is less absorbed by hemoglobin. These properties allow greater transmission of ICG fluorescence compared with that of fluorescein and are of particular value in the following circumstances:

- Detection of occult or poorly defined CNV.

- Distinguishing serous from vascularized portions of a fibrovascular RPE detachment (Figure 2.19).

- CNV associated with overlapping hemorrhage, pigment or exudate.

- Recurrent CNV adjacent to an old photocoagulation scar.

Prognosis

In the majority of cases the prognosis is poor because of the following complications:

1. **Hemorrhagic RPE detachment**, which is caused by rupture of blood vessels within the CMV. Initially, the blood is confined to the sub-RPE space and appears as a elevated mound.

2. **Hemorrhagic sensory detachment**, which most frequently develops within 1–2 weeks of a hemorrhagic detachment of the RPE as the blood breaks through into the subretinal space and assumes a more diffuse outline and a lighter red color which may surround the RPE detachment (Figure 2.20).

b. Subfoveal in which the center of the FAZ is involved either by extension from an extrafoveal area or by originating directly under the center of the fovea (Figure 2.18). It has been shown that about 70% of CNV extend to a subfoveal position within one year. The visual prognosis of these eyes is very poor.

c. Juxtafoveal in which the CNV is closer than 200 μm from the center of the FAZ but not involving the center itself.

- *Occult CNV* is a poorly defined membrane which has less precise features on the early frames but gives rise to late leakage.

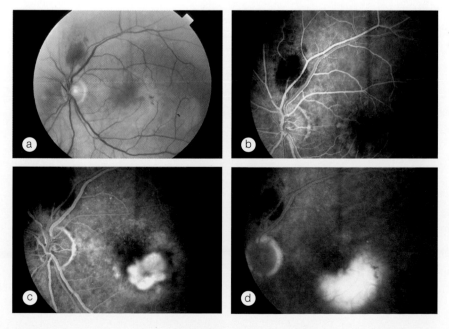

Figure 2.17 FA of classic CNV (see the text). An incidental choroidal nevus is also present above the disk.

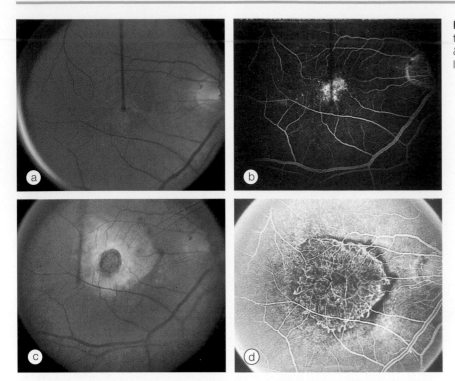

Figure 2.18 Progression of subfoveal CNV in the same eye: (a) & (b) Initial appearance; (c) & (d) appearance one year later showing a large fibrovascular scar

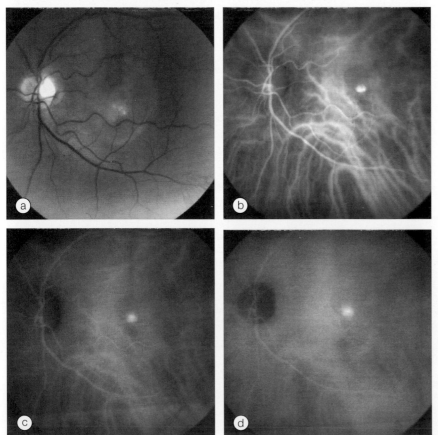

Figure 2.19 ICG of a fibrovascular detachment of the RPE: (a) Red free; (b), (c) & (d) hypofluorescence of the detachment associated with a focal area of hyperfluorescence ('hot spot') corresponding to CNV

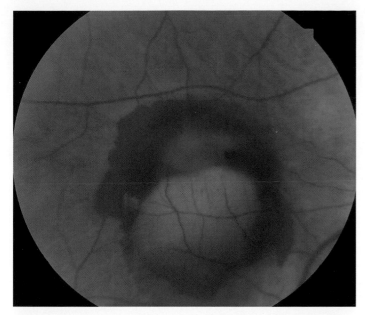

Figure 2.20 Hemorrhagic detachment of the RPE associated with CNV surrounded by a more diffuse and redder subretinal hemorrhage

3. **Vitreous hemorrhage** may rarely occur when blood under a sensory hemorrhagic detachment breaks through into the vitreous cavity (Figure 2.21).

4. **Subretinal (disciform) scarring** follows the hemorrhagic episode in which there is a gradual organization of the blood, and further ingrowth of new vessels from the choroid (Figure 2.22). Eventually, a fibrous disciform scar at the fovea causes permanent loss of central vision (Figure 2.23).

5. **Massive exudation** both intra- and subretinal may develop in some eyes with disciform scars as a result of chronic leakage from the CNV (Figure 2.24).

6. **Exudative retinal detachment** is caused by profuse leakage (Figure 2.25). It is a rare but devastating condition because the subretinal fluid may spread beyond the macula so that not only central but also peripheral vision is lost.

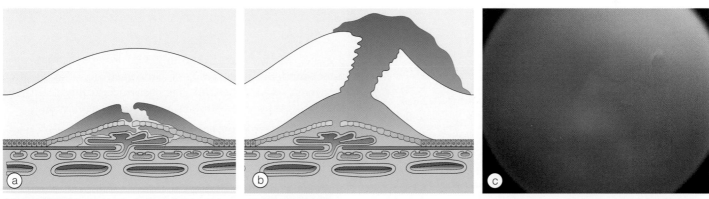

Figure 2.21 Mechanism of vitreous hemorrhage arising from CNV

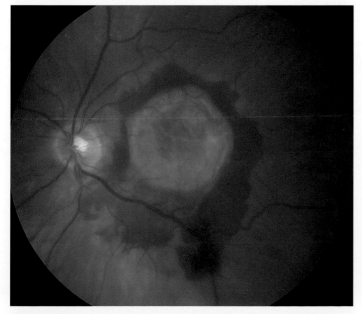

Figure 2.22 Severe subretinal scarring surrounded by subretinal hemorrhage

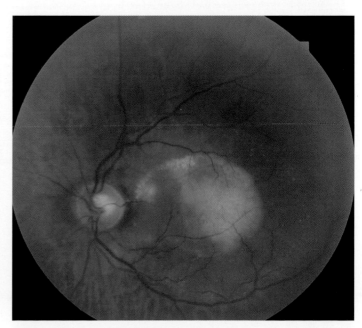

Figure 2.23 Severe subretinal scarring with early hard exudate formation due to chronic leakage from CNV

29

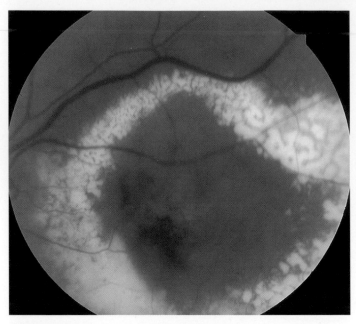

Figure 2.24 Extensive subretinal hard exudates due to chronic leakage from CNV

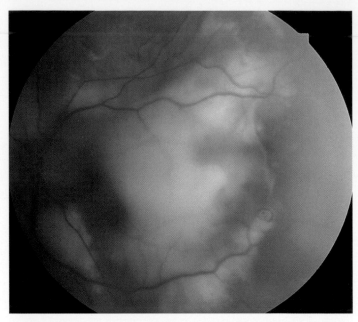

Figure 2.25 Extensive subretinal exudates and exudative retinal detachment due to chronic leakage from CNV

Argon laser photocoagulation

Argon laser photocoagulation of CNV can reduce the risk of severe visual loss in selected cases. The aim of treatment is to destroy the CNV, avoiding damage to the foveola. Because a lesion is more likely to be treatable if detected early, it is important that it is identified promptly by the daily use of the Amsler grid in patients at risk.

1. Potential indications

- *Extrafoveal* or *juxtafoveal CNV* may, in some cases, be treatable if they have well-defined margins.

- *Subfoveal CNV* may occasionally be treated if they are small and classic.

2. Contraindications

- *Poorly defined CNV*, either because the membrane is occult as previously defined or because it is obscured by blood and/or serous RPE detachment. In these cases, treatment, if attempted, may be incomplete because the extent of the CNV cannot be accurately determined.

- *Poor visual acuity* of 6/36 or less is a contraindication because the CNV is likely to be subfoveal. In fact, only about 10% of eyes are suitable for treatment at first presentation.

3. Technique

It is extremely important to emphasize to the patient that the main aim of treatment is not to improve vision, but to prevent further deterioration. The patient must also understand the importance of continued observation after treatment, even if the CNV has been successfully destroyed. The following are the steps of laser photocoagulation:

- Visual acuity is measured for near and distance.

- The area of the scotoma or visual distortion is documented on the Amsler grid.

- A good quality FA, not more than 72 hours old, should be available.

- Selected frames of the FA are projected onto a screen so that the CNV can be precisely localized in relation to visible retinal landmarks.

- The perimeter of the lesion is treated with overlapping 200 μm (0.2–0.5 second) burns and then the entire area is covered with high energy burns. The treatment must extend beyond the margins of the membrane and produce a confluent, intense white burn.

- A post-treatment fundus photograph is taken to document the extent of treatment.

4. Follow-up should be meticulous so that persistent or recurrent CNV is detected early.

- Initial examination is after 1–2 weeks and a FA performed to ensure that treatment has been adequate.

- Re-treatment is indicated if there is true persistence or recurrence of an extrafoveal CNV located more than 200 μm from the center of the fovea.

- Because recurrences can occur several years after the initially successful treatment, it is important for the patient to continue to monitor progress with the regular use of the Amsler grid and to have periodic follow-up examinations.

5. Results are frequently disappointing for the following reasons:

- Using FA as a guide, only a very small proportion of eyes are eligible for treatment.

- Among eligible eyes with extrafoveal or juxtafoveal lesions that are treated, the recurrence rate is greater than 50% and most recurrent lesions are subfoveal.

- Among eligible eyes, at least 50% have subfoveal lesions, which if treated, result in immediate and irreversible loss

of central vision as a result of thermal damage to the sensory retina overlying the CNV.

Photodynamic therapy

1. Principles

Verteporfin, which is a photosensitizer or light-activated compound, is injected intravenously. It is then activated focally by illumination with light from a diode laser source at a wavelength (689 nm) that corresponds to an absorption peak of the compound. The main advantage of photodynamic therapy is the ability for selective tissue damage, in part attributable to preferential localization of the photosensitizer to the CNV complex. The CNV is irradiated with light levels far lower than those required for thermal destruction by argon laser therapy enabling treatment of subfoveal CNV.

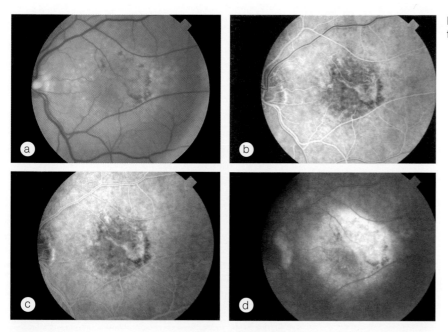

Figure 2.26 Juxtafoveal CNV prior to treatment (see the text)

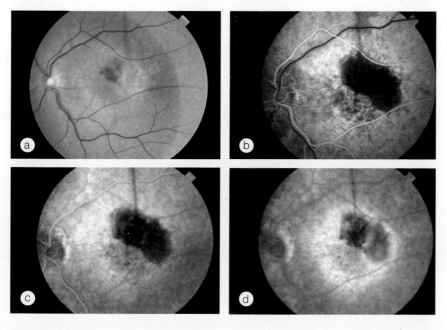

Figure 2.27 The same eye two weeks following successful laser photocoagulation (see the text)

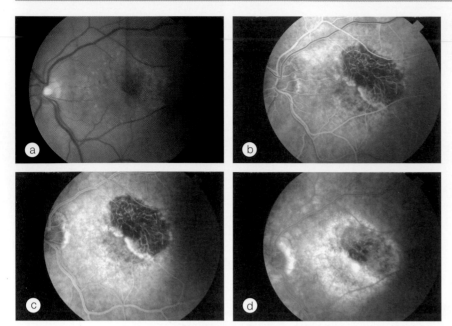

Figure 2.28 The same eye six weeks later showing recurrent CNV involving the fovea (see the text)

Case study 1

1. History

A 69-year-old man presented with five week history of blurring of central vision of his left eye.

2. Examination

Right eye
- Visual acuity was 6/9–1.
- Fundus examination showed multiple macular drusen.

Left eye
- Visual acuity was 6/18.
- Fundus examination showed multiple macular drusen. There was also retinal edema and hemorrhage associated with a large area of CNV (Figure 2.26a).

3. FA left eye

- *Arteriovenous phase* showed a large area of 'lacy' hyperfluorescence (Figure 2.26b).
- *Later phases* showed diffuse hyperfluorescence due to leakage (Figure 2.26c and 2.26d).

4. Diagnosis

- Left supero-temporal, juxtafoveolar CNV just involving the edge of the FAZ.

5. Treatment

- Laser photocoagulation was applied to the CNV. However, prior to treatment the patient was informed of the possible risks and benefits of treatment as well as the possibility of recurrence. He was also made aware that there will also be a permanent scotoma inferior to fixation.

6. Course

- Two weeks later visual acuity was 6/18.
- Fundus examination showed a laser scar and residual hemorrhage (Figure 2.27a).

- FA showed a large hypofluorescent area with no evidence of CNV (Figure 2.27b, 2.27c and 2.27d).

7. Outcome

- Six weeks later the patient reported deterioration of vision (3/60).
- FA showed recurrence of CNV, the inferior margin of which had extended into the fovea (Figure 2.28).

8. Comment

This patient shows recurrence of CNV involving the fovea following initially successful treatment of CNV. This occurs in about 50% of cases

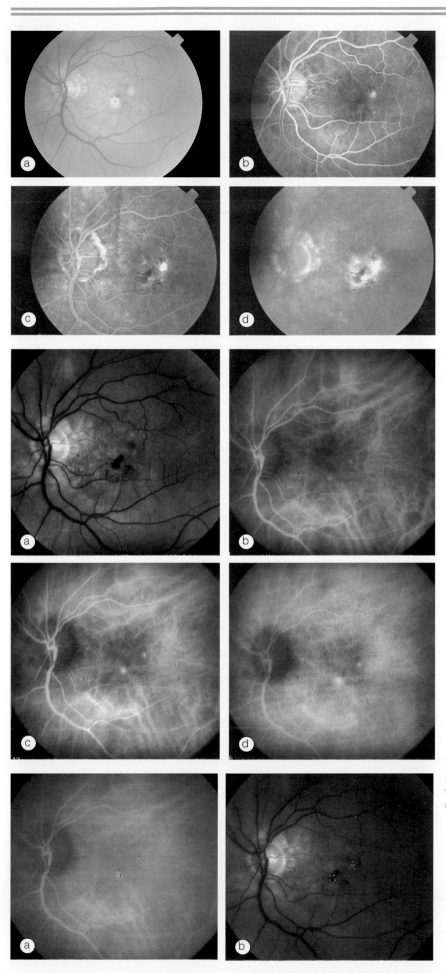

Figure 2.29 Fibrovascular RPE detachment (see the text)

Figure 2.30 ICG of the same eye two 'hot spots' (see the text)

Figure 2.31 Locating CNV by tracing transfer from the ICG (a) to the red free photograph (b) (see the text)

Case study 2

1. History

A 72-year-old man presented with a four week history of blurred and distorted vision in his left eye.

2. Examination

Right eye

- Visual acuity was 6/12.

- Fundus examination showed multiple drusen and mild atrophic AMD.

Left eye

- Visual acuity was 6/60.

- Fundus examination showed multiple drusen, irregular elevation of the RPE and multiple small subretinal hemorrhages at the fovea (Figure 2.29a)

3. FA left eye

- *Early venous phase* showed a small hyperfluorescent spot supero-temporal to the fovea and multiple hypofluorescent spots at the fovea corresponding to the hemorrhages (Figure 2.29b).

- *Later phases* showed increase in intensity but not in area of the hyperfluorescent spot and progressive diffuse hyperfluorescence involving the entire fovea (Figure 2.29c and 2.29d).

4. ICG left eye

- Two small hyperfluorescent 'hot spots' which appear at 7.07 minutes (Figure 2.30b) and persist in the late frames at 12.01 minutes (Figure 2.30c and 2.30d).

- Tracing transfer from the ICG (Figure 2.31a) to the red free photograph (Figure 2.31b) showed that the spots were extrafoveal.

5. Diagnosis

- Extrafoveal fibrovascular RPE detachment.

6. Treatment

- ICG-guided photocoagulation was applied to the CNV using red dye laser to penetrate the blood and yellow dye laser to treat areas not associated with hemorrhage.

7. Outcome

- Four months later visual acuity had improved to 6/18 and the RPE detachment had flattened and there was no leakage.

8. Comment

This patient shows successful treatment of CNV which was identified by ICG but not FA.

2. Results

Photodynamic therapy can safely reduce the risk of moderate to severe visual loss in eyes with predominantly classic (>50%) subfoveal CNV although there appears to be no benefit in eyes without predominantly classic lesions. However, some patients still lose vision in the longterm.

Experimental therapies

1. Surgery

- *Submacular surgery* involves the surgical removal of submacular blood or CNV, or both. At present, the exact indications and benefits for this type of surgery are unknown. Preliminary results show that there is a high rate of recurrent CNV, and the procedure carries a significant risk of complications resulting in visual loss and further surgical intervention.

- *Macular translocation* involves moving the fovea away from the CNV. The procedure consists of chorioscleral folding, vitrectomy, subretinal infusion of balanced salt solution to induce a temporal retinal detachment, fluid-air exchange followed by postoperative up-right positioning. If appropriate, CNV can be treated by photocoagulation without risk of foveal damage. The success of the procedure is dependent on the ability to effectively move the fovea away from the diseased CNV complex and the degree of preoperative neurosensory foveal function. The exact indications for this type of surgery are still evolving.

- *Pneumatic displacement of submacular hemorrhage* involves injection of gas into the vitreous cavity in order to displace the blood away from the fovea. This procedure can also be done with the use of a a fibrinolytic agent called tissue plasminogen activator (tPA).

2. Other modalities

- *Radiotherapy* involves destruction of CNV by external proton beam radiation. Most large studies have reported disappointing results with none or minimal benefit.

- *Transpupillary thermotherapy* involves the use of a diode laser (810 nm) to treat eyes with predominantly occult CNV. It has been speculated that this will have some effect on the deeper choroidal vessels with sparing of the neurosensory retina. At present there are no data to support this hypothesis.

- *Antiangiogenesis drugs* for the prophylaxis of exudative AMD are currently under investigation. These include thalidomide with and without concurrent laser photocoagulation, and intravitreal triamcinolone. Unfortunately, reports using subcutaneous interferon α-2a showed no benefit and found evidence of serious systemic and ocular adverse effects.

FURTHER READING

Bird AC, Bressler NM, Bressler SB, et al. An international classification and grading system for age-related maculopathy and age-related macular degeneration. *Surv Ophthalmol* 1995;39:367–374.

Choroidal Vascularization Prevention Trial Research Group. Choroidal neovascularization in the choroidal neovascularization prevention trial. *Ophthalmology* 1998a;105:1364–72.

Choroidal Neovascularization Prevention Trial Research Group. Laser treatment in eyes with large drusen. Short-term effects seen in a pilot randomized clinical trial. *Ophthalmology* 1998b;105:11–23.

Chuang EL, Bird AC. The pathogenesis of tears of the retinal pigment epithelium. *Am J Ophthalmol* 1988;105:385–390.

Ciulla TA, Danis RP, Harris A. Age-related macular degeneration: a review of experimental treatments. *Surv Ophthalmol* 1998;43:134–146.

Curcio CA, Millican CL. Basal linear deposits and large drusen are specific for age-related maculopathy. *Arch Ophthalmol* 1999;117:329–339.

Fine SL. Photodynamic therapy with verteporfin is effective for selected patients with neovascular age-related macular degeneration. *Arch Ophthalmol* 1999;117:1400–1402.

Gross-Jendroska M, Owens SL, Flaxel CJ, et al. Prophylactic laser treatment to fellow eyes of unilateral retinal pigment epithelial tears. *Am J Ophthalmol* 1998;126:77–81.

Klein R, Klein BEK, Jensen SC, et al. The five-year incidence and progression of age-related maculopathy: The Beaver Dam Eye Study. *Ophthalmology* 1997;104:7–21.

Lafaut BA, Bartz-Schmidt KU, Vanden Broecke C, et al. Clinicopathological correlation in exudative age related macular degeneration: histological differentiation between classic and occult choroidal neovascularization. *Br J Ophthalmol* 2000;84:239–243.

Lewis H, Kaiser PK, Lewis S, et al. Macular translocation for subfoveal choroidal neovascularization in age-related macular degeneration: a prospective study. *Am J Ophthalmol* 1999;128:135–146.

Macular Photocoagulation Study Group. Laser photocoagulation of subfoveal neovascular lesions in age-related macular degeneration. *Arch Ophthalmol* 1991;109:1220–1231.

Macular Photocoagulation Study Group. Laser photocoagulation of subfoveal neovascular lesions of age-related macular degeneration. Updating findings from two clinical trials. *Arch Ophthalmol* 1993;111:1200–1209.

Macular Photocoagulation Study Group. Laser photocoagulation of juxtafoveal choroidal neovascularization: five year results from randomized clinical trial. *Arch Ophthalmol* 1994;112:500–9.

Macular Photocoagulation Study Group. Risk factors for choroidal neovascularization in the second eye of patients with juxtafoveal or subfoveal choroidal neovascularization secondary to age-related macular degeneration. *Arch Ophthalmol* 1997;115:741–747.

Merrill PT, LoRusso FJ, Lomeo MD, et al. Surgical removal of subfoveal choroidal neovascularization in age-related macular degeneration. *Ophthalmology* 1999;106:782–789.

Pieramici DJ, De Juan Jr E, Fujii GY, et al. Limited inferior macular translocation for the treatment of subfoveal choroidal neovascularization secondary to age-related macular degeneration. *Am J Ophthalmol* 2000;130:419–428.

Regallo CD, Blade KA, Custis PH, et al. Evaluation of persistent and recurrent choroidal neovascularization. *Ophthalmology* 1998;105:1821–26.

Sandberg MA, Weiner A, Miller S, et al. High-risk characteristics of fellow eyes of patients with unilateral neovascular age-related macular degeneration. *Ophthalmology* 1998;105:441–447.

Sarks JP, Sarks SH, Killingsworth MA. Evolution of geographic atrophy of the retinal pigment epithelium. *Eye* 1988;2:552–557.

Stevens TS, Bressler NM, Maguire MG, et al. Occult choroidal neovascularization in age-related macular degeneration. A natural history study. *Arch Ophthalmol* 1997;115:345–350.

Submacular Surgical Trials Pilot Study Investigators. Submacular surgery trials randomized pilot trial of laser photocoagulation versus surgery for recurrent choroidal neovascularization secondary to age-related macular degeneration: ophthalmic outcomes. *Am J Ophthalmol* 2000;130:387–407.

Sunness JS, Gonzalez-Baron J, Applegate CA, et al. Enlargement of atrophy and visual loss in the geographic atrophy form of age-related macular degeneration. *Ophthalmology* 1999;106:1768–1779.

Treatment of Age-related Macular Degeneration With Photodynamic Therapy (TAP) Group. Photodynamic therapy of subfoveal choroidal neovascularization in age-related macular degeneration with verteporfin. One-year results of 2 randomized clinical trials – TAP report 1. *Arch Ophthalmol* 1999;117:1329–1345.

Senile macular hole

Pathogenesis

Senile (ideopathic) macular holes develop and subsequently enlarge as a result of progressive tangential vitreoretinal traction at the fovea. The process can be classified into the stages listed below (Figure 2.32).

1. **Stage 1a** is an impending macular hole which is rarely seen clinically and is usually first detected in a patient with a fully developed macular hole in the opposite eye. It is characterized by a yellow foveolar spot with loss of the foveal depression (Figure 2.33) which is thought to represent cystic changes rather than a true detachment of the sensory retina as previously proposed.

2. **Stage 1b** is an occult macular hole which results from centrifugal displacement of the foveolar retina and xanthophyll. It is characterized by a yellow ring with a bridging interface of vitreous cortex. These findings may be associated with a recent mild decrease in visual acuity or metamorphopsia. About 50% of stage 1 holes resolve following spontaneous vitreofoveolar separation.

3. **Stage 2** is an early full-thickness macular hole which is characterized by an eccentric, oval, crescent, or horseshoe retinal defect less than 400 μm in diameter with or without an overlying prefoveal opacity (pseudo-operculum). It is important to point out that true opercula are very rare and the pseudo-operculum is formed by the contracted prefoveolar cortical vitreous. Progression from stage 1 to stage 2 takes between one week and several months.

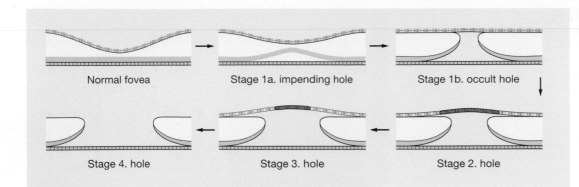

Normal fovea · Stage 1a. impending hole · Stage 1b. occult hole

Stage 4. hole · Stage 3. hole · Stage 2. hole

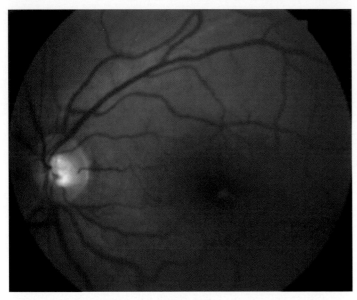

Figure 2.33 Stage 1a senile macular hole

4. **Stage 3** is an established full-thickness macular hole which is characterized by a round retinal defect greater than 400 μm in diameter with an attached posterior vitreous face with or without an overlying pseudo-operculum.

5. **Stage 4** is characterized by enlargement of the round defect which is surrounded by a cuff of subretinal fluid with complete posterior vitreous separation from the posterior pole and optic disc. The presence of a Weiss ring is an important sign of posterior vitreous detachment. The ring is an annular opacity consisting of glial tissue detached from the margin of the optic disc.

Diagnosis

Senile macular holes typically affect elderly females. The risk of involvement to the fellow eye at 5 years is about 16%. The features of a full thickness macular hole are as follows:

1. **Presentation** is frequently by chance when the fellow eye is closed. In other cases a macular hole first becomes apparent when vision in the fellow eye becomes impaired due to hole formation or for some other reason.

2. **Visual acuity** is decreased mainly due to the absence of photoreceptors within the central defect which give rise to an absolute central scotoma. In addition, the surrounding cuff of subretinal fluid and secondary retinal elevation cause a relative scotoma surrounding the absolute central scotoma. There is a tendency for visual acuity to deteriorate progressively from the earliest stages before stabilizing at 6/60 or worse as the hole reached its maximal diameter. Some patients may achieve a better level by using eccentric fixation.

3. **Signs** (Figure 2.34)

• Round punched-out area about one-third of a disc in diameter, which is surrounded by a cuff of subretinal fluid and the presence of an overlying prefoveal opacity.

• Tiny yellowish deposits are seen at the level of the RPE within the hole.

4. **Watzke-Allen test** is positive. The test is performed by projecting a narrow slit beam 100 μm in diameter over the center of the hole both vertically and horizontally with a 90 or 78 dioptre lens. A patient with a macular hole will report that the beam is broken or thinned.

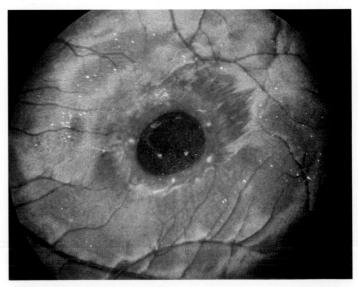

Figure 2.34 Full-thickness senile macular hole

5. Laser aiming beam test is also positive. A 50 μm spot of a laser aiming beam is shone at the center of the hole and the patient is asked whether he can detect the light. A patient with a macular hole will report that the spot has disappeared.

6. FA shows a corresponding area of hyperfluorescence resulting from unmasking of background choroidal fluorescence caused by a RPE 'window defect' (Figure 2.35).

7. Optical coherence tomography (Figure 2.36) is a new technique which employs high-resolution optical sections of the retina and allows for the measurement of the retinal thickness and is effective in the diagnosis and staging of macular holes. It can even measure the volume of a full-thickness macular hole.

Surgical treatment

1. Indications are FTMH associated with a visual acuity worse then 6/18, and a duration less than one year.

2. Technique

- *Conventional vitrectomy* is combined with removal of the internal limiting membrane, gas-fluid exchange followed by strict postoperative face-down positioning. It has been postulated that hole closure is the result of centripetal movement of previously displaced paracentral photoreceptors and not simply reapproximation of the retinal edges to the RPE.

- *'Chemical vitrectomy'* is a new and less complicated method of treating stage 3 macular holes in which an enzyme (plasmin) is injected into the vitreous to chemically disinsert the vitreous from the retina. This results in a posterior vitreous separation without the need for manipulation of the posterior hyaloid. The vitreous is also lavaged with an infusion pipe and vitreous cutter and then 70–80% of the vitreous cavity is filled with 16% C_3F_8. Postoperatively the patient is positioned face-down.

4. Results following successful surgery. Visual improvement is achieved in 80% of eyes, with a final visual acuity of 20/40 or better in up to 65% (Figure 2.37a shows the preoperative appearance and Figure 2.37b shows the postoperative appearance following successful closure).

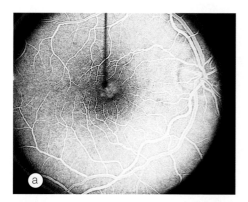

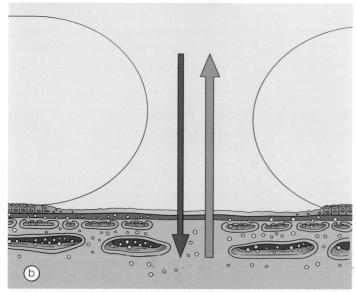

Figure 2.35 FA of a full-thickness senile macular hole

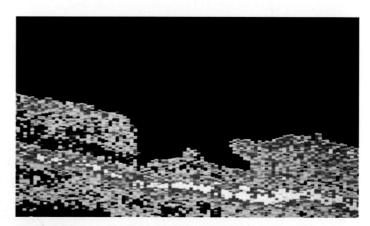

Figure 2.36 Optical coherence tomogram of a macular hole

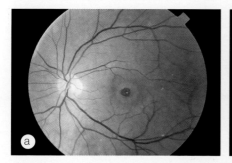

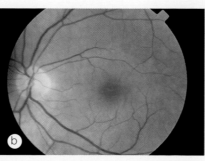

Figure 2.37 Full-thickness senile macular hole: (a) prior to sugery; (b) following successful closure

5. Complications are those associated with vitrectomy, such as retinal detachment and acceleration of cataract. Some patients also develop permanent visual field defects which tend to be inferotemporal.

Differential diagnosis

1. Other macular holes

- *High myopia*, if associated with posterior staphyloma, may be associated with macular hole formation which can lead to retinal detachment. The subretinal fluid is confined to the posterior pole and seldom spreads to the equator.

- *Blunt ocular trauma* may cause a macular hole as a result of either vitreous traction or commotio retinae which leads to subsequent lamellar hole formation.

2. Macular pseudoholes

- *Within premacular fibrosis* (see Figure 2.62).

- *Lamellar hole* associated with severe cystoid macular edema.

- *White dot fovea* is an uncommon asymptomatic condition in which there are white dots on the fovea. The dots may be arranged diffusely or in the form of a ring along the margin of the foveola. The latter pattern gives the appearance of a true macular hole with a cuff of fluid.

FURTHER READING

Asrani S, Zeimer R, Goldberg MF, et al. Serial optical sectioning of macular holes at different stages of development. *Ophthalmology* 1998;105:66–77.

Banker AS, Freeman WR, Kim JW, et al. Vision-threatening complications of surgery for full-thickness macular holes. *Ophthalmology* 1997;104:1442–1453.

Chauhan DS, Antliff RJ, Rai PA, et al. Papillofoveal traction in macular hole formation: the role of optical coherence tomography. *Arch Ophthalmol* 2000;118:32–38.

Chew EY, Sperduto RD, Hiller R, et al. Clinical course of macular holes: the Eye Disease Case-Control Study. *Arch Ophthalmol* 1999;117:242–246.

Ezra E, Wells JA, Gray RH, et al. Incidence of idiopathic full-thickness macular holes in fellow eyes. *Ophthalmology* 1998;105:353–359.

Ezra E. Idiopathic full thickness macular hole; natural history and pathogensis. Perspective. *Br J Ophthalmol* 2001;85:102–108.

Fine SL. Macular hole. A continuing saga. Editorial. *Arch Ophthalmol* 1999;117:248–249.

Gass JDM. Muller cell cone, an overlooked part of the anatomy of the fovea centralis. Hypotheses concerning its role in the pathogenesis of macular hole and foveomacular retinoschisis. *Arch Ophthalmol* 1999;117:821–823.

Gass JDM. Reappraisal of biomicroscopic classification of stages of development of a macular hole. *Am J Ophthalmol* 1995;119:752–759.

Gaudric A, Haouchine B, Massin P, et al. Macular hole formation. New data provided by optical coherence tomography. *Arch Ophthalmol* 1999;117:744–751.

Greven CM, Slusher MM, Czyz CN. The natural history of macular pseudoholes. *Am J Ophthalmol* 1998;125:360–366.

Imai M, Iijima H, Gotoh T, et al. Optical coherence tomography of successfully repaired idiopathic macular holes. *Am J Ophthalmol* 1999;128:621–627.

Kelly NE, Wendel RT. Vitreous surgery for idiopathic macular holes. Results of a pilot study. *Arch Ophthalmol* 1991;109:654–659.

Martinez J, Smiddy WC, Kim J, et al. Differentiating macular holes from macular pseudoholes. *Am J Ophthalmol* 1994;117:762–767.

Scott RAH, Ezra E, West JF, et al. Visual and anatomical results of surgery for longstanding macular holes. *Br J Ophthalmol* 2000;84:150–153.

Tanner V, Williamson TH. Watzke-Allen slit beam test in macular holes confirmed by optical coherence tomography. *Arch Ophthalmol* 2000;118:1059–1063.

Trese MT, Williams GA, Hartzer. A new approach to stage 3 macular holes. *Ophthalmology* 2000;107:1607–1611.

Tsujikawa M, Ohji M, Fujikado T et al. Differentiating full thickness macular holes from impending holes and macular pseudoholes. *Br J Ophthalmol* 1997;81:117–122.

Wendel RT, Patel AC, Kelly NE, et al. Vitreous surgery for macular holes. *Ophthalmology* 1993;100:1671–1676.

Central serous retinopathy

Pathogenesis

Central serous retinopathy (CSR), which is also referred to as central serous chorioretinopathy, is typically a sporadic, self-limited disease of young or middle-aged adult males with type A personality. This fairly common condition is characterized by a usually unilateral, localized detachment of the sensory retina at the macula with or without associated RPE detachment. It is uncertain whether the disease is of the RPE or caused by hyperpermeability of the choroidal vasculature. Factors that have been reported to induce or aggravate CSR include emotional stress, pregnancy, hypertension, systemic lupus erythematosus and the administration of systemic steroids. The two types of CSR are typical and the much less common bullous.

Diagnosis

1. Presentation

- *Typical CSR* presents with a fairly sudden onset of blurred vision in one eye associated with a positive relative scotoma, micropsia and/or metamorphopsia and impaired dark adaptation. Occasionally the condition is extrafoveal and asymptomatic.

- *Bullous CSR* presents with a visual field defect which corresponds to the area of subretinal fluid.

2. Signs

- *Typical CSR*
  a. Visual acuity is usually modestly reduced (6/9 to 6/12) and often correctable to 6/6 with the addition of a weak 'plus' lens. The elevation of the sensory retina

gives rise to an acquired hypermetropia with disparity between the subjective and objective refraction of the eye.

b. Fundus examination shows a round or oval separation of the sensory retina at the posterior pole (Figure 2.38). The subretinal fluid may be clear or turbid and small precipitates may be present on the posterior surface of the sensory detachment. Occasionally, the abnormal area in the RPE, through which fluid has leaked from the choriocapillaris into the subretinal space, can also be detected. In some cases a small RPE detachment can be detected within the serous detachment.

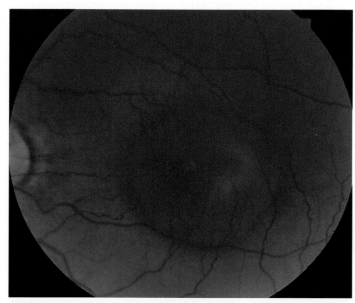

Figure 2.38 Typical central serous retinopathy

• *Bullous CSR* is characterized by large, single or multiple, serous retinal and RPE detachments (Figure 2.39) that are associated with a bullous inferior retinal detachment (Figure 2.40) This appearance may lead to diagnostic difficulties and the inappropriate diagnosis of rhegmatogenous retinal detachment, or exudative retinal detachment from some other cause.

3. **FA** in typical CSR is helpful in providing a definitive diagnosis and in ruling out the presence of CNV in atypical cases. In CSR, there is a breakdown of the outer blood-retinal barrier which allows the passage of free fluorescein molecules into the subretinal space. Two angiographic patterns may be seen:

• *Smoke-stack* appearance which evolves as follows:

a. The early phase shows a small hyperfluorescent spot due to leakage of dye from the choroid (Figure 2.41a). Occasionally more than one leak is present

b. During the late venous phase, the fluid passes into the subretinal space and ascends vertically (like a smoke-stack) from the point of leakage until it reaches the upper border of the detachment (Figure 2.41b).

c. The dye then spreads laterally taking on a 'mushroom' or 'umbrella' configuration, until the entire area of detachment is filled (Figure 2.41c).

• *Ink-blot* appearance, which is less common, evolves as follows:

a. The early phase shows a small hyperfluorescent spot (Figure 2.42a).

b. Subsequently, the spot gradually increases circumferentially until the entire subretinal space is filled with dye (Figure 2.42b and 2.42c).

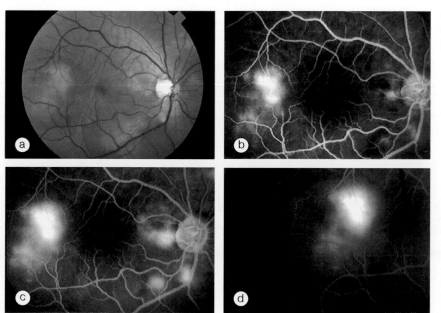

Figure 2.39 Multiple serous retinal detachment in bullous central serous retinopathy (see the text)

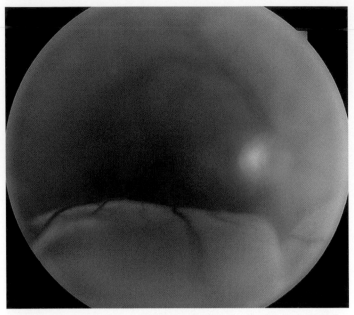

Figure 2.40 Inferior exudative retinal detachment in bullous central serous retinopathy

Prognosis

The natural course of CSR may be as follows:

- *Short course*, in about 80% of cases, with spontaneous resolution of subretinal fluid within 1–6 months and a return to normal, or near normal, visual acuity. Figure 2.43a, 2.43b and 2.43c shows active CSR. Figure 2.43d, 2.43e and 2.43f shows spontaneous resolution of fluid after two months.

- *Prolonged course*, in about 20% of cases, lasting longer than 6 months but with spontaneous resolution within 12 months. Even if visual acuity returns to normal, some degree of subjective visual impairment such as micropsia can persist, but seldom causes any significant disability.

- *Chronic course*, in a small minority of cases, lasting longer than 12 months which is characterized by progressive RPE

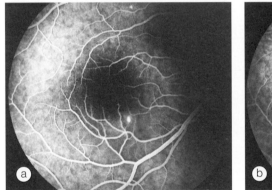
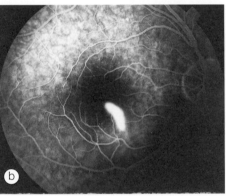
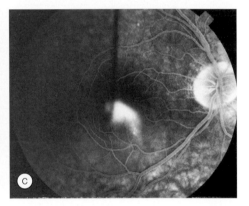

Figure 2.41 FA of central serous retinopathy showing the classic smoke-stack appearance

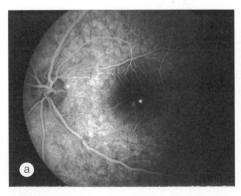
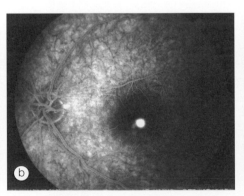
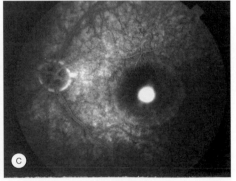

Figure 2.42 FA of central serous retinopathy showing the less common 'ink-blot' appearance

changes (Figure 2.44a) associated with a permanent impairment of visual acuity and occasionally the development of CNV. FA shows granular hyper-fluorescence containing one or more leaks (Figure 2.44b, 2.44c and 2.44d). This may be a consequence of either multiple recurrent attacks or prolonged detachment although a minority of patients do not have a past history of typical CSR, and in some the changes are bilateral.

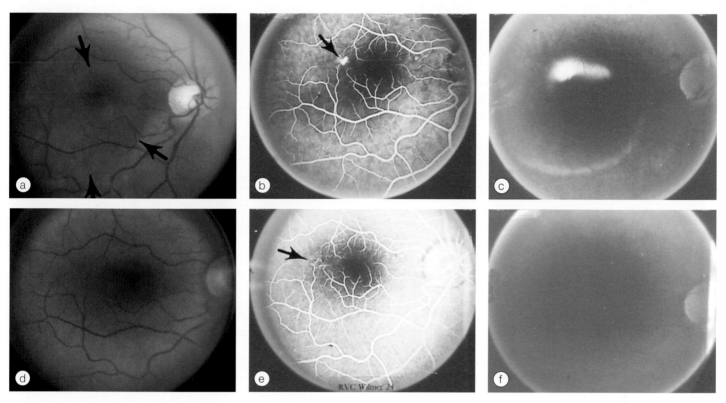

Figure 2.43 Typical central serous retinopathy (a), (b) & (c); spontaneous resolution two months later (d), (e) & (f)

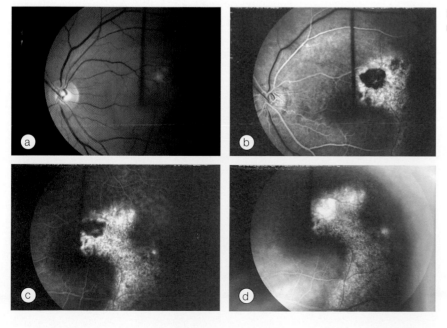

Figure 2.44 Chronic central serous retinopathy (see the text)

Laser photocoagulation

1. Indications

Treatment to the site of RPE leak or RPE detachment achieves a speedier resolution, lowers recurrence rate but does not influence the final visual outcome. In general, about 4 months should elapse before considering treatment of the first attack and one month for recurrent disease. Treatment is contraindicated if the site of leakage is near to or within the FAZ.

2. Technique

Treatment, if deemed appropriate, consists of two or three burns applied directly to the leakage site, using a 200 μm spot size, with an exposure of 0.2 second and low-moderate intensity to produce mild greying of the RPE. Figure 2.45a shows FA of a leaking point prior to laser photocoagulation and Figure 2.45b shows successful closure. Careful follow-up is required as between 2–5% of treated eyes subsequently develop CNV.

Differential diagnosis

The differential diagnosis consists of the following conditions which may also cause a sensory retinal detachment at the macula.

1. **Congenital optic disc anomalies**, most frequently optic disc pit (see Figure 2.101) and occasionally tilted disc, may be associated with serous macular detachments. Unless the optic disc is examined carefully in eyes with suspected CSR the causative disc lesion may be missed.

2. **Choroidal tumors** which have a predilection for the posterior pole such as circumscribed choroidal hemangioma and metastatic carcinoma.

3. **Unilateral acute idiopathic maculopathy**, which is a rare self-limiting condition that typically causes a sudden unilateral visual loss in a young person (see Figure 4.98).

4. **Choroidal neovascularization**, particularly if idiopathic.

5. **Harada disease** during the stage of multifocal detachments of the sensory retina may be mistaken for multifocal CSR (see Figure 4.60).

FURTHER READING

Burumcek E, Mudum A, Karacorlu S, et al. Laser photocoagulation for persistent central serous retinopathy. Results of a long-term follow-up. *Ophthalmology* 1997;104:616–622.

Gass JDM. Central serous chorioretinopathy and white subretinal exudation during pregnancy. *Arch Ophthalmol* 1991;109:677–681.

Gass JDM, Little H. Bilateral bullous exudative retinal detachment complicating idiopathic central serous chorioretinopathy. *Ophthalmology* 1995;102:737–747.

Gilbert CM, Owens SL, Smith PD, et al. Long-term follow-up of central serous chorioretinopathy. *Br J Ophthalmol* 1984;68:815–820.

Haimovici R, Gragoudas ES, Duker JS, et al. Central serous chorioretinopathy associated with inhaled or intranasal corticosteroids. *Ophthalmology* 1997;104:1653–1660.

Ie D, Yannuzzi LA, Spaide RF, et al. Subretinal exudative deposits in central serous chorioretinopathy. *Br J Ophthalmol* 1993;77:349–353.

Muzzaca D, Benson W. Central serous retinopathy: variants. *Surv Ophthalmol* 1986;31:170–174.

Spaide RF, Campeas L, Haas A, et al. Central serous chorioretinopathy in younger and older adults. *Ophthalmology* 1996;103:2070–2080.

Sahu DK, Namperumalsamy P, Hilton GF, et al. Bullous variant of idiopathic central serous chorioretinopathy. *Br J Ophthalmol* 2000;84:485–492.

Cystoid macular edema

Pathogenesis

Cystoid macular edema (CME) is the result of accummulation of fluid in the outer plexiform and inner nuclear layers of the retina centred about the foveola which results in the formation of cystic changes. In the short term,

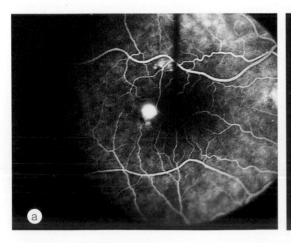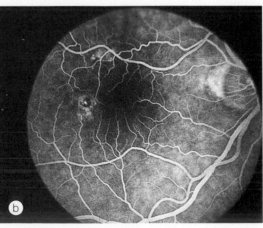

Figure 2.45 Laser treatment of central serous retinopathy: (a) FA prior to treatment showing the site of leakage; (b) appearance following successful closure of the leak

CME is usually innocuous, although long-standing cases usually lead to coalescence of the fluid-filled microcysts into large cystic spaces (Figure 2.46a) and subsequent lamellar hole formation at the fovea (Figure 2.46b) with irreversible damage to central vision. CME is a common and non-specific disease that may occur with any type of macular edema.

Diagnosis

1. **Presentation** varies according to the cause. In some cases visual acuity may already be poor from a pre-existing disease such as branch vein occlusion. In other cases without pre-existing disease as in post-cataract extraction CME, the patient complains of impairment of central vision associated with a small positive central scotoma.

2. **Signs**

- Visual acuity is reduced according to presence or absence of other disease as well as the severity and duration of CME.

- Slitlamp biomicroscopy shows loss of the foveal depression, thickening of the retina and multiple cystoid areas in the sensory retina (Figure 2.47 and Figure 2.48a). However, in early cases the cystic changes may be difficult to discern and the main finding is the presence of a yellow spot at the foveola.

3. **FA**

- The early venous phase shows the start of focal leakage into the parafoveal area (Figure 2.48b).

- The late venous phase shows increasing hyperfluorescence and coalescence of the focal leaks (Figure 2.48c).

- The late phase shows a 'flower-petal' pattern of hyperfluorescence (Figure 2.48d). This is caused by the accumulation of dye within microcystic spaces in the outer plexiform layer of the retina, with its radial arrangement of fibres about the centre of the foveola (Henle layer).

Causes and treatment

1. **Retinal vascular disease** (see Chapter 3)

- *Causes* include: diabetic retinopathy, retinal vein occlusion, idiopathic retinal telangiectasia, retinal artery macroaneurysm and radiation retinopathy.

- *Treatment* by laser photocoagulation may be appropriate in selected cases.

2. **Intraocular inflammatory diseases** (see Chapter 4)

- *Causes* include: intermediate uveitis, bacterial endophthalmitis, birdshot retinochoroidopathy, multifocal choroiditis with panuveitis, toxoplasmosis, cytomegalovirus retinitis, Behçet disease and scleritis.

- *Treatment* is aimed at controlling the inflammatory process with steroids or immunosuppressive agents. However, systemic carbonic anhydrase inhibitors may be beneficial in CME associated with intermediate uveitis.

3. **Post-cataract extraction CME** is rare following uncomplicated surgery, occurring in 1–2% of cases and frequently resolves spontaneously.

- *Risk factors* for the development of significant and persistent post-cataract extraction CME are anterior chamber intraocular lens implantation, secondary lens

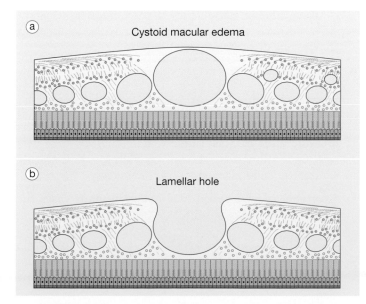

Figure 2.46 Severe chronic cystoid macular edema (a) resulting in lamellar hole formation (b)

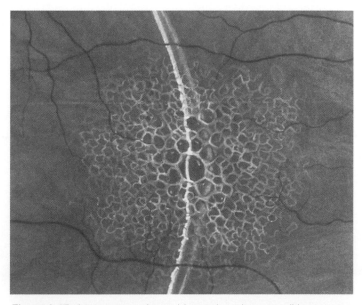

Figure 2.47 Appearance of cystoid macular edema on slitlamp biomicroscopy

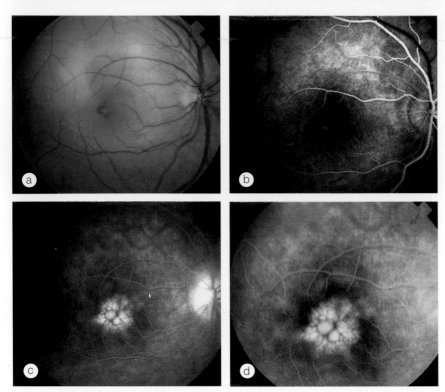

Figure 2.48 Cystoid macular edema (see the text)

implantation, and operative complications such as posterior capsular rupture, vitreous loss and vitreous incarceration into the incision site (Figure 2.49). The peak incidence of CME is 6–10 weeks, although in some cases the interval may be much longer.

- *Treatment* involves identification and correction of the underlying cause, if possible. For example, vitreous incarceration in the anterior segment may be amenable to anterior vitrectomy or YAG laser disruption of vitreous adhesions and as a last resort it may be necessary to remove an anterior chamber intraocular lens. If a correctable predisposing cause is not present, treatment may be difficult although many cases resolve

spontaneously within six months. Treatment of severe and persistent CME may respond to one or more of the following measures:

a. Systemic carbonic anhydrase inhibitors.

b. Steroids, given topically or by posterior periocular injections, combined with non-steroidal anti-inflammatory drugs (NSAIDS) such as ketorolac 0.5% (Acular) administered four times daily may be beneficial even in severe and long-standing cases. Unfortunately, in many cases the CME recurs when treatment is discontinued so that long-term medication may be required.

c. Pars plana vitrectomy may be useful in cases resistant to medical therapy even in eyes without apparent vitreous disturbance.

4. Post-surgical

- *Causes* include: YAG laser capsulotomy, peripheral retinal cryotherapy or laser photocoagulation. The risk of CME is reduced if capsulotomy is delayed for 6 months or more after cataract surgery. Rarely, CME may also develop following scleral buckling, penetrating keratoplasty and glaucoma filtration surgery.

- *Treatment* is unsatisfactory although in many cases the CME is mild and self-limited.

5. Drug induced

- *Causes* include: topical adrenaline 2% if used in an aphakic eye, topical latanoprost and systemic nicotinic acid.

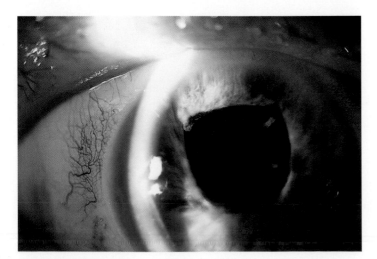

Figure 2.49 Vitreous incarceration into the incision site following vitreous loss at the time of cataract extraction

- *Treatment* involves cessation of medication.

6. Retinal dystrophies (see Chapter 5)

- *Causes* include: retinitis pigmentosa, gyrate atrophy and dominantly inherited CME (see Chapter 5).

- *Treatment* with systemic carbonic anhydrase inhibitors may be beneficial in CME associated with retinitis pigmentosa.

7. Vitreomacular traction syndrome is an uncommon condition characterized by partial peripheral vitreous separation with persistent posterior attachment to the macula resulting in anteroposterior and tangential traction vectors. Chronic CME resulting from anteroposterior traction is very common and may respond to vitrectomy.

8. Macular epiretinal membranes may occasionally cause CME by disrupting the perifoveal capillaries. Surgical excision of the membrane may be beneficial in selected cases.

Differential diagnosis

The following conditions give rise to subtle foveal lesions that may be mistaken for CME on cursory examination.

1. Stage 1 macular hole is characterized by a small yellow foveolar spot or ring (see Figure 2.33).

2. Solar retinopathy is characterized by a small yellow foveolar spot (see Figure 2.94). The diagnosis is usually evident from the history.

3. Retinal pigment epitheliitis is characterized by a blunted foveolar reflex and small foveolar lesions (see Figure 4.96).

4. X-linked retinoschisis has a 'bicycle-wheel' configuration (see Figure 5.19) reminiscent of CME. The condition is bilateral and associated with peripheral retinoschisis in 50% of cases.

5. Butterfly dystrophy is characterized by bilateral yellow lesions at the fovea (see Figure 5.58).

Case study

1. History

A 77-year-old female underwent bilateral uncomplicated extracapsular cataract extractions without intraocular lens implantation 23 years previously. Five years ago she had secondary anterior chamber intraocular lens implantations. She presented with a 6 week's history of progressive blurring of central vision in her right eye.

2. Examination right eye

- Visual acuity was 6/18.

- The intraocular lens was well centered, the pupil was normal and there was no vitreous herniation into the anterior chamber.

- Fundus examination showed CME (see Figure 2.48a).

3. FA right eye (see Figure 2.48b, 2.48c and 2.48d).

4. Diagnosis

- Pseudophakic CME.

5. Treatment

- Topical prednisolone and ketorolac 0.5% (Acular) drops both four times daily.

6. Course

- After three months visual acuity improved to 6/9. Treatment was discontinued but the CME recurred.

- Treatment was re-started and the CME resolved after four months and did not recur.

7. Comment

This case illustrates the development of CME following uncomplicated secondary lens implantation. It is, however, unusual for the time interval to be so long but fortunately the outcome was favorable.

FURTHER READING

Cox SN, Bird AC. Treatment of chorionic cystoid macular edema with acetazolamide. *Arch Ophthalmol* 1988;106:1190–1195.

Flach AJ, Jampol LM, Weinberg D, et al. Improvement in visual acuity in chronic aphakic and pseudophakic cystoid macular edema after treatment with topical 0.5% ketorolac tromethamine. *Am J Ophthalmol* 1991;112:514–519.

Kent D, Vonores SA, Campochario PA. Macular edema: the role of soluble mediators. Perspectives. *Br J Ophthalmol* 2000;84:542–545.

Moroi SE, Gottfredsdottir MS, Schteingart MT, et al. Cystoid macular edema associated with latanoprost therapy in a case series of patients with glaucoma and ocular hypertension. *Ophthalmology* 1999;106:1024–1029.

Pendergast SD, Margherio RR, Williams GA, et al. Vitrectomy for chronic pseudophakic cystoid macular edema. *Am J Ophthalmol* 1999;128:317–323.

Rosetti L, Chaudhuri J, Dickersin K. Medical prophyaxis and treatment of cystoid macular edema after cataract surgery: the results of meta-analysis. *Ophthalmology* 1998;105:397–405.

Thach AB, Dugel PU, Findall RJ, et al. A comparison of retrobulbar versus sub-Tenon's corticosteroid injection for cystoid macular edema refractory to topical therapy. *Ophthalmology* 1997;104:2003–2008.

Myopic maculopathy

Pathogenesis

High myopia is associated with progressive, excessive elongation of the globe which may be followed by degenerative changes involving the sclera, choroid, Bruch's membrane, RPE and sensory retina. Fundus changes usually occur when the degree of myopia is 6D or more and the axial length 25 mm or over.

Diagnosis

1. Chorioretinal changes

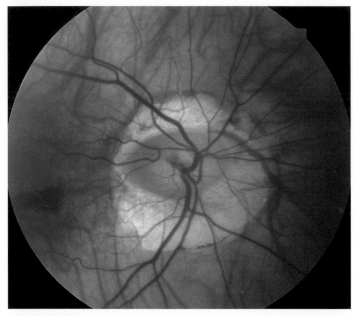

Figure 2.50 Tilted optic disc with peripapillary chorioretinal atrophy in high myopia

- A pale tesselate appearance due to attenuation of the RPE.

- Peripapillary chorioretinal atrophy which may occasionally surround a tilted optic disc (Figure 2.50).

- Severe chorioretinal atrophy involving the posterior pole which is characterized by visibility of the larger choroidal vessels and eventually the sclera (Figure 2.51).

- Peripheral chorioretinal (pavingstone) atrophy (Figure 2.52).

2. 'Lacquer cracks' develop in about 5% of highly myopic eyes. They consist of large breaks in Bruch's membrane and are characterized by fine, irregular, yellow lines, often branching and criss-crossing at the posterior pole (Figure 2.53).

3. **Maculopathy** may take one of the following forms:

- *Geographic atrophy* of the RPE and choriocapillaris involving the macula (Figure 2.54).

- *CNV* which may develop in association with 'lacquer cracks'. The prognosis for central vision is, however, better than in exudative AMD because CNV in highly myopic eyes tends to be relatively self-limited and not associated with the subsequent formation of subretinal fibrovascular scarring.

- *Foerster-Fuchs* spot is a raised, circular, pigmented lesion that may develop after the macular hemorrhage has absorbed (Figure 2.55).

- *Subretinal 'coin' hemorrhages*, which may be intermittent, may develop from lacquer cracks in the absence of CNV (Figure 2.56).

- *Macular hole*.

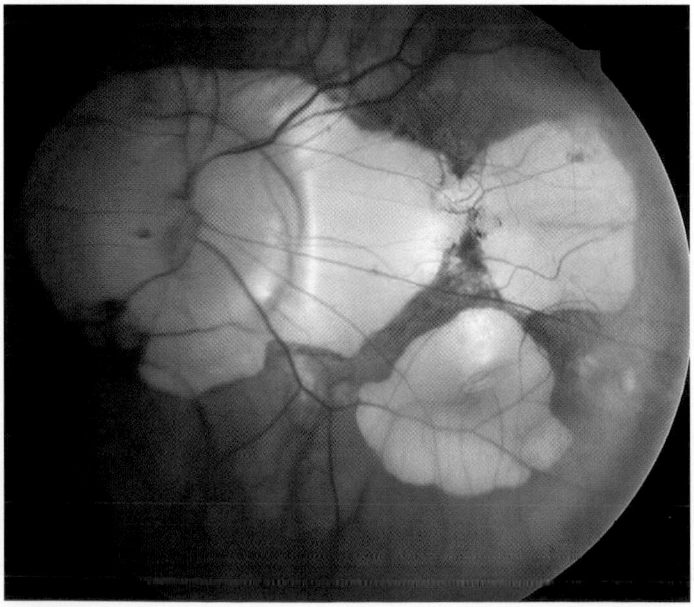

Figure 2.51 Severe chorioretinal atrophy involving the macula in high myopia

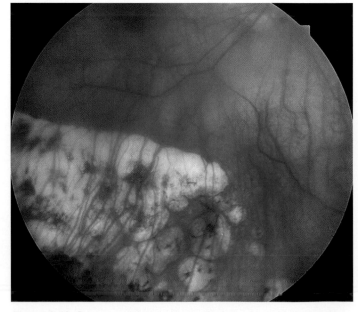

Figure 2.52 Severe peripheral chorioretinal atrophy in high myopia

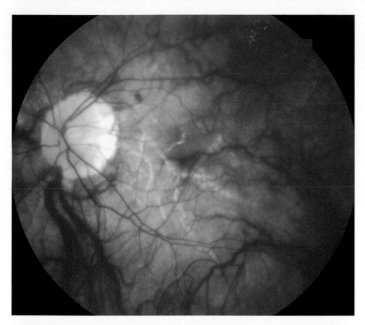

Figure 2.53 Lacquer cracks in high myopia

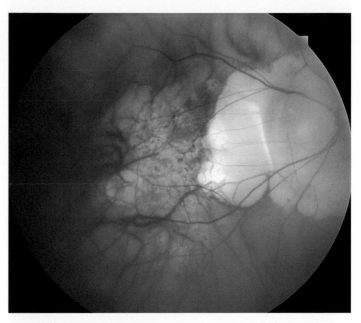

Figure 2.54 Geographic atrophy of the macula in high myopia

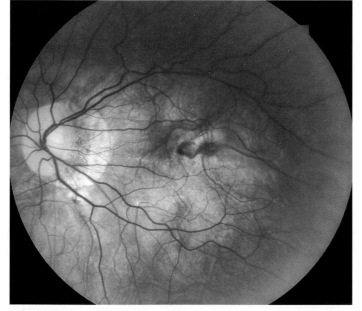

Figure 2.55 Foerster-Fuchs spot in high myopia

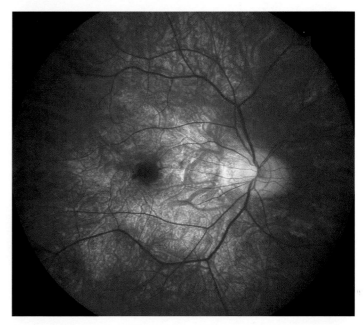

Figure 2.56 Small 'coin' hemorrhage at the fovea in high myopia

4. Retinal detachment may occur due to vitreous degeneration associated with macular hole formation, lattice degeneration associated with atrophic holes (Figure 2.57) and occasionally giant retinal tears (Figure 2.58) which typically occur in patients with very high myopia.

Associations of high myopia

1. Ocular

* *Cataract*, which may be either posterior subcapsular or early onset nuclear sclerosis.

* *Increased prevalence* of primary open-angle glaucoma, pigmentary glaucoma and steroid responsiveness.

* *Retinopathy of prematurity* may be associated with the subsequent development of myopia.

2. Systemic associations include: Stickler syndrome, Marfan syndrome, Ehlers-Danlos syndrome and Pierre-Robin syndrome.

Differential diagnosis

Other disorders characterized by extensive chorioretinal atrophy include the following:

1. Choroideremia

* *Differences* – nyctalopia, absence of peripapillary changes and macula is spared till late (see Figure 5.39).

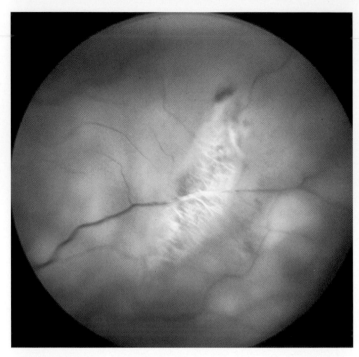

Figure 2.57 Lattice degeneration

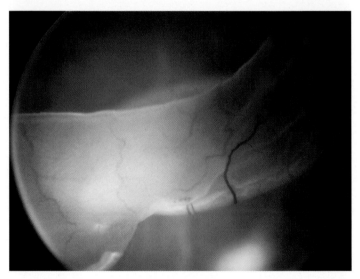

Figure 2.58 Retinal detachment caused by a giant retinal tear

Case study

1. History

A highly myopic 16-year-old boy presented with a 2 month's history of seeing a blank spot in the central vision of his left eye.

2. Examination left eye

- Visual acuity was 3/60 (−7.75DS).

- Fundus examination showed a round, slightly raised chorioretinal scar just temporal to the fovea with a hyperpigmented outline which itself was surrounded by a larger halo of RPE loss which involved the fovea (Figure 2.59a). Diffuse myopic changes with visibility of the choroidal vessels.

3. FA left eye

- *Arteriovenous phase* showed a round area of hyperfluorescence encircled by a hypofluorescent ring which itself was surrounded by a larger area of hyperfluorescence (Figure 2.59b).

- *Late phase* showed more intense hyperfluorescence of the round area and the larger surrounding area, but no increase in size (Figure 2.59c). The choroiodal vessels are easily visible due to diffuse thinning of the RPE.

4. Diagnosis

- Old CNV (Foerster-Fuchs spot).

5. Management

- The patient was advised to check the vision in both eyes with the Amsler grid because of an increased risk of CNV. Seven years later visual acuity was still 3/60 and his right eye remained normal.

6. Comment

This case illustrates that CNV in myopes may occur at a relatively young age, but unlike that associated with exudative AMD it tends to remain localized.

2. Gyrate atrophy

- *Differences* – early onset, lesions have typically scalloped edges and macula is spared till late (see Figure 5.44).

3. Diffuse choroidal atrophy

- *Differences* – chorioretinal changes are diffuse and not punched out as in myopia (see Figure 5.62).

4. Progressive bifocal chorioretinal atrophy

- *Differences* – early onset, specific atrophic areas confined to the macular and nasal fundus (see Figure 5.64).

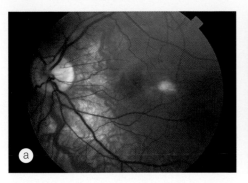
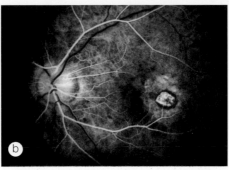
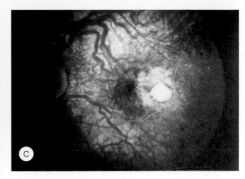

Figure 2.59 High myopia and CNV (see the text)

FURTHER READING

Curtin BJ. Myopia: a review of its etiology, pathogenesis and treatment. *Surv Ophthalmol* 1970;15:1–17.

Grossniklaus HE, Green WR. Pathologic findings in pathologic myopia. *Retina* 1992;12:127–133.

Jalkh AE, Weiter JJ, Trempe CL, et al. Choroidal neovascularization with degenerative myopia: role of laser photocoagulation. *Ophthalmic Surg* 1987;18:721–725.

Johnson DA, Yannuzzi LA, Shakin JL, et al. Lacquer cracks following laser treatment of choroidal neovascularization in pathologic myopia. *Retina* 1998;18:118–124.

Steidl SM, Pruett RC. Macular complications associated with posterior staphyloma. *Am J Ophthalmol* 1997;123:181–187.

Stripe M, Michels RG. Retinal detachment in highly myopic eyes due to macular holes and epiretinal traction. *Retina* 1990;10:113–114.

Tabandeh H, Flynn HW Jr, Scott IU, et al. Visual acuity outcomes of patients 50 years of age or older with high myopia and untreated neovascularization. *Ophthalmology* 1999;106:2063–2067.

Takano M, Kishi S. Foveal schisis and retinal detachment in severely myopic eyes with posterior staphylomas. *Am J Ophthalmol* 1999;128:472–476.

Macular epiretinal membrane

Pathogenesis

Macular epiretinal membranes that develop at the vitreoretinal interface consist of proliferation of retinal glial cells which have gained access to the retinal surface through breaks in the internal limiting membrane. It has been postulated that these breaks may be created when the posterior vitreous detaches from the macula. The causes are as follows:

1. **Idiopathic membranes** predominantly affects otherwise healthy elderly individuals and are bilateral in about 10% of cases.

2. **Secondary membranes** may be associated with the following conditions:

- *Retinal procedures* such as detachment surgery, photocoagulation and cryotherapy may either induce or worsen a pre-existing macular epiretinal membrane. Untreated, these membranes usually cause a variable but permanent reduction of vision. Very occasionally, however, the membrane may separate spontaneously from the retina.

- *Other causes* include: retinal vascular disease, intraocular inflammation and ocular trauma.

Classification

The clinical appearance of epiretinal membranes depends on their density and any associated distortion of the retinal vasculature. It is convenient to divide the condition into: (a) *cellophane maculopathy* and (b) *macular pucker*.

Cellophane maculopathy

Cellophane maculopathy is caused by a thin layer of epiretinal cells. It is common and usually idiopathic.

1. **Presentation** may be with mild metamorphopsia although frequently the condition is asymptomatic and discovered by chance.

2. **Signs**

- Visual acuity may be normal or slightly reduced (6/9).

- The macula shows an irregular light reflex or sheen at the macula.

- The membrane itself is translucent and is best detected using 'red-free' light, but as it thickens and contracts it becomes more obvious and causes fine striae on the retinal surface and distortion of blood vessels (Figure 2.60a) which is highlighted on FA (Figure 2.60b).

3. **Treatment** is not appropriate.

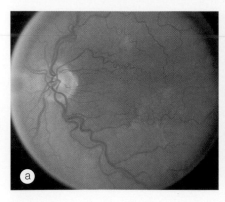

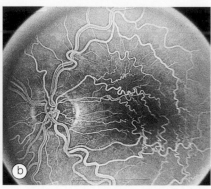

Figure 2.60 Cellophane maculopathy (see the text)

Macular pucker

Macular pucker is caused by thickening and contraction of the membrane. It is much less common than cellophane maculopathy and may be idiopathic or secondary.

1. **Presentation** is with metamorphopsia and blurring of central vision.

2. **Signs**

- Visual acuity is reduced to 6/12 or worse, depending on severity.

- The macula shows severe distortion of the blood vessels, retinal wrinkling and white striae which may obscure underlying blood vessels (Figure 2.61).

- Associated findings are a macular pseudo-hole within the membrane (Figure 2.62) and occasionally secondary chronic CME.

3. **Treatment** by surgical removal of the membrane usually improves or eliminates distortion, and improves visual acuity in about 50% of cases.

FURTHER READING

Appiah AP, Hirose T. Secondary causes of premacular fibrosis. *Ophthalmology* 1989;96:386–392.

de Bustros S, Thompson JT, Michels RG, et al. Vitrectomy for idiopathic epiretinal membranes causing macular pucker. *Br J Ophthalmol* 1988;72:692–695.

Heilskov TW, Massicotte SJ, Folk JC, et al. Epiretinal macular membranes in eyes with attached posterior cortical vitreous. *Retina* 1996;16:279–284.

Margheiro RR, Cox MS Jr, Trese MT, et al. Removal of epiretinal membranes. *Ophthalmology* 1985;92:1075–1083.

McLeod D, Hiscott PS, Grierson I. Age-related cellular proliferation at the vitreoretinal junction. *Eye* 1987;1:263–281.

Mitchell P, Smith W, Chey T, et al. Prevalence and associations of epiretinal membranes. The Blue Mountains Eye Study, Australia. *Ophthalmology* 1997;104:1033–1040.

Rice TA, de Bustros S, Michels RD, et al. Prognostic factors in vitrectomy for epiretinal membranes of the macula. *Ophthalmology* 1986;93:602–610.

Smiddy WE, Maguire AM, Green WR, et al. Idiopathic epiretinal membranes; ultrastructural characteristics and clinicopathologic correlation. *Ophthalmology* 1989;96:811–821.

Uemura A, Ideka H, Nagasaki H, et al. Macular pucker after retinal detachment surgery. *Ophthalmic Surg* 1992;23:116–119.

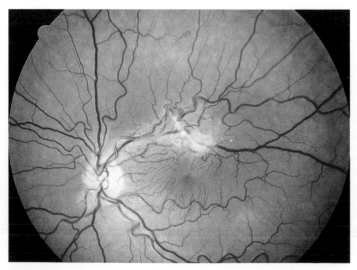

Figure 2.61 Severe macular pucker

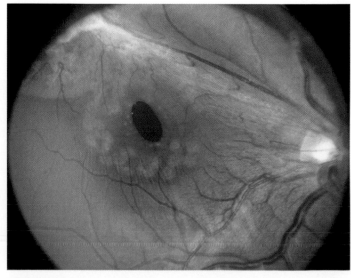

Figure 2.62 Severe macular pucker with a pseudo-hole

Angioid streaks

Pathogenesis

Angioid streaks are the result of crack-like dehiscences in a thickened, calcified and brittle Bruch's membrane with secondary changes in the RPE and choriocapillaris.

Diagnosis

1. Signs

- Linear, grey or dark-red lesions with irregular serrated edges lying beneath the normal retinal blood vessels which may initially be very subtle and easily overlooked (Figure 2.63).

- Later they become more obvious due to secondary RPE atrophy or hypertrophy (Figure 2.64).

- The streaks intercommunicate in a ring-like fashion around the optic disc and then radiate outwards from the peripapillary area (Figure 2.65).

2. FA shows hyperfluorescence caused by RPE window defects over the streaks (see Figure 2.74).

3. Associated findings

- *'Peau d'orange'* consisting of mottled pigmentation of the posterior pole most apparent temporal to the macula (Figure 2.66), which may occasionally antedate the appearance of angioid streaks.

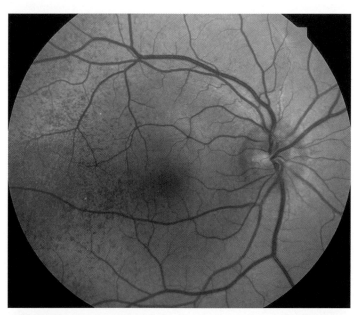

Figure 2.63 Mild angioid streaks

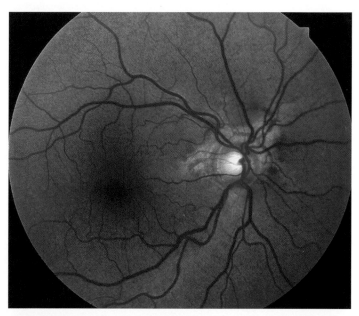

Figure 2.64 Moderate angioid streaks

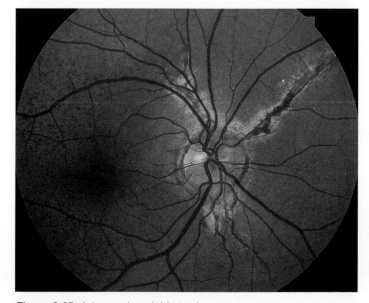

Figure 2.65 Advanced angioid streaks

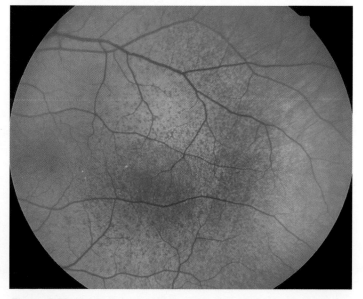

Figure 2.66 Mottled pigmentation 'peau d'orange' in an eye with angioid streaks

- *Salmon spots* consisting of peripheral, focal chorioretinal scars (Figure 2.67).

- *Optic nerve drusen* (Figure 2.68) are found more frequently in eyes with angioid streaks than in those without.

Prognosis

Visual impairment occurs in over 70% of patients as a result of one or more of the following:

1. **CNV** with subsequent serous and hemorrhagic detachment of the fovea and scarring is the most serous complication (see Figure 2.74). Treatment of early CNV by laser photocoagulation may be appropriate in selected cases but the recurrence rate is high.

2. **Choroidal rupture**, which may occur following relatively trivial ocular trauma and result in a subfoveal hemorrhage (Figure 2.69) and subsequent scarring (Figure 2.70). This is because eyes with angioid streaks are very

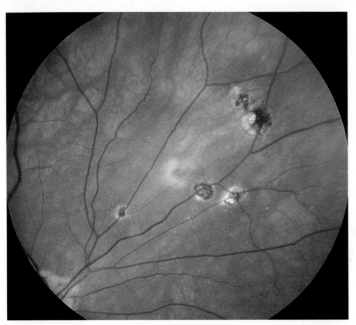

Figure 2.67 Peripheral, focal, chorioretinal scars ('salmon spots') in an eye with angioid streaks

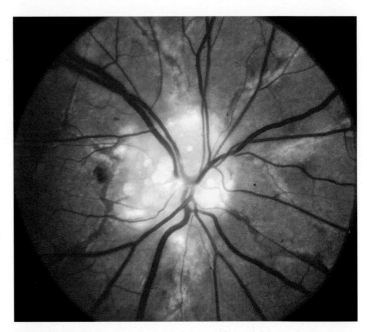

Figure 2.68 Optic disc druse in an eye with angioid streaks

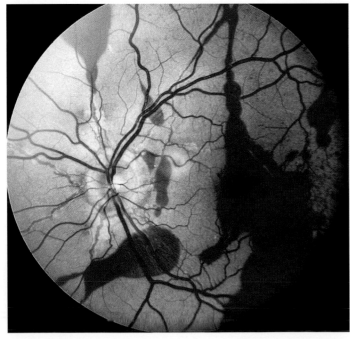

Figure 2.69 Hemorrhage caused by traumatic choroidal rupture in an eye with angioid streaks

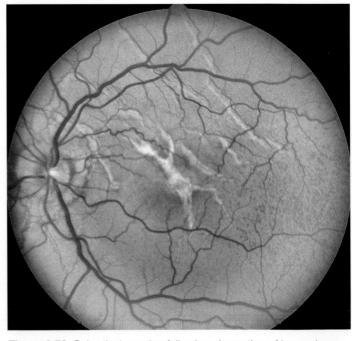

Figure 2.70 Subretinal scarring following absorption of hemorrhage in an eye with angioid streaks

fragile and patients should be warned against participating in contact sports.

3. **Foveal involvement by a streak**.

Systemic associations

Approximately 50% of patients with angioid streaks have no associated systemic disorder. The remainder have one of the following conditions.

1. **Pseudoxanthoma elasticum** (PXE) is by far the most common association of angioid streaks. Approximately 85% of patients develop ocular involvement, usually after the second decade of life. The combination of the two is referred to as 'Groenblad-Strandberg syndrome'. PXE is an uncommon, inherited, generalized disorder of connective tissue. It affects the elastin in the dermis, arterial walls and Bruch's membrane, resulting in abnormal mineralization and deposition of phosphorus in the fibrils. There are four main types, of which two are dominant and two recessive with varying severity of systemic and ocular manifestations. The following are the main clinical features of PXE:

- *Skin lesions* consist of yellow papules arranged in a linear or reticulate pattern giving rise to a 'chicken-skin' appearance. The lesions are most frequently located on the neck, antecubital fossae, axillae, groins, and the paraumbilical area. The affected areas of skin are loose (Figure 2.71), and may also be delicate and hyperelastic. Occasionally the condition is subclinical and can be diagnosed only by skin biopsy.

- *Cardiovascular disease*, which is characterized by accelerated atherosclerosis resulting in coronary artery disease and intermittent claudication, hypertension from renovascular disease, and mitral incompetence.

- *Gastrointestinal hemorrhage*, which may occur within the first decade of life and be life-threatening.

2. **Ehlers–Danlos syndrome type 6** (ocular sclerotic) is a rare, usually dominantly inherited, disorder of collagen caused by deficiency of procollagen lysyl hydroxylase. There are 11 subtypes but only type 6 is associated with angioid streaks. Systemic features include the following:

- The *skin* is thin, hyperelastic and heals poorly.

- The *joints* are hypermobile with lax ligaments (Figure 2.72). This may lead to recurrent dislocation, repeated falls, hydroarthrosis and pseudotumor formation over the knees and elbows.

- *Cardiovascular disease* consists of a bleeding diathesis, dissecting aneurysms, spontaneous rupture of large blood vessels and mitral prolapse.

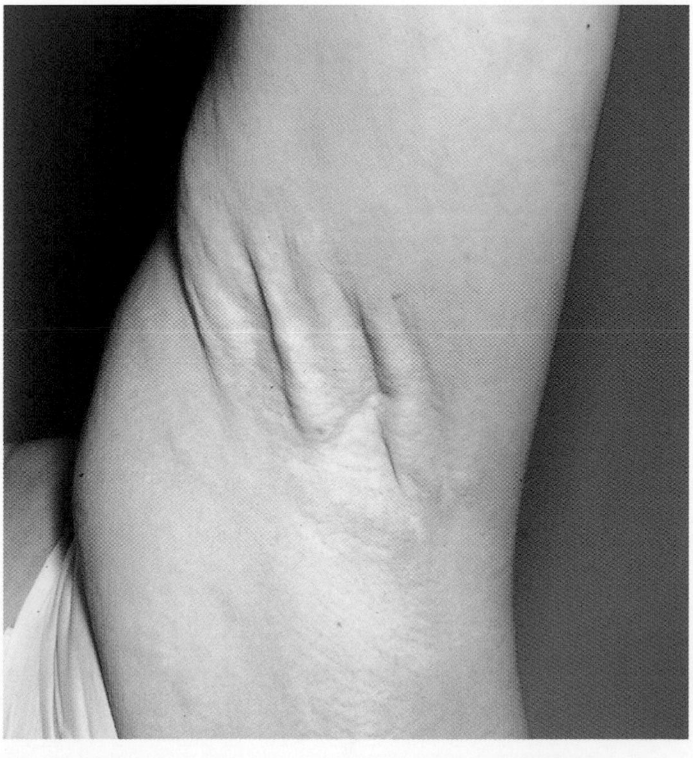

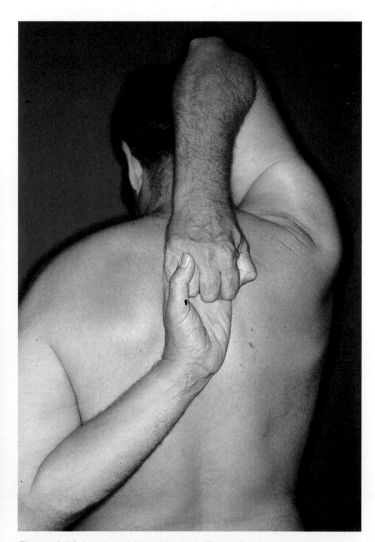

Figure 2.71 Loose axillary skin in pseudoxanthoma elasticum

Figure 2.72 Hypermobility of joints in Ehlers-Danlos syndrome

- *Other systemic problems* include: scoliosis, diaphragmatic hernias and diverticula of the gastrointestinal and respiratory tracts.

- *Other ocular features* include: epicanthic folds, ocular fragility to trauma, keratoconus, high myopia, retinal detachment, blue sclera and lens subluxation.

3. **Paget disease** is a chronic, progressive metabolic bone disease characterized by excessive and disorganized resorption and formation of bone. Angioid streaks are uncommon occurring in only about 2% cases. Systemic features include the following:

- *Bone deformities*, such as enlargement of the skull and anterior bowing of the tibias (Figure 2.73).

- *Systemic complications* include: deafness, arthropathy, kyphoscoliosis, fractures, compression of spinal and cranial nerves, heart failure and increased risk of osteosarcoma.

- *Other ocular features* include: optic atrophy, proptosis and ocularmotor nerve palsies.

4. **Hemoglobinopathies** are occasionally associated with angioid streaks are: homozygous sickle-cell disease (HbSS), sickle-cell trait (HbAS), sickle-cell thalassemia (HbS thalassemia), sickle-cell hemoglobin C disease (HbSC), hemoglobin H disease (HbH), homozygous β-thalassemia major, β-thalassemia intermedia and β-thalassemia minor.

FURTHER READING

Clarkson JG, Altman RD. Angioid streaks. *Surv Ophthalmol* 1982;26:235–246.

Dabbs TR, Skjodt K. Prevalence of angioid streaks and other ocular complications of Paget's disease of bone. *Br J Ophthalmol* 1990;74:579–582.

Lim JI, Bressler NM, Marsh MJ, et al. Laser treatment of choroidal neovascularization in patients with angioid streaks. *Am J Ophthalmol* 1993;116:414–423.

Shields JA, Federman JL, Tomer TL, et al. Angioid streaks. I. Ophthalmoscopic variations and diagnostic problems. *Br J Ophthalmol* 1975;59:257–266.

Case study

1. History

A 31-year-old man presented with a 2 month's history of the sudden onset of blind spots in the temporal aspect of his right vision. The patient's brother developed a problem with his vision two years ago. The patient, his brother and sister have leathery thickening involving the skin of their necks.

2. Examination

Right eye

- Visual acuity was 6/6.

- Fundus examination showed widespread streaks radiating outwards in a spoke-like manner from the peripapillary zone (Figure 2.74a). Finger-like projections of RPE atrophy surrounded a particular streak traversing just inferior to the fovea.

- There was a small subretinal hemorrhages infero-nasal to the fovea and two, small, grayish subretinal lesions in the papillomacular bundle probably consisting of CNV.

- Other fundus findings were widespread mid-peripheral granular pigmentary changes (peau d'orange) and multiple, small, punched out peripheral chorioretinal scars.

Left eye

- Visual acuity was 6/6.

- The fundus findings were similar but there were neither hemorrhages nor focal subretinal lesions.

3. FA

Right eye

- *Arteriovenous phase* showed three small localized areas of lacy hyperfluorescence and transmitted choroidal fluorescence corresponding to RPE atrophy associated with the streaks (Figure 2.74b).

- *Later phases* showed increasing hyperfluorescence from the three small localized areas, especially the larger area in infero-nasal to the fovea. (Figure 2.74c).

Left eye

- Transmitted choroidal hyperfluorescence corresponding to RPE atrophy associated with the streaks.

4. Diagnosis

- Pseudoxanthoma elasticum, bilateral angioid streaks, and right CNV.

5. Treatment

- Focal argon laser photocoagulation was applied to the three areas of CNV.

6. Outcome

- Two years later, visual acuity was 6/6 with no evidence of recurrence of CNV.

7. Comment

This patient had PXE which is the most frequent systemic association of angioid streaks. He had a favorable outcome following treatment of three areas of CNV.

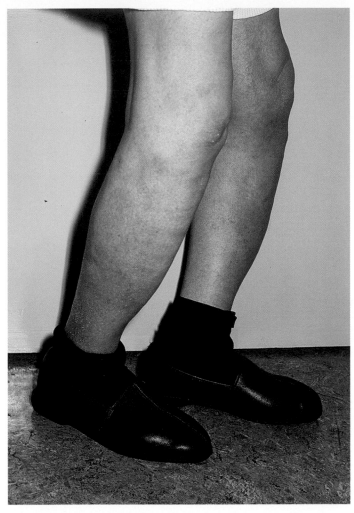

Figure 2.73 Anterior bowing of the tibias in Paget disease

Choroidal folds

Causes

Choroidal folds are parallel grooves or striae involving inner choroid, Bruch's membrane, RPE and may also involve the outer sensory retina. Possible mechanisms include choroidal congestion, scleral folding and contraction of Bruch's membrane. The main causes are the following:

1. **Idiopathic** folds may occur for no apparent reason in both eyes of healthy hypermetropic patients with normal or near-normal visual acuity.

2. **Orbital diseases** such as retrobular tumors and thyroid ophthalmopathy, may cause choroidal folds that impair visual acuity.

3. **Choroidal tumors** such as melanomas may mechanically displace the surrounding choroid and cause folding.

4. **Ocular hypotony**, which may occur following filtration surgery, if severe and prolonged, may be associated with choroidal folds.

5. **Miscellaneous** uncommon causes include: chronic papilledema, posterior scleritis and scleral buckle for repair of retinal detachment.

Diagnosis

1. **Presentation** may be with metamorphopsia, although the patient may be asymptomatic. Initially visual dysfunction is caused by distortion of overlying retinal receptors, but in long-standing cases, permanent changes may develop in the RPE and sensory retina.

2. **Signs**

- Visual acuity may be normal or variably impaired.

- The fundus shows parallel lines, grooves or striae, usually horizontally orientated but they may occasionally be

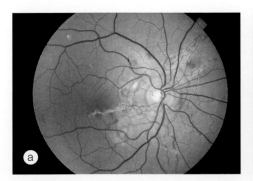
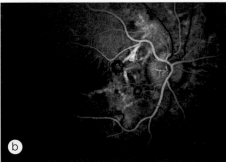
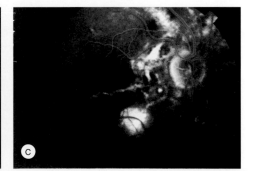

Figure 2.74 Angioid streaks with CNV (see the text)

vertical, oblique or irregular usually situated at the posterior pole (Figure 2.75a).

- The crest (elevated portion) of a fold is yellow and less pigmented as a result of stretching and thinning of the RPE.

- The trough of a fold is darker due to compression of the RPE.

3. FA shows alternating hyperfluorescent and hypofluorescent streaks at the level of the RPE (Figure 2.75b, 2.75c and 2.75d).

- The hyperfluorescence corresponds to the crests as a result of increased background choroidal fluorescence showing through the stretched and thinned RPE, and the

hypofluorescence corresponds to the troughs due to blockage of choroidal fluorescence by the compressed and thickened RPE (Figure 2.76).

FURTHER READING

Cassidy LM, Sanders MD. Choroidal folds and papilloedema. *Br J Ophthalmol* 1999;83:1139–1143.

Griebel SP, Kosmorsky GS. Choroidal folds associated with increased intracranial pressure. *Am J Ophthalmol* 2000;129:513–516.

Leahey AB, Brucker AK, Wyszynski RE, et al. Chorioretinal folds. A comparison of unilateral and bilateral cases. *Arch Ophthalmol* 1993;111:357–359.

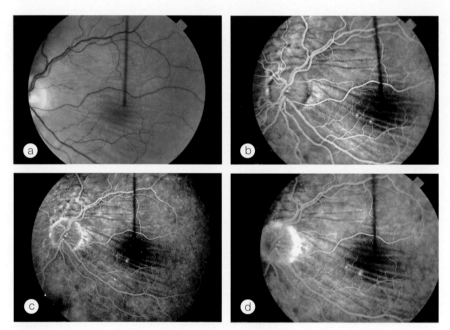

Figure 2.75 Choroidal folds (see the text)

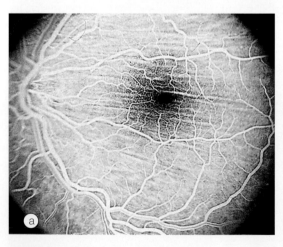

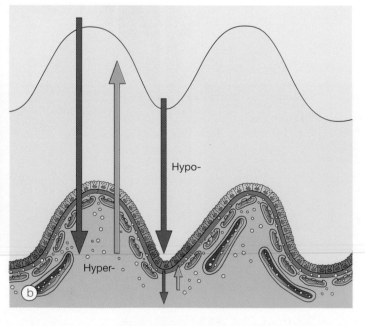

Figure 2.76 Mechanisms of hypo- and hyperfluorescence in choroidal folds

Idiopathic choroidal neovascularization

Diagnosis

Idiopathic CNV is an uncommon condition which affects patients under the age of 50 years. The diagnosis is one of exclusion of other possible associations of CNV such as AMD, angioid streaks, high myopia and presumed ocular histoplasmosis. Idiopathic CNV carries a better visual prognosis than that associated with AMD and in some cases spontaneous evolution may occur.

FURTHER READING

Cohen SY, Laroche A, Leguen Y, et al. Etiology of choroidal neovascularization in young patients. *Ophthalmology* 1995;102:782–889.

Ho AC, Yannuzzi LA, Pisciano K, et al. The natural history of idiopathic subfoveal neovascularization. *Ophthalmology* 1995;102:782–789.

Lindblom B, Andersson T. The prognosis of idiopathic choroidal neovascularization in persons younger than 50 years of age. *Ophthalmology* 1998;105:1816–1820.

Macular Photocoagulation Study Group. Argon laser photocoagulation for idiopathic neovascularization. Results of a randomized clinical trial. *Arch Ophthalmol* 1983;101:1358–1361.

Macular Photocoagulation Study Group. Krypton laser photocoagulation for idiopathic neovascular lesions. Results of a randomized clinical trial. *Arch Ophthalmol* 1990;108:832–837.

Case study

1. History

A 47-year-old female presented with a one day history of blurred and distorted vision in her right eye.

2. Examination right eye

- Visual acuity was 3/60.

- Fundus examination showed retinal edema about one disc in diameter nasal to the fovea associated with a small hemorrhage and hard exudates (Figure 2.77a).

3. FA right eye

- *Arterial phase* showed lacy hyperfluorescence on the nasal side of the fovea and a small area of hypofluorescence above the fovea corresponding to the hemorrhage (Figure 2.77b).

- *Later phases* showed extensive hyperfluorescence at the fovea (Figures 2.77c and 2.77d).

4. Diagnosis

- Idiopathic, juxtafoveal CNV based on the relatively young age of the patient and the absence of other disorders that may be associated with CNV.

5. Treatment

- Focal laser photocoagulation (32 burns, 200 µm, 0.5 seconds, 300 mW) was applied to the CNV.

6. Outcome

- Seven years later visual acuity was 6/12.

- Fundus examination showed a laser scar just nasal to fixation (Figure 2.78a).

- FA showed early hypofluorescence of the laser scar (Figure 2.78b) and later gradual hyperfluorescence at the edge of the scar (Figure 2.78c) which was associated with late staining (Figure 2.78d). There was no evidence of recurrent CNV.

7. Comment

This patient has done extremely well following laser treatment with no evidence of recurrent CNV with improvement and preservation of good visual acuity for 7 years. This is in contrast to the results of laser treatment in AMD in which recurrence of CMV is very common.

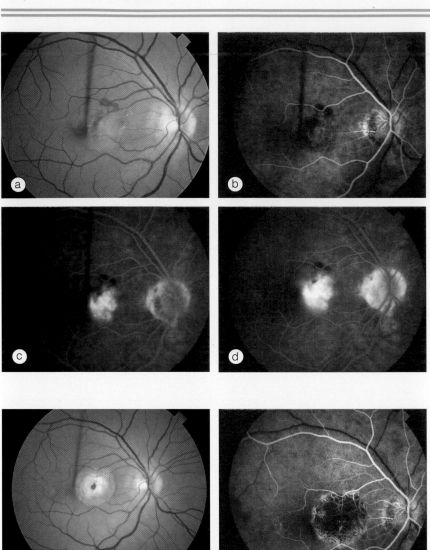

Figure 2.77 Idiopathic CNV prior to laser photocoagulation (see the text)

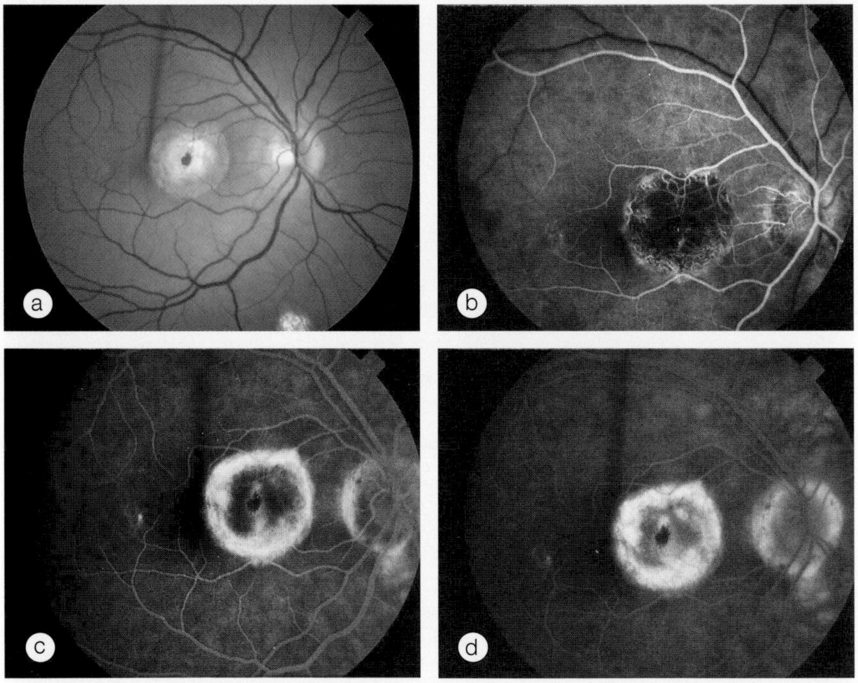

Figure 2.78 The same eye after successful laser photocoagulation (see the text)

Drug-induced maculopathies

Antimalarials

Chloroqine (Nivaquine, Avlocor) and hydroxychloroquine (Plaquenil) are quinolone antimalarial drugs which are used in the prophylaxis and treatment of malaria as well as in the treatment of certain rheumatological disorders (e.g., rheumatoid arthritis, juvenile chronic arthritis, systemic lupus erythematosus). The use of chloroquine has also been advocated in the treatment of calcium abnormalities of sarcoidosis. Antimalarials are excreted from the body very slowly and are melanotropic drugs that become concentrated in melanin-containing structures of the eye such as the RPE and choroid. The two main potential ocular side-effects of antimalarials are retinotoxicity and corneal deposits. Although uncommon, the retinal changes are potentially serious and the corneal changes (vortex keratopathy) which are extremely common, are innocuous (Figure 2.79).

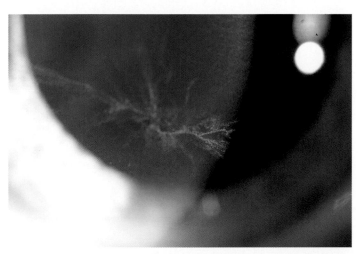

Figure 2.79 Vortex keratopathy

1. **Chloroquine** retinotoxicity is related to the total cumulative dose. The normal daily dose is 250 mg. If the cumulative dose is less than 100 g or the duration of treatment is under one year, it is rarely associated with retinal damage. The risk of toxicity increases significantly when the cumulative dose exceeds 300 g (i.e. 250 mg daily for 3 years). However, there have been reports of patients receiving cumulative doses exceeding 1000 g who did not develop retinotoxicity. If possible, chloroquine should be used only if other agents are ineffective.

2. **Hydroxychloroquine** is much safer than chloroquine, and if the daily dose does not exceed 400 mg, the risk of retinotoxicity is negligible. Physicians should therefore be encouraged to use hydroxychloroquine instead of chloroquine whenever possible.

Diagnosis

Chloroquine maculopathy can be divided into the following stages:

1. **Premaculopathy** is characterized by normal visual acuity and a scotoma to a red target between 4° and 9° from fixation. Amsler grid testing may also show a defect. However, the most sensitive test is assessment of colour vision to detect both mild blue-yellow and protan red-green defects. The two most sensitive tests for detecting these defects are the Adams Desaturation-15 test and the American Optical Hardy Rand Ritter test. Other color vision tests such as the Ishihara do not appear to be as sensitive. If the drug is discontinued, the scotoma usually disappears.

2. **Early maculopathy** is the next stage, if treatment is not discontinued. It is characterized by a modest reduction of visual acuity (6/9–6/12). Fundus examination shows a subtle 'bull's eye' macular lesion characterized by central foveolar pigmentation surrounded by a depigmented zone of RPE atrophy which is itself encircled by a hyperpigmented ring (Figure 2.80a). The lesion may be more obvious on FA than ophthalmoscopy, because the RPE atrophy gives rise to a RPE 'window' defect (Figure 2.80b and 2.80c). This stage may progress even if the drug is stopped.

3. **Moderate maculopathy** is characterized as moderate reduction of visual acuity (6/18–6/24) and an obvious 'bull's eye' macular lesion (Figure 2.81).

4. **Severe maculopathy** is characterized by marked reduction of visual acuity (6/36 to 6/60) with widespread RPE atrophy surrounding the fovea (Figure 2.82).

5. **End-stage maculopathy** is characterized by severe reduction of visual acuity and marked atrophy of the RPE with unmasking of the larger choroidal blood vessels (Figure 2.83). The retinal arterioles may also become attenuated and pigment clumps develop in the peripheral retina.

Screening

Routine screening of patients on hydroxychloroquine is unnecessary. In clinical practice chloroquine can also be administered safely to patients without the need for repetitive routine examinations by ophthalmologists or the use of complicated tests. Recording of visual acuity and ophthalmoscopy by the prescribing doctor is all that is required. The patient can be given an Amsler grid to use once a week. If an abnormality is found, then the opinion of an ophthalmologist should be sought. The ophthalmologist can, if necessary, perform more sophisticated tests such as visual fields, macular threshold, color vision testing as described above, contrast sensitivity, FA and electro-oculography.

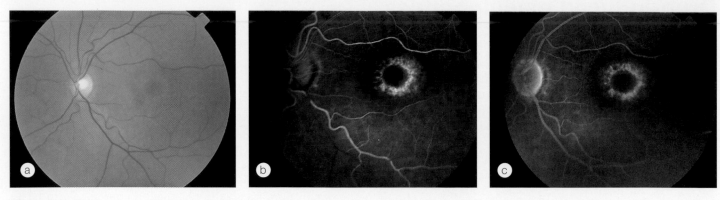

Figure 2.80 Bull's eye maculopathy (see the text)

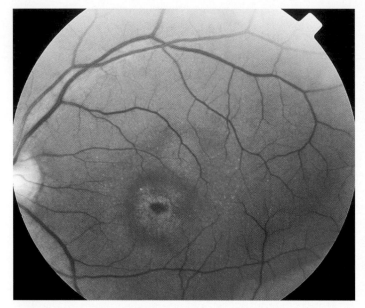

Figure 2.81 Moderately severe chloroquine maculopathy

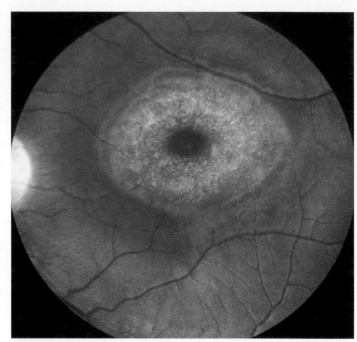

Figure 2.82 Very severe chloroquine maculopathy

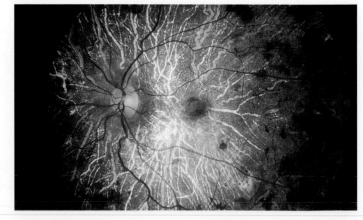

Figure 2.83 End-stage chloroquine maculopathy

Phenothiazines

Thioridazine

Thiodirazine (Melleril) is used to treat schizophrenia and related psychoses. The normal daily dose is 150–600 mg. Higher doses which exceed 800 mg/day for just a few weeks may be sufficient to cause reduced visual acuity and impairment of dark adaptation. The clinical signs of progressive retinotoxicity are as follows:

- Salt-and-pepper pigmentary disturbance involving the mid-periphery and posterior pole.

- Coarse plaque-like pigmentation and focal loss of the RPE and choriocapillaris (Figure 2.84).

- Diffuse loss of the RPE and choriocapillaris (Figure 2.85 and Figure 2.86).

Chlorpromazine

Chlorpromazine (Largactil) is used as a sedative and to treat schizophrenia. The normal daily dose is 75–300 mg. Retitoxicity may occur if very much larger doses are used over a prolonged period. It is characterized by non-specific pigmentary granularity and clumping. Other innocuous ocular side-effects include yellowish-brown granules on the anterior lens capsule and corneal endothelial deposits.

Crystalline maculopathies

Tamoxifen

Tamoxifen (Nolvodex, Emblon, Noltan, Tamofen) is a specific anti-estrogen used in the treatment of selected patients with breast carcinoma. It has few systemic side-effects and ocular complications are uncommon. The normal daily dose is 20–40 mg. Retinotoxicity may develop in some patients on higher doses and rarely in patients on normal doses. It is characterized by relatively innocuous bilateral, multiple, yellow, crystalline, ring-like deposits at the maculae (Figure 2.87). Other rare ocular side-effects are vortex keratopathy (see Figure 2.79) and optic neuritis, which are reversible on cessation of therapy.

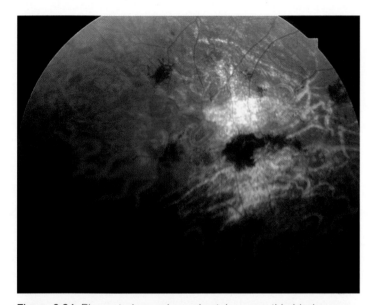

Figure 2.84 Pigment plaques in moderately severe thioridazine toxicity

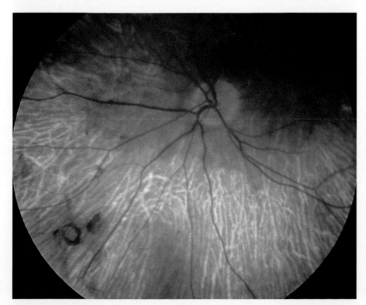

Figure 2.85 Diffuse atrophy of the RPE and choriocapillaris in very severe thioridazine toxicity

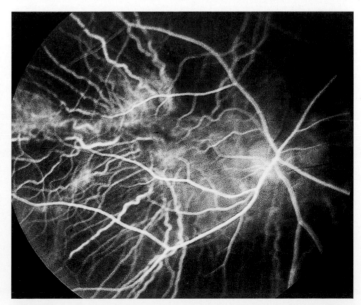

Figure 2.86 FA of very severe thioridazine toxicity showing loss of choriocapillaris with preservation of larger choroidal and retinal vessels

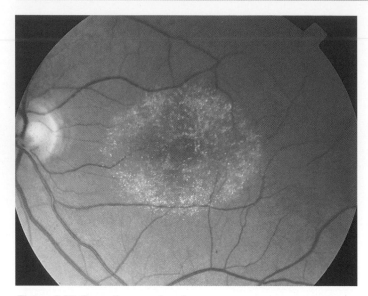

Figure 2.87 Tamoxifen maculopathy

Canthaxanthin

Canthaxanthin is a carotenoid used to enhance suntanning. If used over prolonged periods of time it may cause the deposition of bilateral, tiny, glistening, yellow deposits, arranged symmetrically in a doughnut shape at the posterior poles (Figure 2.88). The deposits are located in the superficial retina and are innocuous.

Methoxyflurane

Methoxyflurane (Penthrane) is an inhalant general anesthetic. It is metabolized to oxalic acid which combines with calcium to form an insoluble salt which is deposited in tissues including the RPE. Prolonged administration may lead to renal failure and secondary hyperoxalosis. It may also

result in the formation of innocuous crystals within the retinal vasculature.

Further reading

Block JA. Hydroxychloroquine and retinal safety. *Lancet* 1998;315:771.

Blyth C, Lane C. Hydroxychloroquine retinopathy: is screening necessary? *Br Med J* 1998:916:710–717.

Fielder A, Graham E, Jones S, et al. Royal College of Ophthalmologist guidelines: Ocular toxicity and hydroxychloroquine. *Eye* 1998;12:907–909.

Johnson MW, Vine AK. Hydroxychloroquine therapy in massive total doses without retinal toxicity. *Am J Ophthalmol* 1987;104:139–144.

Vu LBL, Easterbrook M, Hovis JK. Detection of color vision defects in chloroquine retinopathy. *Ophthalmology* 1999;106:1799–1804.

Weiner A, Sandberg MA, Gaudio AR, et al. Hydroxychloroquine retinopathy. *Am J Ophthalmol* 1991;112:528–534.

Traumatic maculopathies

Commotio retinae

1. **Pathogenesis** – concussion of the sensory retina resulting in cloudy swelling.

2. **Signs** – the involved retina has a grey appearance which most frequently affects the temporal fundus but may also involve the macula (Figure 2.89).

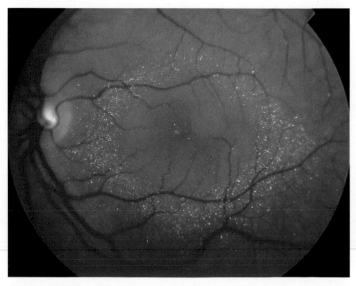

Figure 2.88 Canthaxanthin maculopathy

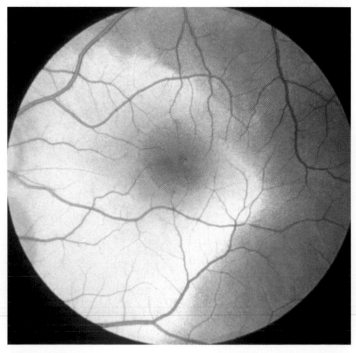

Figure 2.89 Commotio retinae involving the macula

3. Prognosis in mild cases is good with spontaneous resolution within a few weeks without sequelae. More severe involvement may be associated with intraretinal hemorrhage and the subsequent development of atophic changes including macular hole formation.

Choroidal rupture

1. Pathogenesis – tearing involving the choroid, Bruch's membrane and RPE caused by either blunt or penetrating ocular trauma. Choroidal ruptures can be either direct or indirect. Large ruptures may be associated with subretinal hemorrhage, and in some cases the blood may break through the internal limiting membrane and result in subhyaloid or vitreous hemorrhage.

2. Clinical types

- *Direct ruptures* are located anteriorly to the site of impact and oriented parallel with the ora serrata.

- *Indirect ruptures* occur opposite to the site of impact.

3. Sign of indirect rupture

- A *fresh rupture* is a crescent-shape, vertical lesion concentric with the optic disc which frequently involves the macula. Its exact location and extent may be difficult to determine because of masking by subretinal hemorrhage (Figure 2.90a).

- An *old rupture* is characterized by a white crescentic streak of exposed underlying sclera (Figure 2.91)

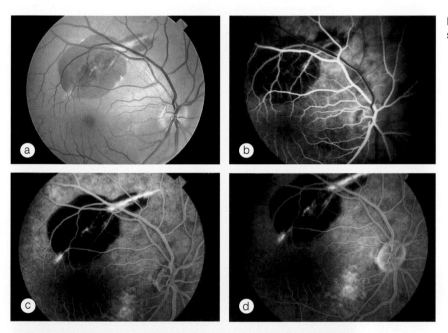

Figure 2.90 Fresh choroidal rupture and subretinal haemorrhage (see the text)

4. FA during the acute stage may not be helpful if the rupture is obscured by subretinal hemorrhage (see Figure 2.90b, 2.90c and 2.90d).

5. ICG may show the extent of the lesion.

6. Prognosis depends on the absence or presence (Figure 2.92) of fovea involvement. An uncommon late complication is secondary CNV which may result in bleeding and further visual deterioration.

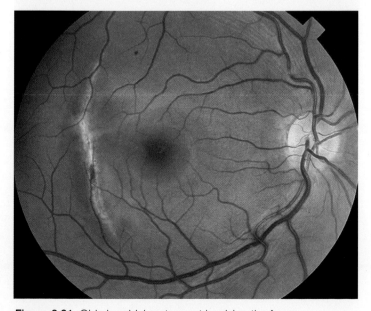

Figure 2.91 Old choroidal rupture not involving the fovea

Valsalva maculopathy

1. Pathogenesis – transmission of a sudden and severe increase in intrathoracic or intra-abdominal pressure to the eye resulting in intraocular bleeding.

2. Signs – small, unilateral or bilateral, macular hemorrhages which are most frequently pre-retinal (Figure 2.93).

3. Prognosis is excellent with spontaneous resolution without sequelae.

Solar maculopathy

1. Pathogenesis – retinal injury caused by photochemical effects of solar radiation as a result of directly or indirectly viewing the sun (eclipse retinopathy).

2. Presentation is between 1–4 hours of solar exposure with unilateral or bilateral impairment of central vision, metamorphopsia or central scotomas.

3. Signs

* Visual acuity is variable according to the extent of damage.

* Initially there are small, unilateral or bilateral, yellow foveolar spots with a gray margin (Figure 2.94).

* This is followed about 2 weeks later by circumscribed RPE mottling (Figure 2.95) or a lamellar hole.

4. Treatment with systemic steroids has no proven benefit.

5. Prognosis is usually good in most cases with improvement of visual acuity to normal or near-normal levels within 6 months although mild symptoms may persist.

FURTHER READING

Aguilar JP, Green WR. Choroidal rupture: a histopathologic study of 47 cases. *Retina* 1984;4:269–275.

Kempster RC, Green WR, Finkelstein D. Choroidal rupture: clinicopathologic correlation of an unusual case. *Retina* 1996;16:57–63.

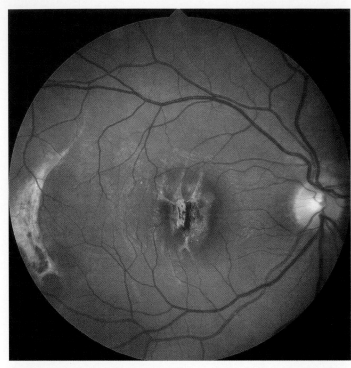

Figure 2.92 Two old choroidal ruptures one of which had involved the fovea

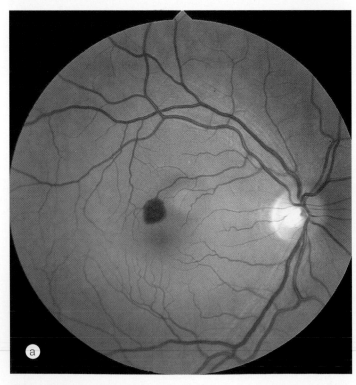

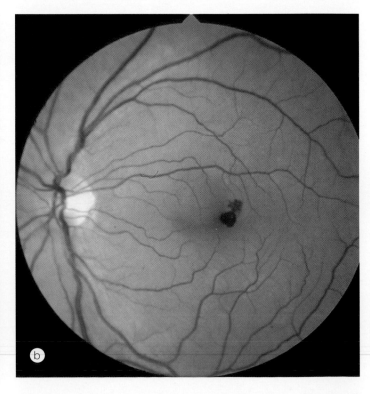

Figure 2.93 Bilateral valsalva maculopathy

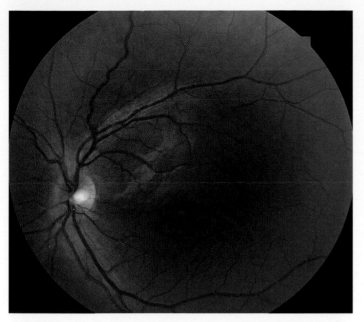

Figure 2.94 Early solar maculopathy showing a small yellow foveolar spot

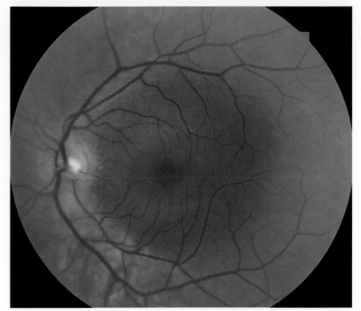

Figure 2.95 Late solar maculopathy showing mild RPE mottling

Kohno T, Miki T, Hayashi K. Choroidopathy after blunt trauma to the eye; a fluorescein and indocyanine green angiographic study. *Am J Ophthalmol* 1998;126:248–260.

Kohno T, Miki T, Shiraki K, et al. Indocynine green angiographic features of choroidal rupture and choroidal vascular injury after contusion ocular injury. *Am J Ophthalmol* 2000;129:38–46.

Yannuzzi LA, Fisher YL, Krueger A, et al. Solar retinopathy; a photobiological and geophysical analysis. *Trans Am Ophthalmol Soc* 1987;85:120–128.

Maculopathies associated with congenital optic disc anomalies

Optic disc drusen

Optic disc drusen are composed of hyaline-like calcific material within the substance of the optic nerve head (Figure 2.96a). Clinically, disc drusen are present in 0.3% of the general population and are frequently bilateral and familial.

1. Signs

- Visual acuity is normal in the absence of complications.

- In early childhood drusen lie beneath the disc tissue and cause an elevation of the disc (Figure 2.96b.

- The disc itself has a pink or yellow color and its margins have a 'lumpy' appearance.

- There is no physiological cup.

- The emerging blood vessels show anomalous premature branching patterns.

- During the early 'teens' the drusen usually emerge to the disc surface and can be recognized as waxy, pearl-like deposits (Figure 2.97).

2. FA

- Prior to dye injection drusen show the phenomenon of 'autofluorescence' (Figure 2.98a).

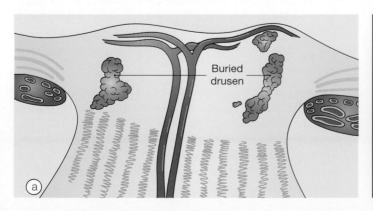

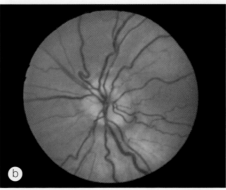

Figure 2.96 Buried optic disc drusen: Schematic showing their location (a); clinical appearance (b)

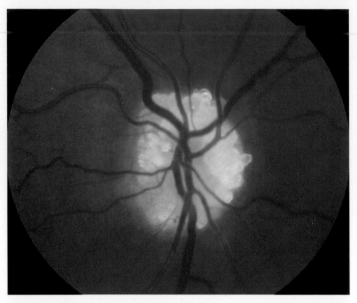

Figure 2.97 Exposed optic disc drusen

- During the venous phase the disc becomes increasingly hyperfluorescent but there is no leakage (Figure 2.98b).

- During the late phases the disc remains hyperfluorescent due to staining (Figure 2.94c).

3. **Maculopathy** secondary to juxtapapillary CNV develops in a small percentage of eyes with disc drusen (Figure 2.99). Because the CNV does not usually involve the fovea, the results of treatment by laser photocoagulation are favorable.

Optic disc pit

Diagnosis

An optic disc pit is a rare and usually unilateral congenital lesion.

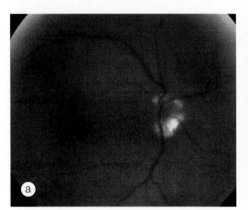 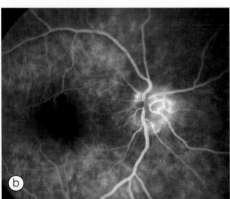 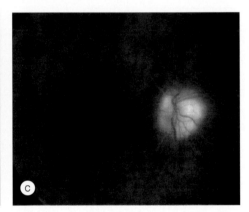

Figure 2.98 Optic disc drusen: (a) Autofluorescence; (b) & (c) FA showing increasing hyperfluorescence

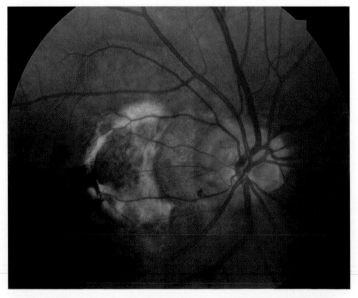

Figure 2.99 Peripapillary scarring due to old CNV associated with optic disc drusen

1. **Signs**

- Visual acuity is normal in the absence of complications.

- The optic disc is larger than normal and contains a round or oval pit of variable size (Figure 2.100).

- The pit is usually located in the temporal aspect of the disc, but may occasionally be central.

- Visual field defects are common and may mimic those due to glaucoma.

2. **FA** of the pit shows early hypofluorescence and late hyperfluorescence.

3. **Maculopathy** in the form of serous detachment develops in about 45% of eyes with non-central disc pits, most frequently at about puberty (Figure 2.101a). The subretinal fluid is thought to be derived either from the vitreous or the subarachnoid space. A less likely source is leakage from abnormal vessels within the base of the pit (Figure 2.101b).

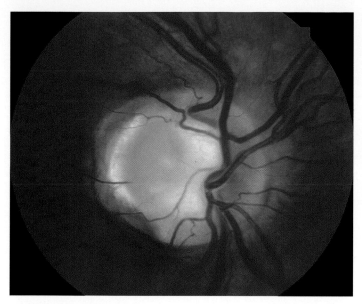

Figure 2.100 Optic disc pit

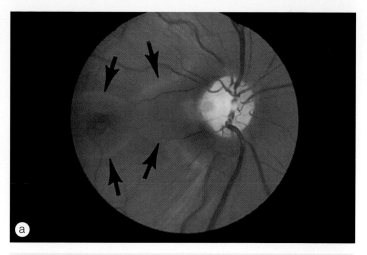

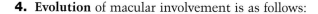

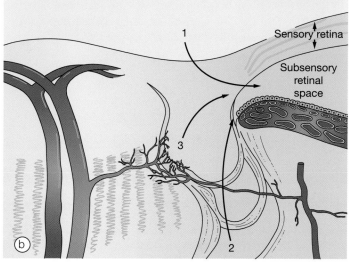

Figure 2.101 (a) Optic disc pit and serous macular detachments; (c) possible mechanisms of access of fluid into the subretinal space

4. Evolution of macular involvement is as follows:

- Initially, there is a schisis-like separation of the inner layers of the retina which communicates with the pit.

- This is followed by serous detachment of the outer retinal layers from the RPE. This appearance may be mistaken for central serous retinopathy, and it is therefore important to examine the optic disc carefully in all patients with suspected central serous retinopathy.

Treatment options

1. Observation at 3-monthly intervals for evidence of spontaneous resolution of the detachment which occurs in up to 25% of cases.

2. Laser photocoagulation may be considered if visual acuity is deteriorating. The burns are applied along the temporal aspect of the disc. The success rate is 25–35%.

3. Vitrectomy with air-fluid exchange, postoperative prone positioning and subsequent laser photocoagulation may be considered if laser alone was unsuccessful. The success rate is 50–70%.

4. Gas injectors (C_2F_6) without virectomy may also be successful.

FURTHER READING

Apple DJ, Raab MF, Walsh PM. Congenital anomalies of the optic disc. *Surv Ophthalmol* 1982;27:3–41.

Brodsky MC. Congenital optic disc anomalies. *Surv Ophthalmol* 1994;39:89–112.

Brown GC, Brown MM. Treatment of retinal detachment associated with congenital excavation defects of the optic dic. *Ophthalmic Surg* 1995;26:11–15.

Cohen SY, Quentel G, Guiberteau B, et al. Macular serous retinal detachment caused by subretinal leakage in tilted disc syndrome. *Ophthalmology* 1998;105:1831–1834.

Cox MS, Witherspoon CD, Morris RE, et al. Evolving techniques in the treatment of macular detachment caused by optic nerve pits. *Ophthalmology* 1988;95:889–896.

Rutledge BK, Puliafito CA, Duker JS, et al. Optical coherence tomography of macular lesions associated with optic nerve head pits. *Ophthalmology* 1996;103:1047–1053.

Sobol WM, Blodi CF, Folk JC, et al. Long-term visual outcome in patients with optic nerve pits and serous retinal detachment of the macula. *Ophthalmology* 1990;97:1539–1542.

Case study

1. History

A 16-year-old girl presented with slightly blurred vision in her right eye, particularly when reading, of several months duration.

2. Examination right eye

- Visual acuity was 6/12.

- Fundus examination showed an optic disc pit with an adjacent teardrop-shaped serous retinal detachment involving the macula (Figure 2.102a). Also present was a macular cyst or hole just temporal to fixation through which choroidal vasculature was visible. There were also small cystic spaces surrounding the cyst or hole. The area of macular detachment was associated with RPE atrophy.

3. FA

- *Early venous phase* showed hypofluorescence of the pit and transmitted choroidal fluorescence at the macula corresponding to RPE atrophy (Figure 2.102b).

- *Later phases* showed hyperfluorescence of the disc pit but no leakage and fading of transmitted choroidal fluorescence (Figure 2.102c and 22.102d).

4. Diagnosis

- Serous macular detachment associated with an optic disc pit. The detachment was thought to be longstanding because of the presence of associated RPE atrophy.

5. Management

- The patient was observed without intervention because visual acuity was good despite the long-standing nature of the detachment.

- Sixteen months later the detachment had spontaneously flattened and visual acuity was still 6/12.

6. Comment

This patient is very fortunate because the detachment resolved spontaneously and she retained surprisingly good visual acuity despite the chronicity of the problem.

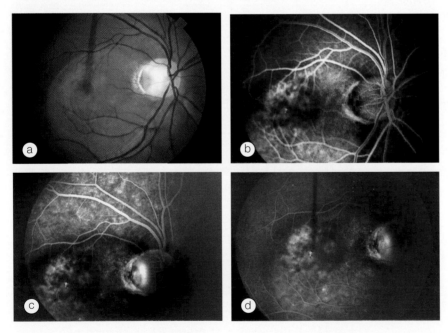

Figure 2.102 Optic disc pit and serous macular detachment (see the text)

Idiopathic polypoidal choroidal vasculopathy

Idiopathic polypoidal choroidal vasculopathy, also described as posterior uveal bleeding syndrome or multiple serosanguinous RPE detachment syndrome, is an uncommon condition that has a predilection for non-white individuals.

1. Pathogenesis

An abnormality of the inner choroidal vessels consisting of a dilated network and multiple terminal aneurysmal protrubences in a polypiodal configuration that have a predilection for the macula and less frequently the peripapillary area. These polypoidal lesions appear to be responsible for episodic leakage and bleeding under the RPE and sensory retina.

2. Presentation

is with sudden unilateral visual impairment.

3. Signs

* Serosanguinous detachments of the RPE which may be multiple and variable in size.

* In some cases bullous retinal detachments and vitreous hemorrhage may also occur.

4. ICG

shows the presence of large choroidal vascular complexes with localized terminal polyp-like bulbs that fill slowly and then leak intensely (Figure 2.103).

5. Treatment

by laser photocoagulation is occasionally required if serosanguinous leakage threatens the fovea.

6. Prognosis

is good in most cases, with spontaneous resolution of exudation and hemorrhage.

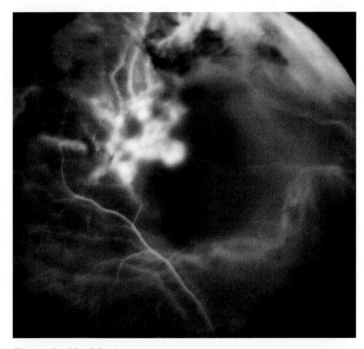

Figure 2.103 ICG of idiopathic polypoidal choroidal vasculopathy showing hyperfluorescence of the dilated terminal polyp-like bulbs and blocked fluorescence by blood

FURTHER READING

Ahuja RA, Stanga PE, Vingerling JR, et al. Polypoidal vasculopathy in exudative and haemorrhagic pigment epithelial detachments. *Br J Ophthalmol* 2000;84:479–484.

Moorthy RS, Lyon AT, Rabb MF, et al. Idiopathic polypoidal choroidal vasculopathy of the macula. *Ophthalmology* 1998;105:1380–1385.

Spaide RF, Yannuzzi LA, Slakter JS, et al. Indocyanine green videoangiography of idiopathic polypoidal choroidal vasculopathy. *Retina* 1995;15:100–110.

Yannuzzi LA, Ciardella A, Spaide RF, et al. The expanding clinical spectrum of idiopathic polypoidal choroidal vasculopathy. *Arch Ophthalmol* 1997;115:478–485.

Chapter **3**

Retinal vascular disorders

Diabetic retinopathy

Diabetes mellitus

Classification

Diabetes mellitus is a common metabolic disease characterized by sustained hyperglycemia of varying severity secondary to lack of or diminished efficacy of endogenous insulin. It affects about 2% of the population of the UK. Although there is a certain amount of overlap, the following are the two main types of diabetes:

1. **Insulin-dependent diabetes (IDD)** which is also known as type 1 diabetes. It develops most frequently between the ages of 10 and 20 years, although elderly patients can also be insulin-dependent. It typically presents with an acute-onset of weight loss, polyuria, polydipsia and nocturia.

2. **Non-insulin-dependent diabetes (NIDD)** which is also known as type 2. It develops most frequently between the ages of 50 and 70 years. Most patients remain non-insulin dependent whilst some subsequently develop IDD. Presentation is usually gradual with recurrent infections of the skin, vulva or glans penis. In some cases NIDD is initially asymptomatic and is discovered by a chance finding of fasting plasma glucose concentration equal to or greater than 7.0 mmol/l or a random glucose concentration equal to or greater than 11 mmol/l.

Important chronic complications

1. **Nephropathy** is initially manifest by microscopic proteinuria. Severe renal disease may eventually result in renal failure requiring dialysis or transplantation.

2. **Accelerated atherosclerosis** may affect the coronary or lower limb arteries, or both. In severe cases involvement of the lower limb arteries may give rise to painful ischemic ulceration and gangrene which may necessitate amputation.

3. **Polyneuropathy** most frequently involves the sensory nerves and initially involves the feet. If advanced it may give rise to secondary painless neuropathic perforating ulcers of the feet at pressure points as well as degenerative (Charcot) arthropathy.

Systemic risk factors for diabetic retinopathy

The prevalence of diabetic retinopathy (DR) is higher in IDD (40%) than in NIDD (20%), and DR is the most common cause of legal blindness in individuals between the ages of 20 and 65 years. The following are the main risk factors:

1. **Duration of diabetes** is the most important factor. In patients diagnosed as having diabetes before the age of 30 years, the incidence of DR after 10 years is 50% and after 30 years 90%. It is extremely rare for DR to develop within five years of the onset of diabetes and before puberty, but about 5% of NIDDs have background DR at presentation.

2. **Intensive metabolic control** is beneficial for the following reasons:

   - It delays the onset of DR.

   - It delays the progression of non-proliferative diabetic retinopathy (NPDR).

   - It decreases the rate of conversion of severe NPDR to proliferative diabetic retinopathy (PDR).

   - It delays the onset of macular edema.

   - It decreases the need for laser photocoagulation.

3. Miscellaneous adverse risk factors

- *Pregnancy* is occasionally associated with rapid progression of PDR. Predictive factors are poor pre-pregnancy control of diabetes, too rapid tightening of control during the early stages of pregnancy, and the development of pre-eclampsia and fluid imbalance.

- *Hypertension*, if poorly controlled, is associated with worsening of DR and particularly the development of PDR in both IDD and NIDD.

- *Nephropathy*, if severe, is associated with worsening of DR. Conversely, treatment of renal disease (e.g. renal transplantation) may be associated with improvement of retinopathy and a better response to photocoagulation.

- *Elevated glycosylated hemoglobin levels*.

- *Hyperlipidemia*.

Pathogenesis of diabetic retinopathy

Diabetic retinopathy is a microangiopathy affecting the retinal precapillary arterioles, capillaries and venules. However, larger vessels may also be involved. Retinopathy has features of both microvascular occlusion and leakage. Clinically, DR can be divided into two main types (Figure 3.1):

- *Non-proliferative* DR in which the lesions are intraretinal.

- *Proliferative* DR in which the lesions extend onto or beyond the retinal surface.

Microvascular occlusion

1. Pathogenesis

- *Capillary changes* consist of loss of pericytes, thickening of the basement membrane, endothelial cell damage and proliferation. Figure 3.2 shows a normal capillary bed with equal distribution between pericytes with round dark staining nuclei and endothelial cells with elongated pale staining nuclei. Figure 3.3 shows a diabetic capillary bed in which many capillaries are acellular due to occlusion. The remaining capillaries are dilated and show loss of pericytes and an increase in number of endothelial cells.

- *Deformation of red blood cells*, which leads to decreased oxygen transport.

- *Changes in platelets*, which lead to increased stickiness and aggregation.

2. Consequences of retinal capillary non-perfusion are retinal ischemia which, in turn, causes retinal hypoxia. Initially, the non-perfused area is located in the mid-retinal periphery. The two main effects of retinal hypoxia are the following:

- *Arteriovenous shunts* associated with significant capillary occlusion ('drop-out') which run from arterioles to venules. Because it is unclear whether these lesions represent actual new vessels, they are often referred to as 'intraretinal microvascular abnormalities' (IRMA).

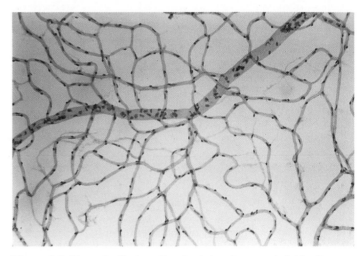

Figure 3.2 Normal retinal capillary bed showing equal distribution between pericytes and endothelial cells

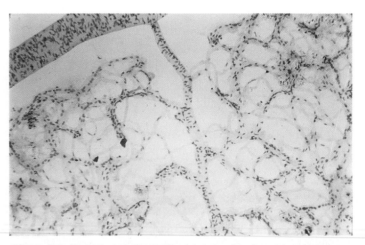

Figure 3.3 Diabetic retinal capillary bed showing loss of pericytes, increase in number of endothelial cells, and many acellular and dilated capillaries

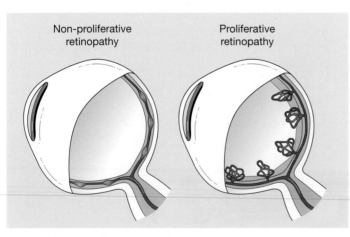

Figure 3.1 Two main types of DR

- *Neovascularization* is thought to be caused by 'vasoformative substances' (growth factors) elaborated by hypoxic retinal tissue in an attempt to revascularize hypoxic areas of the retina. These substances promote neovascularization on the retina and optic nerve head (PDR) (Figure 3.4) and occasionally on the iris (rubeosis iridis) (Figure 3.5). Many growth factors have been identified and the vascular endothelial growth factor appears to be of particular importance.

Microvascular leakage

1. Pathogenesis

The tight junctions between capillary endothelial cells constitute the inner blood-retinal barrier. In diabetes there is a breakdown of the blood-retinal barrier, leading to leakage of plasma constituents into the retina (Figure 3.6).

Microaneurysms are saccular pouches which may form as a result of local capillary distension (Figure 3.7). They may either leak or become thrombosed.

2. **Consequences** of increased vascular permeability are the development of intraretinal hemorrhage and retinal edema which may be diffuse or localized.
   a. *Diffuse retinal edema* is caused by extensive capillary dilatation and leakage.
   b. *Localized retinal edema* is caused by focal leakage from microaneurysms and dilated capillary segments. Chronic localized retinal edema leads to the deposition of hard exudates at the junction of normal and edematous retina (Figure 3.8). The exudates, which are composed of lipoprotein and lipid-filled macrophages, typically surround leaking microvascular lesions in a circinate pattern. With cessation of leakage they absorb spontaneously over a

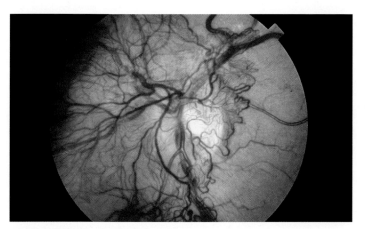

Figure 3.4 Severe proliferative DR

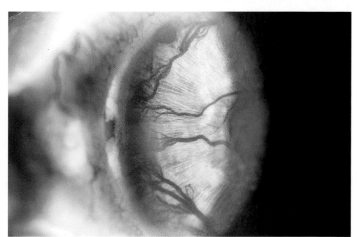

Figure 3.5 Severe rubeosis iridis

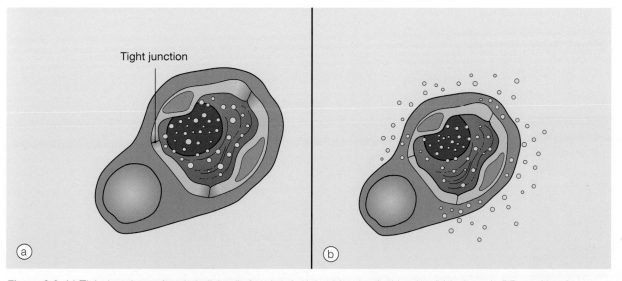

Figure 3.6 (a) Tight junctions of endothelial cells forming the inner blood-retinal barrier; (b) leakage in DR resulting from disruption of the inner blood-retinal barrier

73

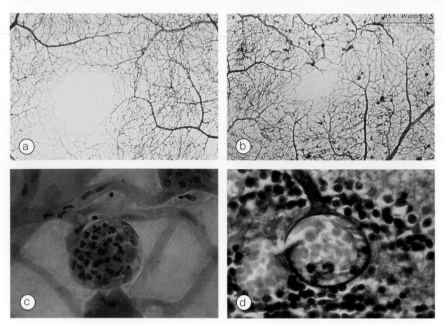

Figure 3.7 (a) Trypsin digest of normal retina; (b) trypsin digest of DR showing perifoveal microaneurysms with a predilection for the temporal zone of the fovea; (c) high power view showing microaneurysms containing many cells; (d) cross-section of a microaneurysm

period of months or years, either into the healthy surrounding capillaries or by phagocytosis of their lipid content. In other cases, more chronic extravasation leads to enlargement of the exudates and sometimes the deposition of cholesterol.

Background diabetic retinopathy

Diagnosis

The main clinical features and the location within the retina of lesions in background DR are shown in Figure 3.9.

1. **Microaneurysms** are located within the inner nuclear layer and are the first clinically detected lesions.

- *Signs* – small round dots, usually temporal to the fovea (Figure 3.10). When coated with blood they may be indistinguishable from dot hemorrhages.

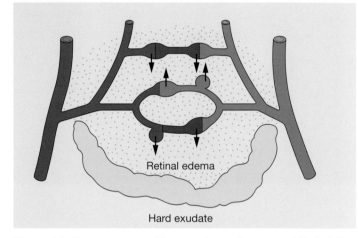

Figure 3.8 Consequences of increased vascular permeability in DR

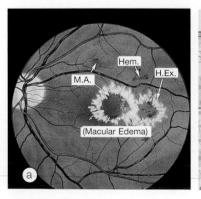

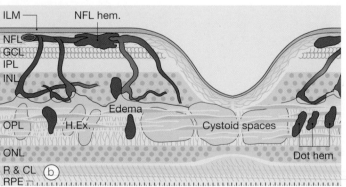

Figure 3.9 Background DR; (a) Clinical features; (b) location of lesions

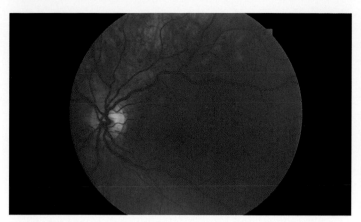

Figure 3.10 Microaneurysms and small dot hemorrhages in very early background DR

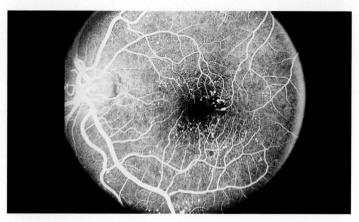

Figure 3.11 FA of microaneurysms showing spotty perifoveal hyperfluorescence

- *FA* of patent microaneurysms shows tiny hyperfluorescent dots (Figure 3.11).

2. **Hard exudates** are located within the outer plexiform layer.

- *Signs* – yellow waxy lesions with relatively distinct margins arranged in clumps and/or rings most frequently at the posterior pole (Figure 3.12). The centres of rings of hard exudates usually contain microaneurysms. With

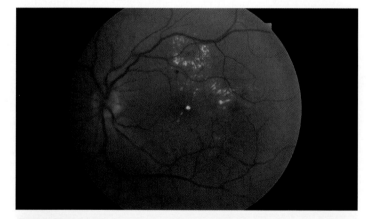

Figure 3.12 Hard exudates in mild background DR

time the number and size of hard exudates tends to increase and may threaten or involve the fovea.

- *FA* shows hypofluorescence due to blockage.

3. **Retinal edema** is initially located between the outer plexiform and inner nuclear layers. Later it may also involve the inner plexiform and nerve fiber layers, until eventually the entire thickness of the retina becomes edematous. With further accumulation of fluid the fovea assumes a cystoid appearance (Figure 3.13b).

- *Signs* – thickening of the sensory retina which obscures the underlying RPE and choroid (Figure 3.14). It is best detected clinically by slitlamp biomicroscopy with either a fundus contact lens or a +78D lens.

- *FA* shows diffuse late hyperfluorescence due to leakage which may assume a flower-petal pattern if CME is present (Figure 3.13a).

4. **Hemorrhages**

- *Intraretinal* hemorrhages arise from the venous end of the capillaries and are located in the compact middle layers of the retina and therefore have a red, 'dot-blot' configuration.

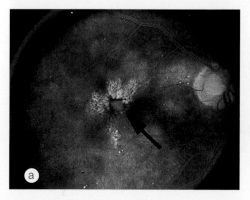

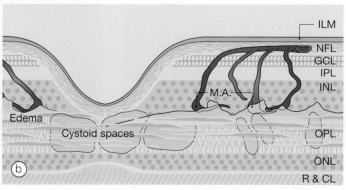

Figure 3.13 (a) FA of cystoid macular edema showing late 'petalloid' hyperfluorescence; (b) location within the outer plexiform layer

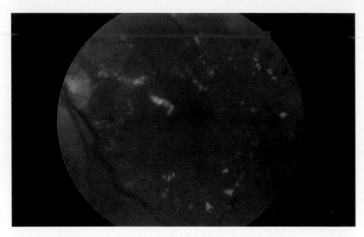

Figure 3.14 Retinal edema in severe background DR

- *Retinal nerve fiber layer* hemorrhages arise from the larger superficial precapillary arterioles and are therefore flame-shaped.

Management

Patients with mild background DR (Figure 3.15) do not require laser treatment. However, they should be reviewed annually and any factors such as associated hypertension, anemia or renal failure corrected, if possible. Patients with more severe background DR (Figure 3.16) should be carefully assessed, if necessary with FA, to determine whether they have clinically significant macular edema (see below).

Differential diagnosis

The diagnosis of simple background DR is usually relatively straightforward, but occasionally the following conditions may give rise to diagnostic problems.

1. **Macular drusen**

- *Similarities* – bilateral, focal yellow spots at the macula which may be mistaken for hard exudates.

- *Differences* – not usually arranged in rings and not associated with retinal microvascular changes (see Figure 2.2).

2. **Hypertensive retinopathy**

- *Similarities* – bilateral retinal edema, hard exudates and flame-shaped hemorrhages.

- *Differences* – hard exudates typically form a macular star figure and are not arranged in clumps or rings (see Figure 3.108).

3. **Old retinal branch vein occlusion**

- *Similarities* – hard exudates, retinal edema and microvascular changes.

- *Differences* – usually unilateral; presence of collaterals (see Figure 3.69).

4. **Retinal artery macroaneurysm**

- *Similarities* – hard exudates, retinal edema and microvascular changes.

- *Differences* – unilateral in 90% of cases: hemorrhage is usually more localized (see Figure 3.123a).

5. **Radiation retinopathy**

- *Similarities* – macular non-perfusion, microvascular changes, hard exudates and hemorrhages.

- *Differences* – unilateral (see Figure 3.140).

6. **Idiopathic juxtafoveolar retinal telangiectasia**

- *Similarities* – hard exudates, retinal edema and microvascular changes.

- *Differences* – usually confined to the fovea (see Figure 3.128).

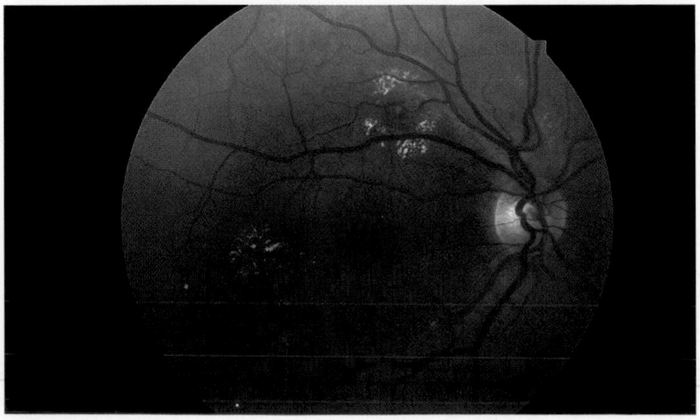

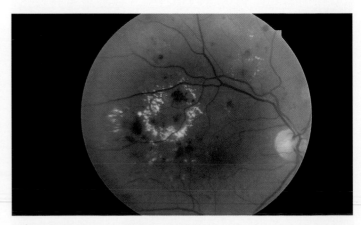

Figure 3.15 Mild background DR not requiring treatment

Figure 3.16 Severe background DR with a ring of hard exudates threatening the fovea

Preproliferative diabetic retinopathy
Diagnosis

Preproliferative DR develops in some eyes that initially show only mild background changes, and it may also subsequently progress to proliferative disease. The underlying cause of preproliferative DR is retinal ischemia which is seen on FA as extensive areas of retinal capillary non-perfusion (dropout). The clinical features and location of the lesions are shown in Figure 3.17. The greater the number of lesions, the greater the risk of progression to proliferative disease.

1. **Cotton-wool spots** (Figure 3.18a) are caused by precapillary arteriolar occlusion within the retinal nerve fiber layer (Figure 3.18c). The interruption of axoplasmic transport caused by the ischemia and subsequent build-up of transported material within the nerve axons, is responsible for the white appearance of these lesions. Figure 3.18d shows disorganization of the nerve fiber and ganglion cell layers following capillary closure.

- *Signs* – small, whitish, fluffy superficial lesions which may obscure underlying blood vessels (Figure 3.19a).

- *FA* shows focal hypofluorescence due to blockage which is frequently associated with an area of adjacent capillary non-perfusion (Figures 3.18b and 3.19b.)

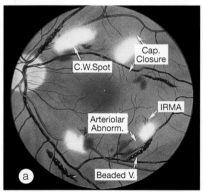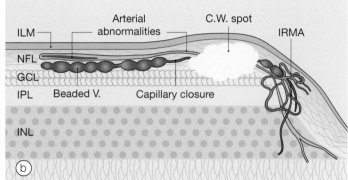

Figure 3.17 Preproliferative DR; (a) Clinical features; (b) location of lesions

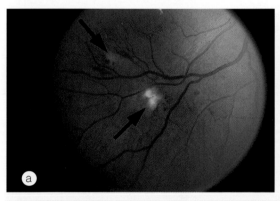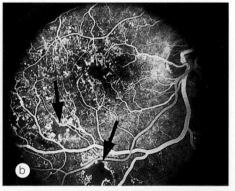

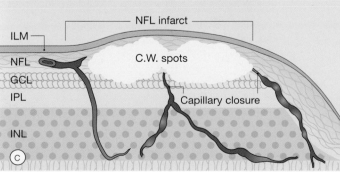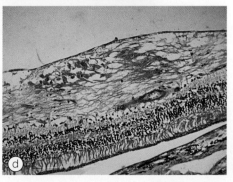

Figure 3.18 (a) Cotton-wool spots; (b) FA showing hypofluorescence due to a combination of blockage by the cotton-wool spots and small adjacent areas of capillary non-perfusion; (c) cotton-wool spot adjacent to an area of capillary closure; (d) low power photomicrograph showing infarction and disorganization of the retinal nerve fiber layer and ganglion cell layer following capillary closure

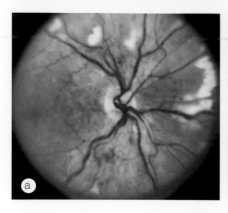

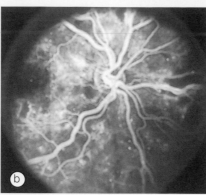

Figure 3.19 (a) Cotton-wool spots; (b) FA showing spotty hyperfluorescence of microaneurysms and areas of hypofluorescence

2. Intraretinal microvascular abnormalities (IRMA)

- *Signs* – capillary changes that are more severe than microaneurysms which may resemble focal areas of flat retinal new vessels. The main distinguishing features of

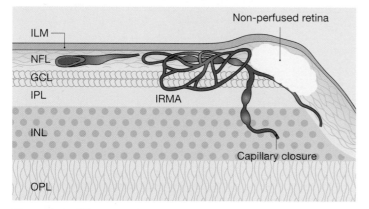

Figure 3.20 IRMA are located in the superficial retina adjacent to areas of non-perfusion

IRMA are their intraretinal location and failure to cross major retinal blood vessels. The location of IRMA is shown in Figure 3.20.

- *FA* shows hyperfluorescence with mild leakage. Figure 3.21a shows IRMA with corresponding leakage and capillary non-perfusion (Figure 3.21b).

3. **Venous changes** consist of 'looping' (Figure 3.22), 'beading' and 'sausage-like' segmentation (Figure 3.23). Figures 3.24a shows a beaded vein. Figure 3.24b shows the beaded vein (small arrow), leakage from IRMA (large arrow) and marked capillary closure.

4. **Arterial changes** consist of narrowing, silverwiring and even obliteration resembling a branch retinal artery occlusion (Figure 3.25). Figure 3.26a shows occluded arterioles (small arrows) and a venous loop (large arrow). Figure 3.26b is the corresponding FA.

5. **Dark blot hemorrhages** (Figure 3.27) which represent hemorrhagic retinal infarcts are located within the middle retinal layers.

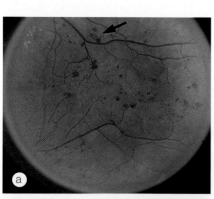

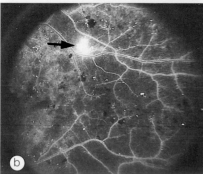

Figure 3.21 (a) IRMA; (b) FA showing focal leakage and extensive capillary non-perfusion

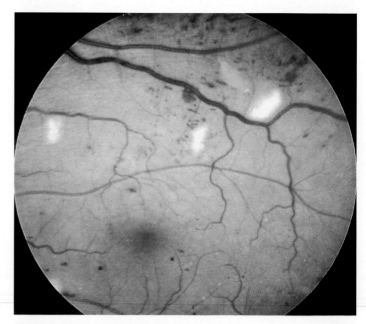

Figure 3.22 Preproliferative DR showing cotton-wool spots, venous tortuosity and looping, and haemorrhages

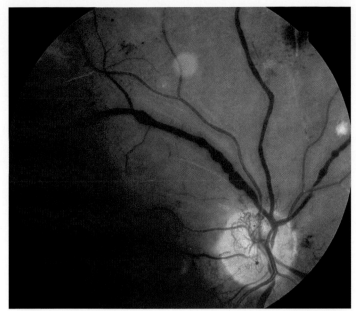

Figure 3.23 Venous segmentation and mild disc new vessels

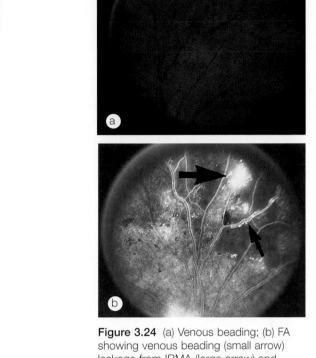

Figure 3.24 (a) Venous beading; (b) FA showing venous beading (small arrow) leakage from IRMA (large arrow) and marked capillary non-perfusion

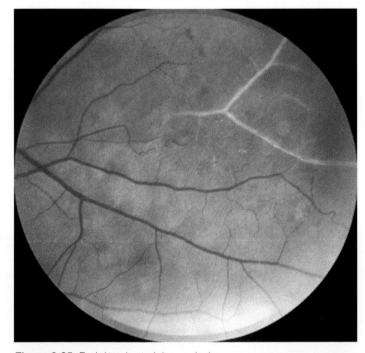

Figure 3.25 Peripheral arteriolar occlusion

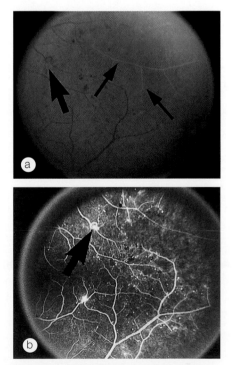

Figure 3.26 (a) Arteriolar occlusions (small arrows) and a venous loop (large arrow); (b) FA showing extensive non-perfusion and filling of the venous loop which does not leak

Management

Patients with preproliferative DR should be watched closely because of the risk of PDR. Figure 3.28a shows a few cotton-wool spots. Two years later (Figure 3.28b) the number of cotton-wool spots has increased and there is early neovascularization (Figure 3.28b). FA shows leakage from the new vessels (arrow) and many areas of capillary closure. (Figure 3.28c). Treatment by photocoagulation is usually not appropriate unless regular follow-up is not possible. This would be particularly applicable to patients who have already lost vision in the fellow eye as a result of the complications of PDR.

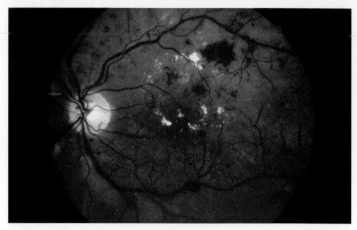

Figure 3.27 Severe preproliferative DR with a venous loop and IRM along the infero-temporal arcade, large blot hemorrhages inside the supero-temporal arcade and hard exudates at the macula

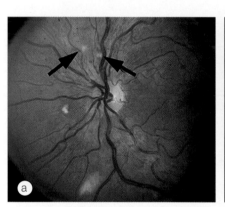
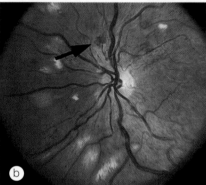
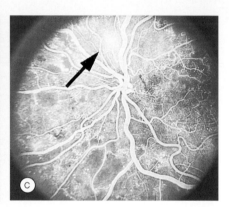

Figure 3.28 Progression of preproliferative to proliferative DR (see the text)

Diabetic maculopathy

Diagnosis

Involvement of the fovea by edema, hard exudates or ischemia (diabetic maculopathy) is the most common cause of visual impairment in diabetic patients, particularly those with NIDD.

1. Focal maculopathy

- *Signs* – well-circumscribed, leaking areas associated with complete or incomplete rings of perifoveal hard exudates. Figure 3.29a shows very mild background DR and normal visual acuity. Three years later there is worsening of DR with the formation of a large hard exudate ring temporal to the fovea (Figure 3.29b).

- *FA* shows late, focal hyperfluorescence due to leakage and good macular perfusion (Figure 3.29c).

- *Treatment* was performed by focal photocoagulation to leaking microaneurysms and other microvascular lesions inside the lipid ring (Figure 3.29d). Four months later there are fewer hard exudates (Figure 3.29e) and seven months after treatment most of the hard exudates have absorbed (Figure 3.29f).

2. Diffuse maculopathy

- *Signs* – diffuse retinal thickening which may be associated with cystoid changes (Figure 3.30a). In severe cases it may be impossible to identify the location of the fovea because landmarks are obliterated by the edema.

- *FA* shows early spotty hyperfluorescence of microaneurysms (Figure 3.30b) and late diffuse hyperfluorescence due to leakage, which is frequently more dramatic than on clinical examination, and may be associated with a flower-petal pattern if CME is present (Figure 3.30c).

- *Treatment* is by grid photocoagulation to areas of retinal thickening (see below).

3. Ischemic maculopathy

- *Signs* – reduced visual acuity in association with a relatively normal appearance of the fovea (Figure 3.31a). Signs of preproliferative DR are also frequently present.

- *FA* shows early spotty hyperfluorescence of microaneurysms and hypofluorescence at the fovea with enlargement and irregularity of FAZ due to retinal capillary non-perfusion (Figure 3.31b). The exact extent

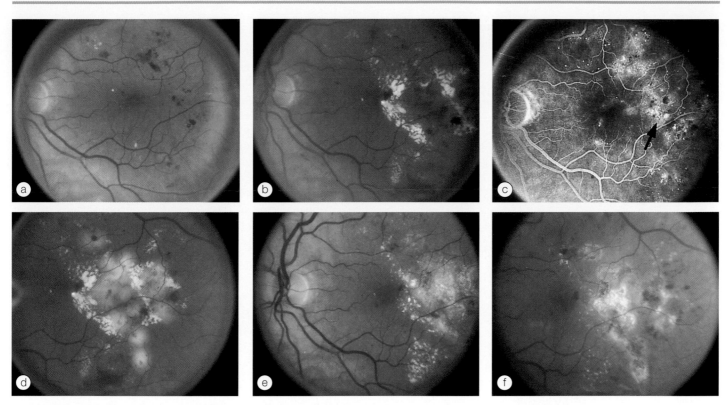

Figure 3.29 Focal diabetic maculopathy: (a) Initial appearance; (b) later formation of a ring of hard exudates associated with edema within its centre; (c) FA shows corresponding focal leakage (arrow); (d) appearance immediately following focal laser photocoagulation; (e) resolving hard exudates; (f) complete resolution of hard exudates and residual laser scars

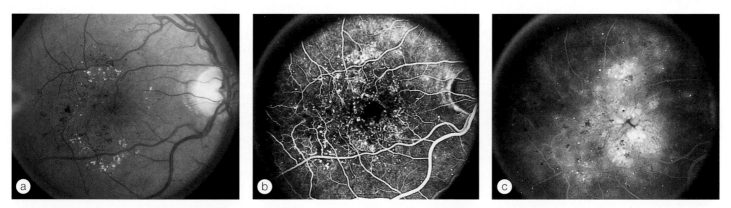

Figure 3.30 (a) Diffuse diabetic maculopathy; (b) early phase FA showing spotty hyperfluorescence of microaneurysms; (c) later phase showing extensive leakage and cystoid macular edema

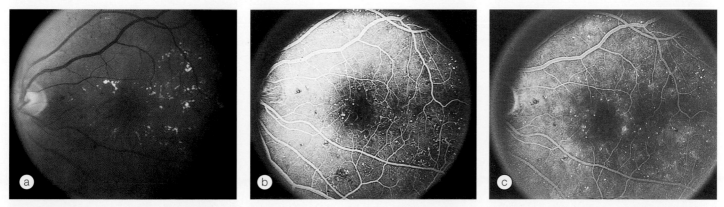

Figure 3.31 (a) Ischemic diabetic maculopathy; (b) early phase FA showing spotty hyperfluorescence of microaneurysms and enlargement and irregularity of FAZ; (c) later phase showing mild leakage

of non-perfusion can only be delineated by FA, but there does not appear to be a direct correlation between the level of visual acuity and the severity of ischemia. Other areas of capillary-non-perfusion are also frequently present at the posterior pole and periphery. The late phase of the FA shows mild hyperfluorescence due to leakage (Figure 3.31c).

- *Treatment* is not appropriate in most cases.

4. Mixed maculopathy is characterized by a combination of diffuse macular edema and ischemia.

Clinically significant macular edema

1. Definition

Clinically significant macular edema (CSME) is defined as the presence of one or more of the following features (Figure 3.32):

- Retinal edema within 500 μm of the center of the fovea (Figure 3.32a).

- Hard exudates within 500 μm of the fovea, if associated with adjacent retinal thickening (which may be outside the 500 μm limit) (Figure 3.32b).

- Retinal edema one disc area (1500 μm) or larger, any part of which is within one disc diameter of the center of the fovea (Figure 3.32c).

2. Indications for treatment

All eyes with CSME should be considered for treatment with laser photocoagulation irrespective of the level of visual acuity, because treatment reduces the risk of visual loss by 50%. FA before treatment is useful in delineating the area and extent of leakage. It is also helpful in detecting the presence of capillary non-perfusion at the fovea (see Figure 3.31c and d) which carries a poor prognosis and may be a contraindication to treatment.

3. Techniques

- *Focal treatment* involves applying laser burns to microaneurysms and microvascular lesions in the center of rings of hard exudates located 500–3000 μm (two disc diameters) from the centre of the fovea. The spot size is 100–200 μm with a duration of 0.10 seconds and sufficient power to obtain a gentle whitening or darkening of the microaneurysm. Treatment of lesions 300–500 μm from the center of the fovea should be considered if CSME persists, in spite of previous treatment and, if visual acuity is less than 6/12. In these cases a shorter exposure time of 0.05 seconds is recommended with a spot size of 50–100 μm.

- *Grid treatment* is used for areas of diffuse retinal thickening located more than 500 μm from the center of the fovea and 500 μm from the temporal margin of the optic disc. The spot size is 100–200 μm and the exposure time 0.10 seconds. The burns should be of very light intensity and one burn width apart.

4. Results

It should be emphasized that the main aim of treatment is to preserve the patient's current visual level. Only 15% of eyes show improvement of visual acuity, and despite treatment, vision subsequently deteriorates in 14% of cases. Because it may take up to 4 months for the edema to resolve in some cases, retreatment should not be considered prematurely.

- *Poor ocular prognostic factors* include the following:
  a. Hard exudates involving the fovea.
  b. Diffuse retinal edema.
  c. Cystoid macular edema.
  d. Impaired macular perfusion.
  e. Severe retinopathy at presentation.

- *Poor systemic prognostic factors* include the following:
  a. Hypertension.
  b. Proteinuria.
  c. Elevated glycosylated hemoglobin levels.

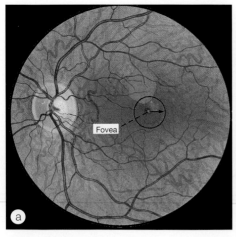
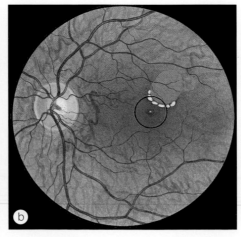
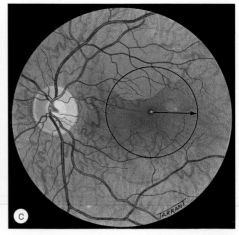

Figure 3.32 Clinically significant macular edema (see the text)

Case study 1

1. History

A 55-year-old man presented with a two month history of slight difficulty in reading. He was diagnosed as having NIDD eight years ago, and his father was also a diabetic.

2. Examination

Right eye

- Visual acuity was 6/18.

- Fundus examination showed circinate hard exudates encroaching within one-half disc diameter of the fovea associated with retinal thickening. Also present were multiple microaneurysms and a few dot-blot hemorrhages (Figure 3.33a).

Left eye

- Visual acuity was 6/6.

- Fundus examination showed mild BDR.

3. FA right eye

- *Venous phase* showed spotty hyperfluorescence of microaneurysms (Figure 3.33b).

- *Later phase* showed hyperfluorescence due to leakage at the macula, particularly superior to the fovea (Figure 3.33c).

4. Diagnosis

- Bilateral background DR, and right clinically significant macular edema with focal maculopathy.

5. Treatment

- Right focal laser photocoagulation was applied to areas of leakage as identified on FA.

6. Outcome

- Three-and-a-half years later.

Right eye

- Visual acuity was 6/18.

- Fundus examination showed laser scars but neither hard exudates nor retinal thickening (Figure 3.34a).

- FA showed early spotty hyperfluorescence of microaneurysms (Figure 3.34b), but no late leakage (Figure 3.34c). The laser scars were hyperfluorescent.

Left eye

- Visual acuity was 6/9.

- Fundus examination showed slight increase in number of hard exudates some of which were very close to the centre of the fovea.

7. Comment

This patient had a good result following treatment of clinically significant macular edema. His visual acuity was stabilized but, as expected, not improved. It is therefore important to inform patients prior to commencing treatment that improvement occurs in only 15% of patients and that 14% subsequently deteriorate despite treatment.

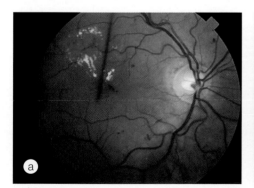
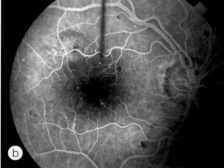
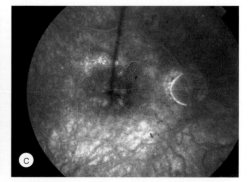

Figure 3.33 Focal diabetic maculopathy prior to treatment (see the text)

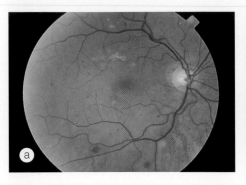 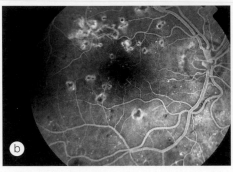 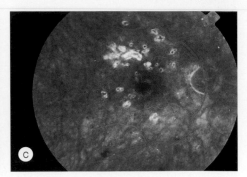

Figure 3.34 Focal diabetic maculopathy after treatment (see the text)

Case study 2

1. History

A 45-year-old female presented with a one year history of gradual visual loss mainly involving the left eye. She developed IDD ten years ago and had her left leg amputated one year ago.

2. Examination

Right eye

- Visual acuity was 6/9.

- Fundus examination showed multiple micro-aneurysms, dot and blot hemorrhages and hard exudate just superior to the fovea.

Left eye

- Visual acuity was 6/24.

- Fundus examination showed multiple micro-aneurysms, hemorrhages, hard exudates with one plaque just below the fovea, and retinal thickening involving the fovea (Figure 3.35a).

3. FA left eye

- *Venous phase* showed spotty hyperfluorescence of microaneurysms and hypofluorescence corresponding to the hard exudates and hemorrhages (Figure 3.35b and 3.35c).

- *Late phase* showed diffuse hyperfluorescence at the macula without CME (Figure 3.35d).

4. Diagnosis

- Bilateral background DR, and left clinically significant macular edema with diffuse maculopathy.

5. Treatment

- Left grid argon laser photocoagulation was applied to areas of retinal leakage as identified on FA.

- The patient subsequently also developed proliferative DR which was treated by PRP.

6. Outcome

- One year later.

Left eye

- Visual acuity was 6/36.

- Fundus examination showed laser scars and mild retinal thickening involving the fovea (Figure 3.36a).

- FA showed mild leakage at the fovea, much less than previously (Figure 3.36b–3.36d).

7. Comment

This patient developed both background and proliferative DR. Not surprisingly, despite extensive treatment her visual acuity deteriorated. The poor prognostic features for central vision were: severe retinopathy at presentation, diffuse retinal edema and hard exudates very near to the fovea. It is also known that treatment of proliferative disease may worsen macular edema.

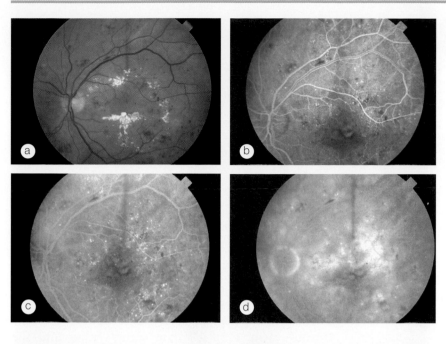

Figure 3.35 Diffuse diabetic maculopathy prior to treatment (see the text)

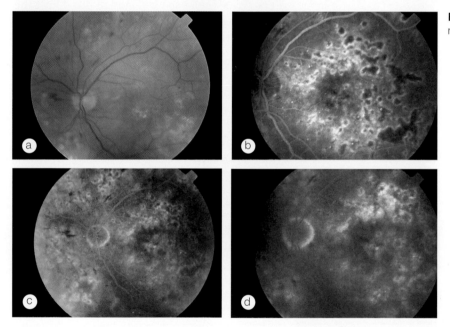

Figure 3.36 Treated diffuse diabetic maculopathy (see the text)

Vitrectomy

In some eyes macular edema may be associated with tangential traction from a thickened and taut posterior hyaloid membrane. In these cases laser therapy is of limited benefit but surgical release of tangential macular traction may be beneficial in some cases.

Proliferative diabetic retinopathy

Diagnosis

Proliferative diabetic retinopathy (PDR) affects 5–10% of the diabetic population. Patients with IDD are at increased risk of PDR with an incidence of about 60% after 30 years.

1. Signs

Neovascularization is the hallmark of PDR (Figure 3.37a). New vessels may proliferate on or within one disc diameter of the optic nerve head (NVD, new vessels at disc), or along the course of the major vessels (NVE, new vessels elsewhere), or both. It has been estimated that over one-quarter of the retina has to be non-perfused before NVD develops. The absence of the internal limiting membrane (ILM) over the optic nerve head may partially explain the predilection for neovascularization at this site. New vessels start as endothelial proliferations, arising most frequently from veins; they then pass through defects in the ILM to lie in the potential plane between the retina and posterior vitreous cortex, using the latter as a 'scaffold' for their growth (Figure 3.37b).

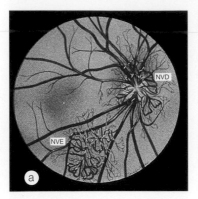

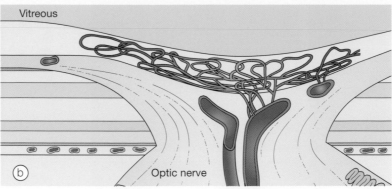

Figure 3.37
Proliferative DR (see the text)

2. **FA**, although not required to make the diagnosis of PDR (Figure 3.38a and 3.38b), will highlight the neovascularization during the early phases of the angiogram and show hyperfluorescence during the later stages due to intense leakage of dye from neovascular tissue (Figure 3.38c and 3.38d).

Natural history

- The fibrovascular network proliferates between the ILM and vitreous gel to which it becomes adherent.

- As a result of the strong attachments of the cortical vitreous gel to areas of fibrovascular proliferation, traction at these sites by contracting vitreous gel causes elevation of the vessels above the plane of the retina. Figure 3.39a shows flat NVE without fibrosis; Figure 3.39b shows elevated NVE with some fibrosis; Figure

3.39c shows elevated NVE associated with partial vitreous separation.

- The fibrovascular tissue then continues to proliferate along the posterior surface of the partially detached vitreous, and is progressively pulled further into the vitreous cavity until bleeding occurs either into the vitreous gel or retrohyaloid space (Figure 3.40). Until the onset of hemorrhage, PDR is completely asymptomatic and can only be detected by screening.

- The burnt-out stage is characterized by a gradual increase in the fibrous component and a decrease in the vascular component of the fibrovascular proliferation, so that the blood vessels become non-perfused and no further proliferation occurs. Figure 3.41a shows very severe PDR with a normal visual acuity because of a round window overlying the macula in fibrous tissue; Figure 3.41b shows mainly avascular tissue.

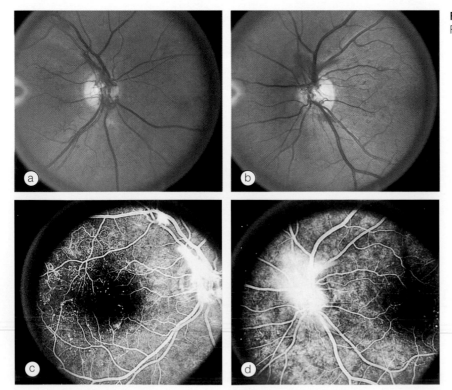

Figure 3.38 (a) & (b) Bilateral NVD; (c) & (d) FA showing leakage

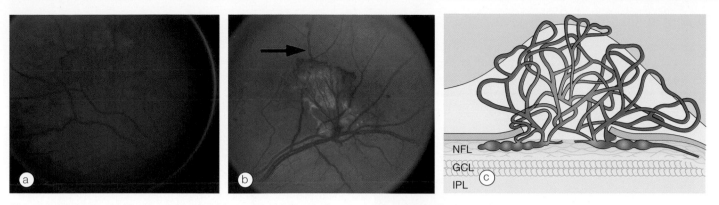

Figure 3.39 (a) Flat NVE without fibrosis; (b) elevated NVE with fibrosis; (c) elevated NVE with partial vitreous separation

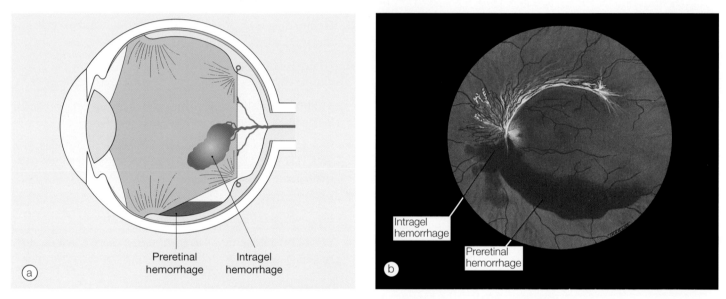

Figure 3.40 Proliferative DR showing the location of preretinal and intragel hemorrhages

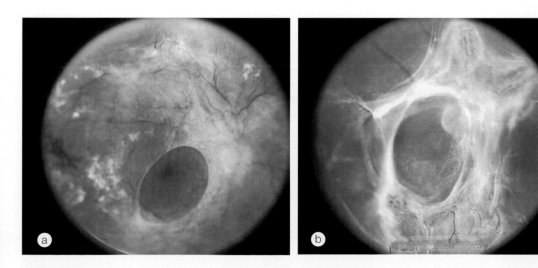

Figure 3.41 (a) Extensive fibrovascular proliferation with a window over the macula; (b) extensive avascular fibrosis

Clinical assessment

1. **Severity** of neovascularization is determined by the area covered with new vessels in comparison to the area of the disc. It should also be noted whether the new vessels are flat or elevated (Figure 3.42) because the latter are less responsive to treatment. The severity of PDR is described as follows:

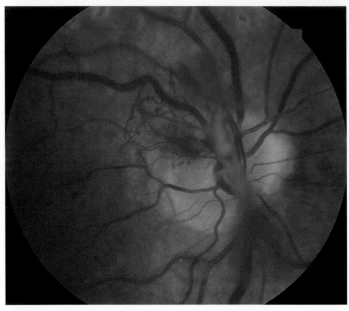

Figure 3.42 Elevated NVD

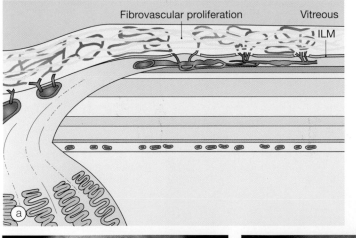

- NVD is mild when the vessels cover less than one third disc area.

- NVD is severe if one-third or more of disc area is covered.

- NVE is mild if less than half disc area in extent.

- NVE is severe if half disc area or more in extent.

2. **Fibrosis** associated with neovascularization is important because eyes with significant fibrous proliferation are less likely to bleed, but carry an increased risk of tractional retinal detachment. Figure 3.43a shows severe fibrovascular proliferation between the ILM and the vitreous; Figure 3.43b shows severe fibrosis but a flat retina; Figure 3.43c shows early tractional retinal detachment associated with fibrosis involving the infero-temporal arcade; Figure 3.43d shows a total tractional retinal detachment.

3. **Hemorrhage** which may be pre-retinal and/or vitreous (Figure 3.44) is an important risk factor for visual loss.

4. **High-risk characteristics** of subsequent severe visual loss within two years without treatment are as follows:

- Mild NVD with hemorrhage carries a 26% risk of visual loss, which is reduced to 4% with treatment.

- Severe NVD without hemorrhage (Figure 3.45) carries a 26% risk of visual loss, which can be reduced to 9% with treatment.

- Severe NVD with hemorrhage carries a 37% risk of visual loss, which is reduced to 20% with treatment.

- Severe NVE (Figure 3.46) with hemorrhage carries a 30% risk of visual loss, which is reduced to 7% with treatment.

Unless the above criteria apply, treatment is usually withheld and the patient is followed up at three-monthly intervals.

Figure 3.43 (a) Fibrovascular proliferation between the internal limiting membrane and the vitreous gel; (b) fibrovascular proliferation and a flat retina; (c) localized tractional retinal detachment (arrows); (d) total tractional retinal detachment

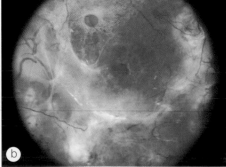
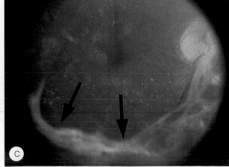
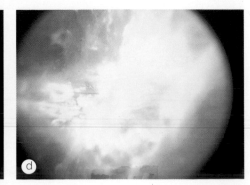

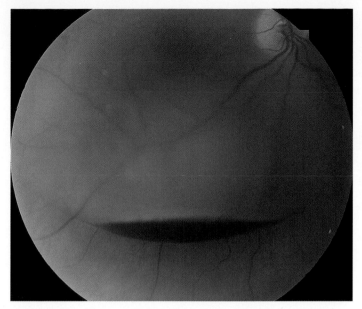

Figure 3.44 A preretinal hemorrhage and a localized mild vitreous hemorrhage

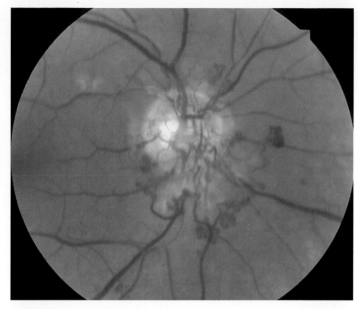

Figure 3.45 Severe NVD

Laser photocoagulation

1. **Aim** of treatment is to induce involution of new vessels, prevent recurrent vitreous hemorrhage and retinal detachment.

2. **Extent** of treatment is dependent on the severity of PDR. The lesions are placed closer together and with greater intensity for severe disease, and further apart and less intensity for milder disease.

3. **Examples**

- Figure 3.47a shows acute burns following moderate treatment; Figure 3.47b is the same eye several months later showing scars that are smaller than the acute burns

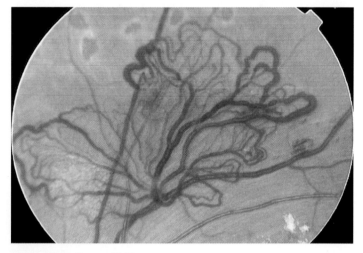

Figure 3.46 Severe NVE

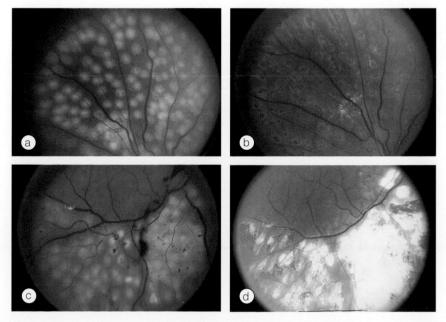

Figure 3.47 Laser PRP for proliferative DR: (a) & (b) Standard; (c) & (d) intensive (see the text)

so that additional treatment between the scars is possible if required.

- Figure 3.47c shows more intensive treatment with less spacing of burns resulting in confluent scarring (Figure 3.47d).

4. Technique

- *Spot size* depends on which contact lens is being used. When using the Goldmann lens, the spot size is set at 500 μm, but when using a panfundoscopic lens it is set at 300–400 μm because of induced magnification.

- *Duration* of the burn is 0.05–0.10 seconds at a power level that produces a gentle burn.

- *Initial treatment* involves the placement of about 2000–3000 burns in a scatter pattern, extending from the posterior fundus to cover the peripheral retina in one or more sessions. PRP completed in one session carries a slightly higher risk of complications. Not infrequently, the amount of treatment during any one session is governed by the patient's pain threshold and ability to maintain concentration. Topical corneal anaesthesia is adequate in most patients.

- *Sequence* of placing burns in PRP is as follows:
  a. Step 1 – close to the disc (Figure 3.48a); below the inferior temporal arcades (Figure 3.48b and 3.48c).
  b. Step 2 – protective barrier around the macula to prevent inadvertent treatment of the fovea (Figure 3.49a); above the supero-temporal arcade (Figure 3.49b and 3.49c).
  c. Step 3 – nasal to the disc (Figure 3.50a and 3.50b); completion of posterior pole treatment (Figure 3.50c).
  d. Step 4 – peripheral treatment (Figure 3.51a and 3.51b) until completion (Figure 3.51c).

Figure 3.48 PRP technique – step 1 (see the text)

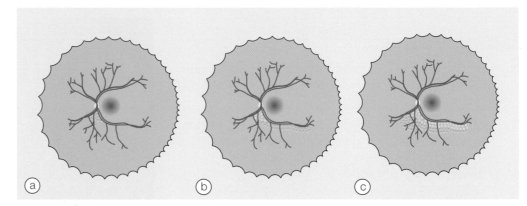

Figure 3.49 PRP technique – step 2 (see the text)

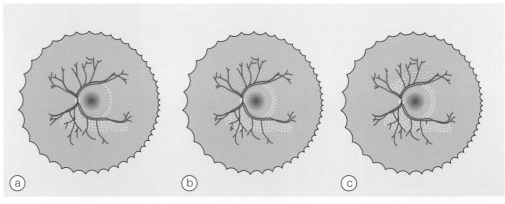

Figure 3.50 PRP technique – step 3 (see the text)

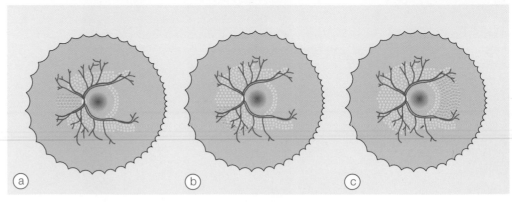

Figure 3.51 PRP technique – step 4 (see the text)

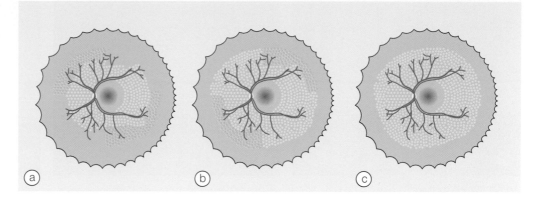

Subsequent management

1. **Follow-up** following PRP should be after four to six weeks. In eyes with severe NVD, several treatment sessions with 5000 or more burns may be required, although in some cases complete elimination of NVD may be extremely difficult and 'early' vitreous surgery should be considered. It should, however, be emphasized that the most important cause of persistent neovascularization is inadequate treatment.

2. **Signs of involution** are regression of neovascularization leaving only 'ghost' vessels or fibrous tissue, decrease in venous dilatation, absorption of retinal hemorrhages and disc pallor. In most eyes, once the retinopathy is quiescent, stability is maintained. In a few eyes, recurrences of PDR occur despite an initial satisfactory response. It is therefore necessary to re-examine the patient at intervals of approximately 6–12 months. It is important to emphasize that photocoagulation influences only the vascular component of the fibrovascular process. Eyes in which the new vessels have regressed leaving only fibrous tissue should not be re-treated.

3. **Examples**

- Figure 3.52a shows mild right NVD; Figure 3.52b shows more severe left NVD with pre-retinal hemorrhage indicating a high risk; Figure 3.52c shows regression of left NVD four weeks after PRP with residual small avascular fibrous tissue; Figure 3.52d 18 months later shows no evidence of recurrence but more prominent laser scars.

- Figure 3.53a shows very severe NVD indicating high risk; Figure 3.53b shows the development of vitreous hemorrhage three days later whilst the patient was awaiting treatment; Figure 3.53c taken nine months later shows resolution of NVD and confluent laser scars following extensive PRP. This case emphasizes the need for urgent treatment of high risk eyes.

4. **Treatment of recurrence** may be with one or both of the following modalities:

- *Further laser photocoagulation*, filling in any gaps between previous laser scars.

- *Cryotherapy* to the anterior retina is particularly useful when further photocoagulation is impossible as a result of inadequate visualization of the fundus caused by opaque media. It also offers a means of treating areas of the retina usually left untreated by photocoagulation.

5. **Example**
Figure 3.54a shows persistent NVD following PRP; Figure 3.54b shows the appearance immediately following further PRP placed between previous laser scars; Figure 3.54c shows regression of NVD.

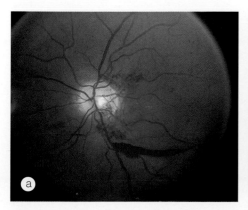
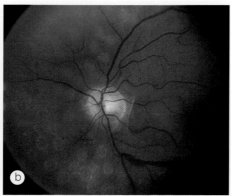
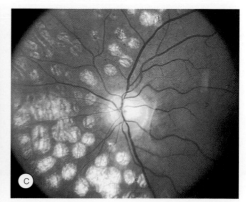

Figure 3.52 PRP of proliferative DR (see the text)

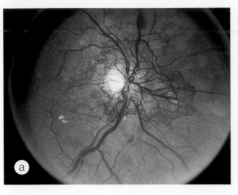
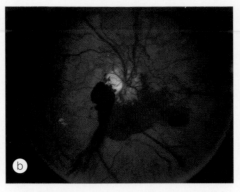
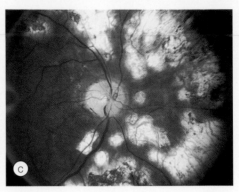

Figure 3.53 PRP of very severe proliferative DR (see the text)

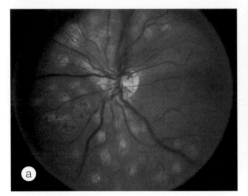
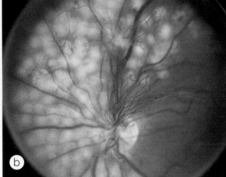
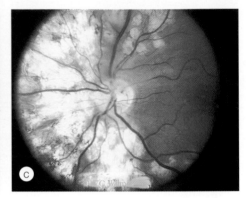

Figure 3.54 PRP for persistent NVD (see the text)

Case study

1. History

A 22-year-old woman presented with a one week history of episodic blurring of vision in her left eye and a large floater. For the last 15 years she has been a poorly controlled IDD.

2. Examination

Right eye
- Visual acuity was 6/12–2.

- Fundus examination showed severe NVD and numerous patches of NVE. The veins were tortuous and irregular. Also present at the macula were blot hemorrhages, small hard exudates and edema (Figure 3.55a).

Left eye
- Visual acuity was 6/24.

- Fundus examination showed very severe NVD with fibrosis extending along the infero-temporal arcade and NVE along the supero-temporal arcade. The veins were tortuous and irregular. Also present at the macula were blot hemorrhages, hard exudates and edema (Figure 3.56a). The vitreous showed a small amount of blood.

3. FA

Right eye
- *Later phases* showed hyperfluorescence due to leakage from new vessels, severe hyperfluorescence at the macula due to leakage and areas of hypofluorescence due to blockage by hemorrhages (Figure 3.55b and 3.55c).

Left eye
- Similar but more severe changes (Figure 3.56b–3.56c).

4. Diagnosis

- Severe bilateral PDR, and bilateral clinically significant macular edema with diffuse maculopathy.

5. Treatment

- Bilateral macular grid laser photocoagulation.

- A few weeks later bilateral PRP was performed in two sessions (right eye, 3000 burns; left eye, 2000 burns).

6. Outcome

- Ten months later the right eye showed some persistent NVE with extensive fibrovascular proliferation nasally (Figure 3.57a).

- The left eye showed proliferation extending nasally and along the arcades but no neovascularization (Figure 3.57b).

- Visual acuity in both eyes was 6/12 and there was no macular edema.

7. Comment

In patients with PDR it is important not to overlook the possible presence of associated maculopathy which should be treated first. In eyes with very severe PDR laser treatment is not always successful in inducing regression and vitrectomy may be required. However, even very advanced cases, such as this, may respond well provided treatment is adequate. Although it may not always be possible to eliminate all neovascularization, as in the right eye of this patient, but this is often compatible with future stability.

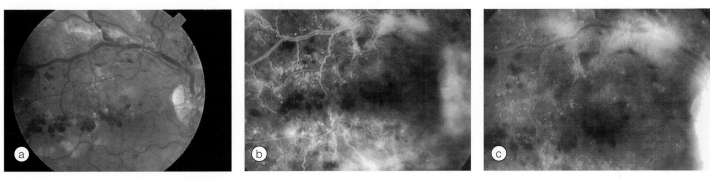

Figure 3.55 Proliferative DR and diffuse maculopathy of the right eye (see the text)

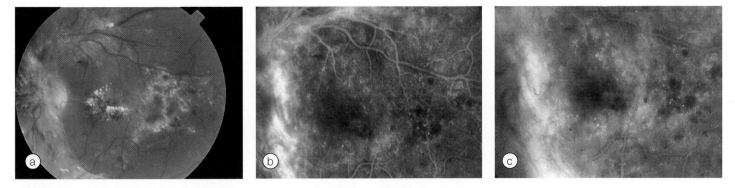

Figure 3.56 Proliferative DR and diffuse maculopathy of the left eye (see the text)

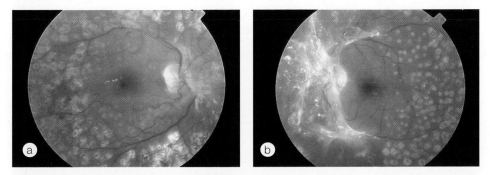

Figure 3.57 (a) Right eye following treatment; (b) left eye following treatment

Advanced diabetic eye disease

Serous vision-threatening complications of diabetic retinopathy (advanced diabetic eye disease) occur in patients who either have not had laser therapy or in whom laser photocoagulation has been unsuccessful or inadequate. One or more of the following complications may be present:

Hemorrhage

Bleeding may occur into the vitreous gel or, more frequently, into the retrohyaloid space (preretinal hemorrhage). A preretinal hemorrhage has a crescentic shape which demarcates the level of posterior vitreous detachment (see Figure 3.44). Occasionally, a preretinal hemorrhage may penetrate the vitreous gel. Intragel hemorrhages usually take longer to clear than preretinal hemorrhages. In some eyes, altered blood becomes compacted on the posterior vitreous face to form an 'ochre membrane'. Patients should be warned that vitreous hemorrhage may occasionally be precipitated by severe physical exertion or straining, hypoglycemia and direct ocular trauma. However, not infrequently, bleeding occurs while the patient is asleep.

Tractional retinal detachment

Tractional retinal detachment (RD) is caused by progressive contraction of fibrovascular membranes over large areas of vitreoretinal adhesion. Posterior vitreous detachment in diabetic eyes is gradual, and because of the strong adhesions of cortical vitreous to areas of fibrovascular proliferation, it is usually incomplete.

1. Pathogenesis

The following are the three types of static vitreoretinal traction that may result in the development of retinal detachment.

- *Tangential* (surface) traction is caused by the contraction of epiretinal fibrovascular membranes resulting in puckering of the retina and distortion of retinal vasculature (Figure 3.58).

- *Anteroposterior* traction is caused by the contraction of fibrovascular membranes extending from the posterior retina, usually in association with the major vascular arcades, to the vitreous base anteriorly (Figure 3.59).

- *Bridging* (trampoline) traction is the result of contraction of fibrovascular membranes that stretch from one part of

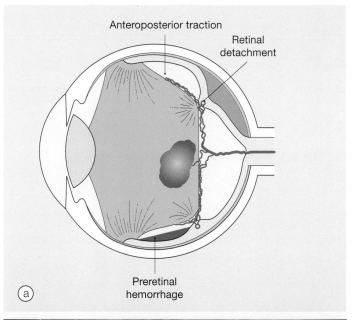

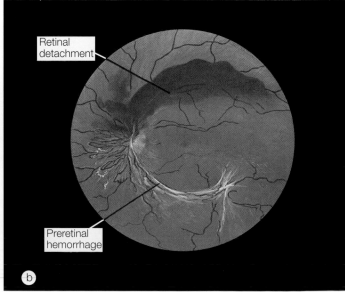

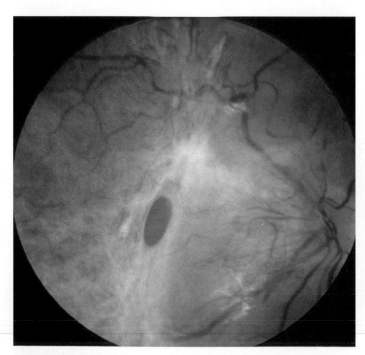

Figure 3.58 Surface fibrovascular proliferation giving rise to tangential traction

Figure 3.59 Antero-posterior vitreoretinal traction giving rise to a superior retinal detachment

the posterior retina to another. This tends to pull the two involved points together and may result in the formation of stress lines as well as displacement of the macula towards the disc or elsewhere depending on the direction of the tractional force (Figure 3.60).

2. Signs

- The RD has a concave configuration with the highest elevation occurring at points of vitreoretinal traction (Figure 3.61).

- The RD is shallow and seldom extends to the equator.

- Retinal mobility is severely reduced and retinal breaks are absent.

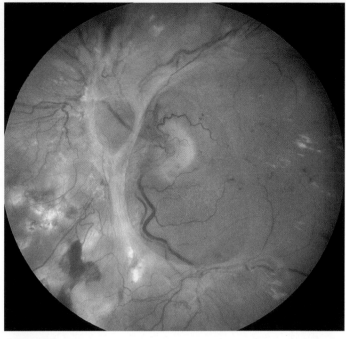

Figure 3.61 Tractional retinal detachment not involving the fovea

Fortunately, diabetic tractional retinal detachments may remain localized for many months without involving the macula. Occasionally, vitreoretinal traction may cause a splitting of the retina into two layers (retinoschisis). In some eyes, traction over areas of fibrovascular adhesion may result in the formation of a retinal break which is usually a small oval hole behind the equator. When this happens, the concave shape characteristic of a tractional retinal detachment assumes a convex bullous configuration (Figure 3.62) typical of a rhegmatogenous retinal detachment. In this event vitreoretinal surgery should be undertaken without delay.

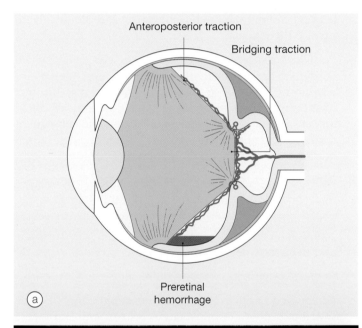

Anteroposterior traction

Bridging traction

Preretinal hemorrhage

(a)

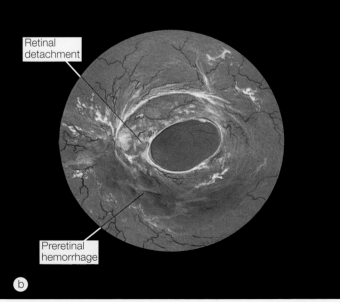

Retinal detachment

Preretinal hemorrhage

(b)

Figure 3.60 Antero-posterior and bridging traction giving rise to a total retinal detachment

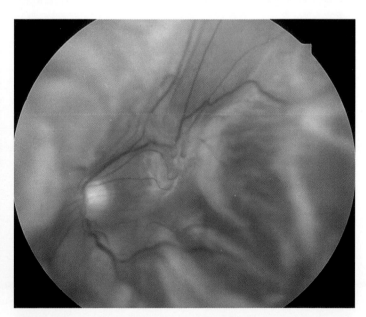

Figure 3.62 Combined tractional and rhegmatogenous retinal detachment

Other complications

1. **Opaque membranes** may develop on the posterior surface of the detached hyaloid and stretch from the superior to the inferior temporal arcades. In some cases the membranes may obscure the macula and further impair visual acuity. More commonly a round or oval hole may be present in the membrane overlying the macula (see Figure 3.58).

2. **Rubeosis iridis** (iris neovascularization) may occur in eyes with PDR, and if severe (see Figure 3.5), may subsequently lead to the development of neovascular glaucoma. Rubeosis is particularly common in eyes with severe retinal ischemia or persistent retinal detachment following unsuccessful pars plana vitrectomy.

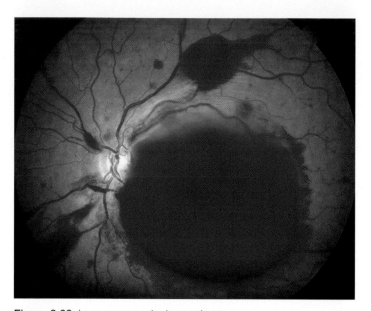

Figure 3.63 Large premacular hemorrhage

Pars plana vitrectomy

1. **Indications**

- *Severe persistent vitreous hemorrhage* is the most common indication for vitrectomy. In these cases the density of the hemorrhage precludes adequate treatment with PRP. In the absence of rubeosis iridis, vitrectomy within three months of the initial vitreous hemorrhage should also be considered in patients with IDD, and at about six months in patients with NIDD.

- *Tractional RD involving the macula* must be treated without delay. However, extramacular tractional detachments may be observed because, in many cases, they remain stationary for prolonged periods of time.

- *Combined tractional and rhegmatogenous RD* should be treated urgently, even if the macula is not involved, because subretinal fluid is likely to spread quickly to involve the macula.

- *Premacular subhyaloid hemorrhage* (Figure 3.63) which is dense and persistent should be considered for vitrectomy because, if untreated, the internal limiting membrane or posterior hyaloid face may act as a scaffold for subsequent fibrovascular proliferation and subsequent tractional macular detachment or macular pucker caused by contraction of epiretinal membranes.

2. **Aims**

- *Removal of vitreous gel* to eliminate the 'scaffold' along which further fibrovascular tissue can proliferate. If this goal is achieved, involution of existing neovascular tissue also frequently occurs.

- *Removal of vitreous blood*, if present.

- *Repair of RD* by excising anteroposterior and bridging tractional membranes (Figure 3.64a) and removing fibrovascular tissue from the retinal surface. Retinal breaks, if present, should also be sealed.

- *Prevention of further neovascularization* by performing laser endophotocoagulation (Figure 3.64b).

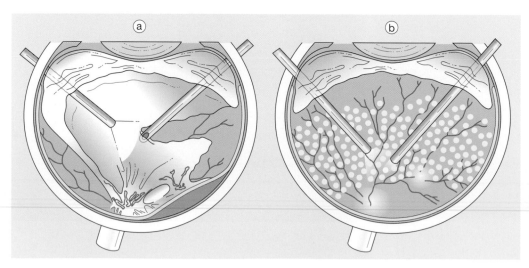

Figure 3.64 Principles of vitreous surgery for advanced diabetic eye disease: (a) Retinal re-attachment by excision of tractional forces; (b) endophotocoagulation

3. Complications

- *Progressive rubeosis iridis* is the most common anterior segment complication resulting in failure. It has an increased incidence in aphakic eyes and in those with residual areas of detached retina. In eyes with total retinal detachments the incidence of rubeosis is virtually 100%.

- *Cataract*, which may be the result of either progression of pre-existing lens opacities or surgical trauma.

- *Glaucoma*, which may be secondary to rubeosis or may be of the ghost cell or red cell type.

- *Recurrent vitreous hemorrhage*, which may be caused by fresh fibrovascular proliferation.

- *Retinal detachment*, which may be caused by intraoperative complications, such as traction on the vitreous base or the inadvertent creation of fresh breaks with the cutter or other instruments. It may also occur later as a result of fresh fibrovascular proliferation.

4. Visual results

Visual results depend on the specific indications for surgery and the complexity of pre-existing vitreoretinal abnormalities. In general, about 70% of cases have visual improvement, about 10% are made worse and the remainder have no change in vision. It appears that the first few postoperative months are vital. If the eye is doing well after six months, then the long-term outlook is favorable because the incidence of subsequent vision-threatening complications is low. Factors associated with a favourable prognosis are:

- Good preoperative visual function.

- Age of 40 years or less.

- Absence of preoperative rubeosis iridis and glaucoma.

- Pre-existing PRP of at least one-quarter of the fundus.

FURTHER READING

Akduman L, Olk RJ. Diode laser (810nm) versus argon green (514nm) modified grid photocoagulation for diffuse diabetic macular edema. *Ophthalmology* 1997;104:1433–1441.

Archer DB. Diabetic retinopathy: some cellular, molecular and therapeutic considerations. Bowman Lecture 1998. *Eye* 1999;13:497–523.

Aylward GW, Pearson RV, Jagger JD, et al. Extensive argon laser photocoagulation in the treatment of proliferative diabetic retinopathy. *Br J Ophthalmol* 1989;73:197–201.

Bailey CC, Sparrow JM, Grey RHB, et al. The National Diabetic Retinopathy Laser Treatment Audit. 1. Maculopathy. *Eye* 1998;12:69–76.

Bailey CC, Sparrow JM, Grey RHB, et al. The National Retinopathy Laser Treatment Audit. 2. Proliferative retinopathy. *Eye* 1998;12:77–84.

Browning DJ, Zhang Z, Benfield JM, et al. The effect of patient characteristics on response to focal laser treatment for diabetic macular edema. *Ophthalmology* 1997;104:466–472.

Cordeiro M, Stanford MR, Phillips PM, et al. Relationship between diabetic microvascular complications to outcome in panretinal photocoagulation treatment of proliferative diabetic retinopathy. *Eye* 1997;11:531–536.

Diabetic Retinopathy Study Research Group. Photocoagulation treatment of proliferative diabetic retinopathy: clinical application of Diabetic Retinopathy Study. DRS report number 8. *Ophthalmology* 1981;88:583–600.

Diabetes Control and Complications Trial Research Group. Progression of retinopathy with intensive versus conventional treatment in the Diabetes Control and Complications Trial. *Ophthalmology* 1995;102:647–661.

Doft B, Metz D, Kelsey S. Augmentation laser for proliferative retinopathy that fails to respond to initial panretinal photocoagulation. *Ophthalmology* 1992;99:1728–1735.

Early Treatment Diabetic Retinopathy Study Research Group. Photocoagulation for diabetic macular edema. Early Treatment Diabetic Retinopathy Study report number 1. *Arch Ophthalmol* 1985;103:1796–1806.

Early Treatment Diabetic Retinopathy Study Research Group. Treatment techniques and clinical guidelines for photocoagulation of diabetic macular edema. Early Treatment Diabetic Retinopathy Study report number 2. *Ophthalmology* 1987;94:761–774.

Early Treatment Diabetic Retinopathy Study Research Group. Techniques for scatter and local photocoagulation treatment of diabetic retinopathy. Early Treatment Diabetic Retinopathy Study report number 3. *Int Ophthalmol Clin* 1987;27:254–264.

Early Treatment Diabetic Retinopathy Study Research Group. Focal photocoagulation treatment of diabetic macular edema, relationship of treatment effect to fluorescein angiographic and other retinal characteristics at baseline: Early Treatment Diabetic Retinopathy Study report number 19. *Arch Ophthalmol* 1995;113:1144–1155.

Ferris III FL. Treating 20/20 eyes with diabetic macular edema. Editorial. *Arch Ophthalmol* 1999;117:675–676.

Fong DS, Ferris III FL, Davis MD, et al. Causes of severe visual loss in the Early Treatment Diabetic Retinopathy Study: ETDRS report no. 24. *Am J Ophthalmol* 1999;127:137–141.

Harbour JW, Smiddy WE, Flynn HW Jr, et al. Vitrectomy for diabetic macular edema associated with a thickened posterior hyaloid membrane. *Am J Ophthalmol* 1996;121:405–413.

Ikeda T, Sato K, Hayashi Y. Improvement of visual acuity following pars plana vitrectomy for diabetic cystoid macular edema and detached posterior hyaloid. *Retina* 2000;20:220–222.

Kylstra JA, Brown JC, Jaffe GJ, et al. The importance of fluorescein angiography in planning laser treatment of diabetic macular edema. *Ophthalmology* 1999;106:2068–2073.

Lee CM, Olk RJ. Modified grid laser photocoagulation for diffuse diabetic macular edema. Long term visual results. *Ophthalmology* 1991;98:1594–1602.

Moss SE, Klein R, Klein BE. Ten-year incidence of visual loss in a diabetic population. *Ophthalmology* 1994;101:1061–1070.

United Kingdom Prospective Diabetes Study, 30. Diabetic retinopathy at diagnosis of non-insulin dependent diabetes mellitus and associated risk factors. *Arch Ophthalmol* 1998;116:297–303.

Vitale S, Maguire MG, Murphy RP, et al. Interval between onset of mild nonproliferative and proliferative retinopathy in type I diabetes. *Arch Ophthalmol* 1997;115:194–198.

Retinal vein occlusion

Classification

1. **Branch retinal vein occlusion (BRVO)**
2. **Central retinal vein occlusion (CRVO)**

- Non-ischemic
- Ischemic
- Papillophlebitis

3. **Hemiretinal vein occlusion**

Pathogenesis

1. **Local factors**

- *Arteriolosclerosis* is an important contributing factor for BRVO. Because retinal arterioles and veins share a common adventitial sheath, the resultant thickening of the arteriole appears to compress the underlying vein if the arteriole is located anterior to the vein. This causes secondary changes which include venous endothelial cell loss, thrombus formation and, eventually, occlusion. Similarly, the central retinal vein and central retinal artery share a common adventitial sheath posterior to the lamina cribrosa so that atherosclerotic changes of the artery may compress the vein and precipitate CRVO. It therefore appears that both arterial and venous disease contributes to retinal vein occlusion. The association with atherosclerosis makes CRVO a common condition in the elderly.

- *Raised intraocular pressure* in patients with primary open-angle glaucoma or ocular hypertension increases the risk of CRVO.

- *Periphlebitis* may occasionally cause BRVO in patients with sarcoidosis and Behçet disease.

2. **Systemic factors**

- *Increased age* is the most important factor, because the largest groups of affected patients are in the sixth and seventh decades of life.

- *Hypertension* is the second most important systemic factor.

- *NIDD.*

- *Hyperlipidemia.*

- *Obesity.*

- *Hyperviscosity* caused by either increased number of circulating cells (e.g. polycythemia, chronic leukemias) or abnormal plasma proteins (e.g. multiple myeloma, Waldenström macroglobulinemia) is an uncommon cause.

- *Thrombophilic disorders*, which may be associated with venous occlusion in young adults, include the following:

a. Inherited defects or deficiencies of a natural anticoagulant such as antithrombin III, protein C or protein S, or resistance to activated protein C (factor V Leiden).

b. Other disorders include hyperhomocysteinemia and antiphospholipid antibody syndrome. Elevated plasma homocysteine concentration is also a risk factor for myocardial infarction, stroke and carotid disease as well as venous occlusion. It is also a risk factor for CRVO, particularly of the ischemic type. Hyperhomocysteinemia is readily reversible in most cases with folic acid.

Note – Factors that appear to decrease the risk of venous occlusion include increased physical activity and moderate alcohol consumption.

Consequences

In the end-artery system of the retina, venous occlusion causes an elevation of venous and capillary pressure with stagnation of blood flow. This stagnation results in hypoxia of the retina drained by the obstructed vein, which in turn, results in damage to the capillary endothelial cells leading to extravasation of blood constituents. The tissue pressure is increased, causing further stagnation of the circulation and hypoxia, so that a vicious cycle is established.

Branch retinal vein occlusion

Classification

BRVO can be classified according to the primary site of occlusion as follows (Figure 3.65):

1. **Major branch occlusion** which may be subdivided as follows:

- Occlusion of a first order branches at the optic disc (Figure 3.65a and see Figure 3.67).

- Occlusion of a first order temporal branches away from the disc but also involving the branches to the macula. (Figure 3.65b).

2. **Minor macular branch occlusion** which involves only a macular branch (Figure 3.65c and 3.66).

3. **Peripheral branch occlusion** which does not involve the macular circulation (Figure 3.65d–3.65f)

Diagnosis of fresh major branch occlusion

1. **Presentation** depends on the amount of macular circulation affected by the occlusion. Patients with macular involvement present with sudden onset of blurred vision and metamorphopsia or a relative visual field defect. Patients with peripheral occlusions may be asymptomatic.

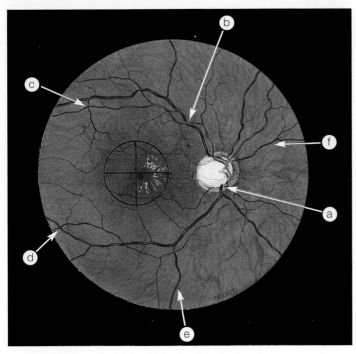

Figure 3.65 Classification of BRVO according to site of blockage (see the text)

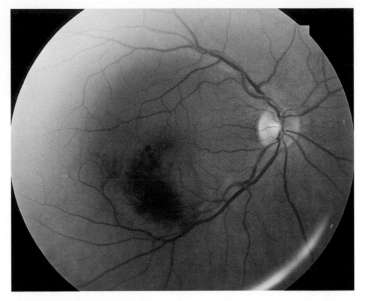

Figure 3.66 Macular BRVO

2. Signs

- Venous dilatation and tortuosity peripheral to the site of occlusion.

- Flame-shaped hemorrhages, 'dot-blot' hemorrhages, retinal edema, and cotton-wool spots affecting the sector of the retina drained by the obstructed vein (Figure 3.67a).

- These acute features take between six and 12 months to resolve.

3. **FA** during the arteriovenous and venous phases show hypofluorerscence due to blockage by hemorrhages (Figure 3.67b and 3.67c). The late phase shows continued blockage by hemorrhages and hyperfluorescence due to leakage from the retinal veins (Figure 3.67d).

Diagnosis of old major occlusion

1. **Presentation** in most patients is with a history of long-standing visual impairment although in some cases the patient may be relatively asymptomatic and the condition is discovered by chance, particularly if the initial occlusion was mild.

Figure 3.67 Major BRVO (see the text)

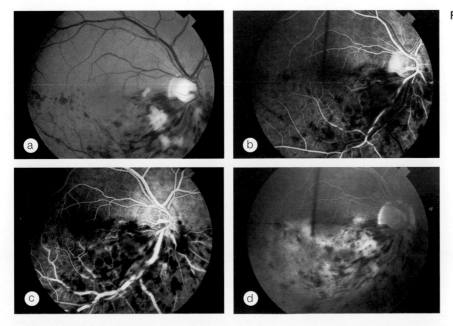

2. Signs

- Venous sheathing and sclerosis peripheral to the site of obstruction and a variable amount of residual hemorrhage (Figure 3.68).

- Venous collateral channels, which are characterized by slightly tortuous vessels which develop locally (Figure 3.69), across the horizontal raphe between the inferior and superior vascular arcades (Figure 3.70), or at the optic disc (Figure 3.71).

- Microaneurysms and hard exudates which may be associated with cholesterol crystal deposition (Figure 3.72).

- The macula may show RPE changes or epiretinal membrane formation (Figure 3.73).

Prognosis

Following a major BRVO, visual acuity may be initially reduced by hemorrhage and macular edema. However, within six months about 50% of eyes develop efficient collaterals, with a return of visual acuity to 6/12 or better. The eventual amount of visual recovery is determined by the amount of venous drainage involved by the occlusion which is determined by the site and size of the occluded vein and the severity of macular ischemia. The two main vision-threatening complications are chronic macular edema and neovascularization.

1. **Chronic macular edema** is the most common cause of persistent poor visual acuity after a BRVO. Some patients

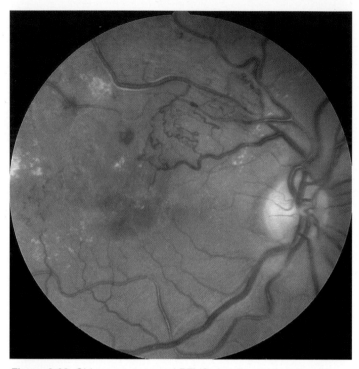

Figure 3.68 Old supero-temporal BRVO showing venous sheathing, collaterals, residual hemorrhages and a few hard exudates

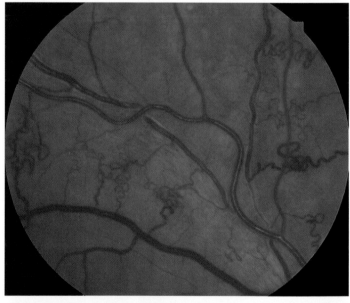

Figure 3.69 Peripheral local collaterals

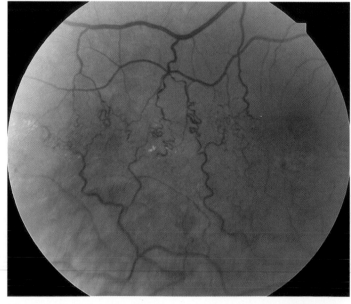

Figure 3.70 Collaterals extending across the horizontal raphe

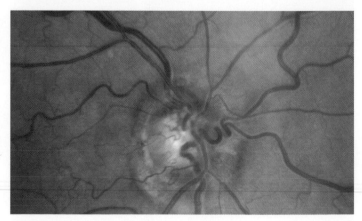

Figure 3.71 Disc collaterals

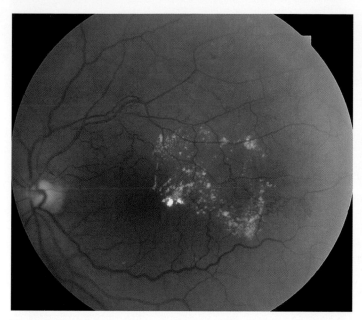

Figure 3.72 Hard exudates associated with an old supero-temporal BRVO

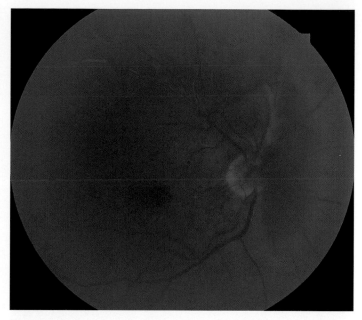

Figure 3.73 Macular epiretinal membrane and vitreous hemorrhage from NVD associated with an old supero-temporal BRVO

with a visual acuity of 6/12 or worse may benefit from laser photocoagulation. However, before recommending treatment, it is important to ensure that the visual loss is caused by macular edema and not ischemia.

2. **Neovascularization** may be either NVD, which develops in about 10% of eyes, or NVE which develops in 20–30% of eyes. However, the incidence of both increases with the severity and extent of involvement. NVE usually develops at the border of the triangular sector of ischemic retina drained by the occluded vein. Neovascularization can develop at any time within the first three years but usually appears during the initial 6–12 months. It is a serious complication because it can lead to recurrent vitreous hemorrhage (Figure 3.73), pre-retinal hemorrhage (Figure 3.74) and occasionally tractional retinal detachment.

Management

1. Evaluation

Wait 6–12 weeks for the retinal hemorrhages to clear sufficiently to enable a good quality FA to be performed and to see whether spontaneous visual improvement occurs. According to the findings further management should be as follows:

- If the FA shows good macular perfusion (Figure 3.75b and 3.75c) and visual acuity is improving then the prognosis is good and no specific treatment is required.

- If the FA shows macular edema associated with good macular perfusion, and visual acuity continues to be 6/12 or worse after three months, treatment by laser photocoagulation should be considered. However, prior to treatment, the FA should be studied carefully to identify the leaking areas. It is also very important to identify

collateral vessels, which do not leak fluorescein, because they must not be treated.

- If FA shows macular non-perfusion and visual acuity is poor, laser treatment will not improve vision. However, if the FA shows five or more disc diameters of non-perfusion (Figure 3.76b–3.76d) the patient should be reviewed at four-monthly intervals for about 18 months because of the risk of neovascularization.

2. Treatment

- *Macular edema* is treated by 'grid' laser photocoagulation (100–200 μm) spaced one burn apart to produce a medium reaction to the area of leakage as defined by the

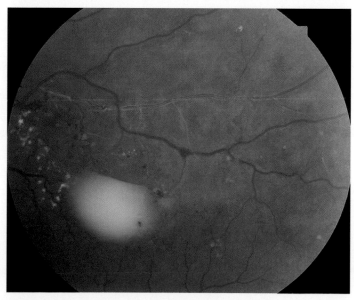

Figure 3.74 Absorbing preretinal hemorrhage associated with an old BRVO

101

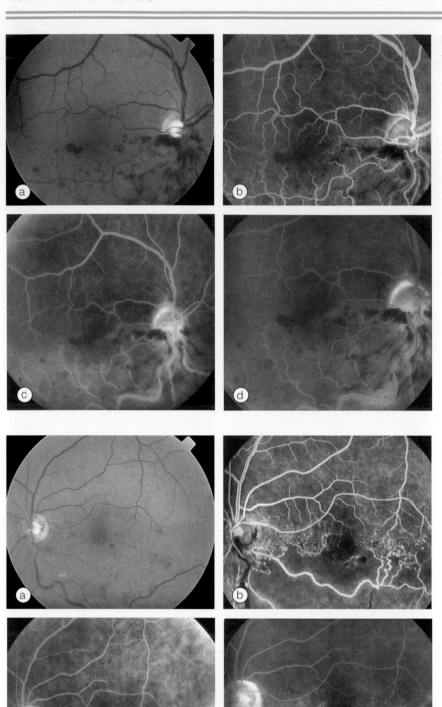

Figure 3.75 Good macular perfusion associated with an infero-temporal BRVO

Figure 3.76 Severe macular non-perfusion associated with an infero-temporal BRVO

FA. The burns should extend no closer to the fovea than the edge of the FAZ and be no more peripheral than the major vascular arcades. Care should be taken to avoid treating over intraretinal hemorrhage. Follow-up should be after two to three months. If macular edema persists re-treatment should be considered although the results may be disappointing.

- *Neovascularization* is treated by 'scatter' laser photocoagulation (200–500 µm) one burn apart to achieve a medium reaction covering the entire involved segment (Figure 3.77) as defined by the colour photograph and FA. Follow-up should be after four to six weeks. If neovascularization persists re-treatment is frequently effective in inducing regression.

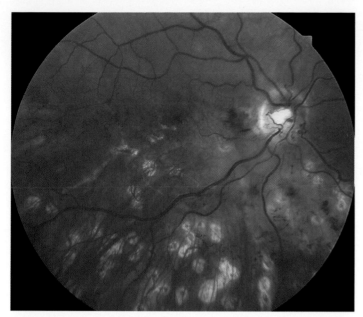

Figure 3.77 Laser scars following treatment of NVD associated with an infero-temporal BRVO

Non-ischemic central retinal vein occlusion

Diagnosis

Non-ischemic CRVO is the most common type accounting for about 75% of all cases.

1. **Presentation** is with a sudden onset of unilateral blurred vision.

2. **Signs**

- Visual acuity is usually moderate to severely reduced.

- Pupillary conduction defect is either absent or mild in contrast to ischaemic CRVO.

- Variable tortuosity and dilatation of all branches of the central retinal vein.

- Mild to moderate retinal hemorrhages ('dot-blot' and flame-shaped), distributed throughout all four quadrants and most numerous in the periphery (Figure 3.78a).

- Variable amount of cotton-wool spots.

- Mild to moderate optic disc and macular edema are common.

Many or all of the acute signs resolve over the next 6–12 months. Residual findings in some cases include disc collaterals, epiretinal membrane formation and RPE changes at the macula.

3. **FA** shows delayed venous return but good retinal capillary perfusion (Figure 3.78b) and late leakage (Figure 3.78c and 3.78d).

Prognosis

Conversion to ischemic CRVO occurs in 15% of cases within four months and 34% of cases within three years. The prognosis in cases that do not subsequently become ischemic, is reasonably good with a return of visual acuity to normal or near normal in about 50%. The main cause for poor visual acuity is chronic CME which may lead to secondary RPE changes. To a certain extent the prognosis depends on the initial visual acuity as follows:

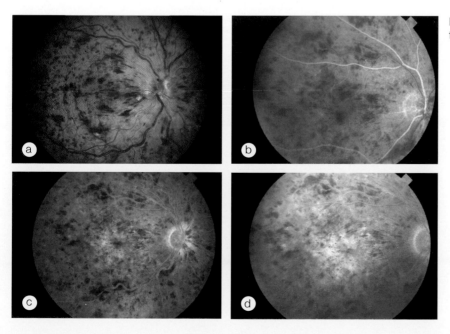

Figure 3.78 Non-ischemic CRVO (see the text)

- If initial visual acuity is 6/18 or better, it is likely to remain good.

- If visual acuity is between 6/24 and 6/60, the clinical course is variable, and vision may subsequently improve, remain the same, or worsen.

- If visual acuity at the onset is worse than 6/60, improvement is unlikely.

Management

1. **Follow-up** should be for about three years to detect the possibility of conversion to ischemic CRVO.

2. **Treatment** by high-intensity laser to create an anastamotic connection between a retinal vein and a choroidal vein, thereby bypassing the site of obstruction to venous outflow may be beneficial in some cases, but is not without potential risks such as fibrous proliferation from the laser site (Figure 3.79) or hemorrhage. Unfortunately, chronic CME is unresponsive to laser therapy.

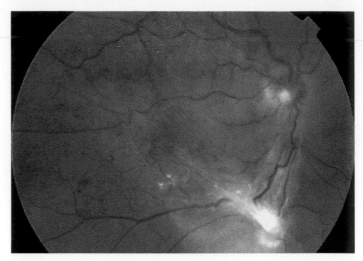

Figure 3.79 Fibrous proliferation at site of laser-induced anastamosis for non-ischaemic CRVO

Case study

1. History

A 75-year-old hypertensive man presented six weeks after developing sudden blurred vision in his right eye.

2. Examination right eye

- Visual acuity was 6/60.

- The pupils reacted briskly to light and there was no rubeosis.

- Fundus examination showed CRVO (see Figure 3.78a).

3. FA right eye

- *Arteriovenous phase* showed delay in venous filling, blockage by hemorrhages and good capillary perfusion (see Figure 3.78b).

- *Later phases* showed macular hyperfluorescence due to leakage (see Figure 3.78c and 3.78d).

4. Diagnosis

- Non-ischemic CRVO on the basis of good retinal capillary perfusion and normal pupillary reactions.

- The patient was followed at monthly intervals because of the potential risk of conversion to ischemic CRVO.

5. Outcome

- One year later visual acuity had improved to 6/18, the hemorrhages had resolved and the optic disc showed collaterals (Figure 3.80a).

- FA showed gradual increasing hyperfluorescence at the macula which had a petalloid appearance characteristic of CME (Figure 3.80c and d).

6. Comment

This patient had two important risk factors for retinal vein occlusion; old age and hypertension. He was fortunate that there was no subsequent conversion to ischemic CRVO and despite initially poor visual acuity this subsequently improved despite the chronic CME.

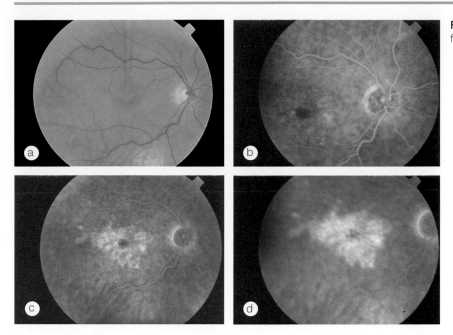

Figure 3.80 Severe cystoid macular edema following non-ischemic CRVO (see the text)

Ischemic central retinal vein occlusion

Diagnosis

Ischemic CRVO is less common than non-ischemic.

1. **Presentation** is with a sudden onset of unilateral severe impairment of vision.

2. **Signs**

- Visual acuity is very severely impaired to counting fingers or less.

- Pupillary conduction defect is marked.

- Marked tortuosity and engorgement of all branches of the central retinal vein.

- Extensive dot-blot and flame-shaped hemorrhages involving the peripheral retina and posterior pole (Figure 3.81a).

- Variable cotton-wool spots.

- Severe optic disc edema and hyperemia, and macular edema.

Many or all of the acute signs resolve over the next 9–12 months. Residual findings in some cases include disc collaterals and macular epiretinal membrane formation and RPE changes. Rarely subretinal fibrosis resembling that associated with end-stage exudative age-related macular degeneration may develop.

3. **FA** shows central masking by retinal hemorrhages (Figure 3.81b), extensive areas of capillary non-perfusion (Figure 3.81c) and late leakage (Figure 3.81d).

Figure 3.81 Acute ischemic CRVO (see the text)

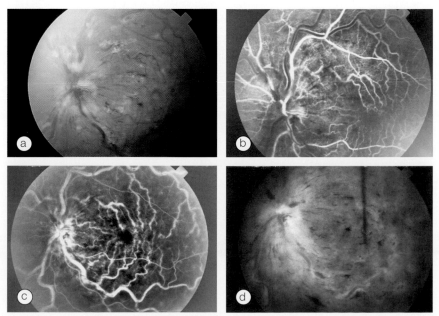

Prognosis

The visual prognosis is extremely poor because of macular ischemia. Rubeosis iridis develops in about 50% of eyes, usually between two and four months (100-day glaucoma), and unless treated there is a high risk of neovascular glaucoma.

Management

1. **Follow-up** should be at monthly intervals for six months in order to detect anterior segment neovascularization. Angle neovascularization, while not synonymous with eventual neovascular glaucoma, is the best clinical predictor of the eventual risk of neovascular glauocoma, because it may occur in the absence of pupil margin neovascularization. It is therefore important that routine gonioscopy of patients at risk should be performed and that mere slitlamp examination of the iris is not adequate.

2. **Treatment** by laser panretinal photocoagulation should be performed without delay in eyes with angle or iris neovascularization. Prophylactic laser therapy is appropriate only in patients who are unable to attend regular follow-up.

Case study

1. **History**

A 67-year-old man presented with a two-day history of severe visual loss in his left eye. Eight years ago he was found to have hypertension and hypercholesterolemia.

2. **Examination left eye**

- Visual acuity was CF at half meter.

- There was a 3+ afferent pupillary defect but no rubeosis.

- Fundus examination showed venous dilatation and tortuosity of all branches of the central retinal vein, severe edema of the macula and optic disc, extensive retinal hemorrahges and cotton-wool spots affecting all quadrants (see Figure 3.81a).

3. **FA left eye**

- *Arteriovenous phase* showed marked delay in venous filling and small areas of hypofluorescence due to blockage by hemorrhage (see Figure 3.81b).

- *Venous phase* showed hypofluorescence at the posterior pole due to retinal capillary non-perfusion (see Figure 3.81c).

- *Late phase* showed extensive diffuse hyperfluorescence due to leakage from the optic disc and retinal capillaries (see Figure 3.81d).

4. **Diagnosis**

- Ischemic CRVO on the basis of very poor visual acuity, afferent pupillary defect and capillary non-perfusion on FA.

- The patient was followed at monthly intervals with fundoscopy, as well as slitlamp examination and gonioscopy to detect rubeosis.

5. **Course**

- Two months later, mild rubeosis was detected at the pupillary border (Figure 3.82) but not the angle. Intraocular pressure was normal.

- Because of the risk of development of neovascular glaucoma laser panretinal photocoagulation was performed (2000 burns, 200 μm).

6. **Outcome**

- Six months later, visual acuity was 3/60. The rubeosis had resolved and the intraocular pressure was normal.

- Fundus examination showed fewer hemorrhages, venous sheathing, laser scars and a pale disc with shunt vessels (Figure 3.83a).

- FA showed severe hypofluorescence due to retinal capillary non-perfusion (Figure 3.83b–3.83d).

7. **Comment**

This patient had two risk factors for CRVO, hypertension and hypercholesterolemia. Because rubeosis was detected early and treated aggressively he did not develop neovascular glaucoma. However, as expected his visual acuity remained severely impaired as a result of macular iscemia.

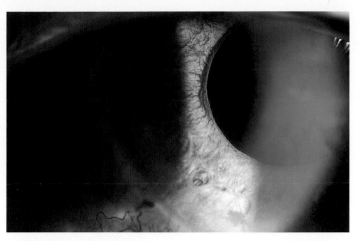

Figure 3.82 Rubeosis iridis

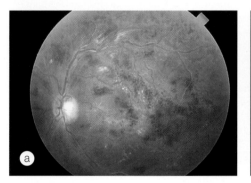
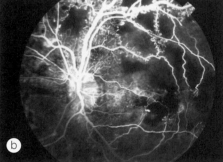
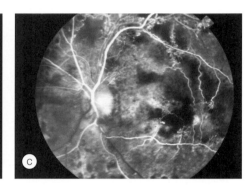

Figure 3.83 Old ischemic CRVO (see the text)

Papillophlebitis

Papillophlebitis, which is also sometimes referred to as optic disc vasculitis, is a relatively uncommon condition which typically affects otherwise healthy individuals who are under the age of 50 years. It is thought that the underlying lesion is optic disc swelling which causes secondary venous congestion rather than venous thrombosis occurring at the level of the lamina cribrosa that occurs in older patients.

1. **Presentation** is with relatively mild blurring of vision which is typically worse on waking.

2. **Signs**

- Visual acuity is good or moderately impaired.

- Normal pupillary reactions.

- Disc edema, which may be associated with cotton-wool spots, is the dominant finding (Figure 3.84).

- Venous dilatation and tortuosity with variable amount of retinal hemorrhages which are usually confined to the peripapillary area and posterior fundus.

- Enlargement of the blind spot.

3. **FA** shows delay in venous filling, hyperfluorescence due to leakage and good capillary perfusion.

4. **Treatment** is of no proven benefit.

5. **Prognosis** is very good in 80% of cases with a final visual acuity of 6/12 or better. The remainder suffer significant and permanent visual impairment as a result of macular edema.

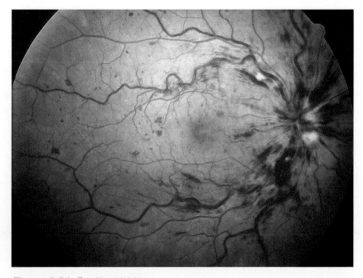

Figure 3.84 Papillophlebitis

Hemiretinal vein occlusion

Classification

Hemiretinal vein occlusion, which is less common than either BRVO and CRVO, is classified into the following two types:

1. **Hemisphere occlusion** of a major branch of the CRV at or near the optic disc.

2. **Hemicentral occlusion**, which is less common, involves one trunk of a dual-trunked CRV which persists in the anterior part of the optic nerve head as a congenital variant present in about 20% of the general population.

Diagnosis

1. **Presentation** is with a sudden altitudinal visual field defect and variable impairment of central vision.

2. **Signs**

- Visual acuity is impaired to a variable extent.

- Venous dilatation and tortuosity involving the superior (Figure 3.85a) or inferior branch of the central retinal vein.

- Extensive hemorrahges and variable amount of cotton-wool spots involving the superior or inferior fundus.

3. **FA** shows early masking by hemorrhages (Figure 3.85b) and late leakage (Figure 3.85c).

Management

The prognosis is variable and is dependent on the severity of macular ischemia and edema. Treatment depends on the severity of retinal ischemia. Patients with extensive retinal ischemia are at risk for rubeosis and neovascular glaucoma and should be managed in the same way as those with ischemic CRVO.

FURTHER READING

Branch Vein Occlusion Study Group. Argon laser photocoagulation for macular edema in branch vein occlusion. *Am J Ophthalmol* 1984;98:271–282.

Branch Vein Occlusion Study Group. Argon laser scatter photocoagulation for prevention of neovascularization and vitreous hemorrhage in branch vein occlusion. A randomized clinical trial. *Arch Ophthalmol* 1986;104:34–41.

Browning DJ, Antoszyk AN. Laser anastamosis for nonischaemic central retinal vein occlusion. *Ophthalmology* 1998;105:670–677.

Browning DJ, Scott AQ, Peterson CB, et al. The risk of missing angle neovascularization by omitting screening gonioscopy in acute central retinal vein occlusion. *Ophthalmology* 1998;105:776–784.

Central Vein Occlusion Study Group. Baseline and early natural history report: the central vein occlusion study. *Arch Ophthalmol* 1993;111:1087–1095.

Central Vein Occlusion Study Group. A randomized clinical trial of early panretinal photocoagulation for ischaemic central vein occlusion. The Central Vein Occlusion Study Group N report. *Ophthalmology* 1995;102:1434–1444.

Central Retinal Vein Occlusion Study Group. Evaluation of grid pattern photocoagulation for macular edema in central vein occlusion. The Central Vein Occlusion Study Group M report. *Ophthalmology* 1995;102:1425–1433.

Central Vein Occlusion Study Group. Natural history and clinical management of central retinal vein occlusion. *Arch Ophthalmol* 1997;115:486–491.

Christofferesen NLB, Larsen M. Pathophysiology and hemodynamics of branch retinal vein occlusion. *Ophthalmology* 1999;106:2054–2062.

Cobo-Soriano R, Sanchez-Ramon S, Aparacio MJ, et al. Antiphospholipid antibodies and retinal thrombosis in patients without risk factors: a prospective case-control study. *Am J Ophthalmol* 1999;128:725–732.

Elman MJ, Bhatt AK, Quinlan PM, et al. The risk for systemic vascular diseases and mortality in patients with central retinal vein occlusion. *Ophthalmology* 1990;97:1543–1548.

Eye Disease Case-Control Study Group. Risk factors for branch vein occlusion. *Am J Ophthalmol* 1993;116:286–296.

Fekrat S, Goldberg MF, Finkenstein D. Laser-induced chorioretinal venous anastamosis with non-ischemic central or branch vein occlusion. *Arch Ophthalmol* 1998;116(1):43–52.

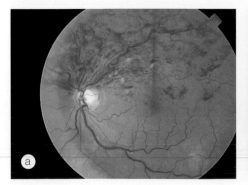
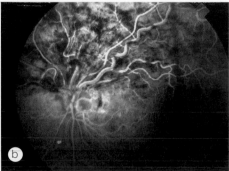
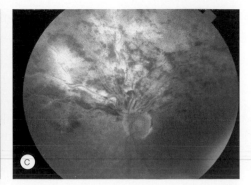

Figure 3.85 Superior hemiretinal vein occlusion (see the text)

Fong ACO, Schatz H. Central retinal vein occlusion in young adults. *Surv Ophthalmol* 1993;37:393–417.

Gottlieb JL, Blice JP, Mestichelli B, et al. Activated protein C resistance, factor V Leiden, and central retinal vein occlusion. *Arch Ophthalmol* 1998;116:577–579.

Hayreh SS. Classification of central retinal vein occlusion. *Ophthalmology* 1983;90:458–474.

Hayreh SS, Hayreh MS. Hemi-central retinal vein occlusion. Pathogenesis, clinical features, and natural history. *Arch Ophthalmol* 1980;98:1600–1609.

Kumar B, Yu D-Y, Morgan WH, et al. The distribution of architectural changes within the vicinity of arteriovenous crossing in branch retinal vein occlusion. *Ophthalmology* 1998;105:424–427.

Lip PL, Blann AD, Jones AF, et al. Abnormalities in haemorhological factors and lipoprotein in retinal vascular occlusion: implications for increased vascular risk. *Eye* 1998;12:245–251.

McAllister IL, Douglas JP, Constable IJ, et al. Laser-induced chorioretinal venous anastamosis for nonischemic central retinal vein occlusion: evaluation of the complications and their risk factors. *Am J Ophthalmol* 1998;126:219–229.

Sandborn GE, Margargal LE. Charactertistics of the hemispheric retinal vein occlusion. *Ophthalmology* 1984;91:1616–1626.

Sperduto RD, Hiller R, Chew E, et al. Risk factors for hemiretinal vein occlusion. Comparison with risk factors for central and branch retinal vein occlusion. The Eye Disease Case Control Study. *Ophthalmology* 1998;105:765–771.

Vine AK. Hyperhomocysteinemia; a risk factor for central retinal vein occlusion. *Am J Ophthalmol* 2000;129:640–644.

Williamson TH. Central retinal vein occlusion; what's the story? Perspectives. *Br J Ophthalmol* 1997;81:698–704.

Williamson TH, Rumley A, Lowe GDO. Blood viscosity, coagulation and activated protein C resistance in central retinal vein occlusion: a population controlled study. *Br J Ophthalmol* 1996;80:203–208.

Retinal artery occlusion

Classification

1. **Branch retinal artery occlusion (BRAO)**

2. **Central retinal artery occlusion (CRAO)**

3. **Cilioretinal artery occlusion**

Pathogenesis

1. **Local factors**

- *Atherosclerotic-related thrombosis* occurring at the level of the lamina cribrosa is by far the most common underlying cause of CRAO accounting for about 80% of cases.

- *Periarteritis* associated with a systemic disease such as dermatomyositis, systemic lupus erythematosus, polyarteritis nodosa, Wegener granulomatosis and Behçet disease may be occasionally responsible for BRAO which may be multiple (Figure 3.86).

- *Retinal migraine*, very rarely, may be responsible for retinal artery occlusion in young individuals. However, the diagnosis should be made only after other more common causes have been excluded.

2. **Cardiac emboli**

Embolism is responsible for about 20% of cases of retinal arterial occlusions and is associated with an increased risk of cerebrovascular disease. Because the ophthalmic artery is the first branch of the internal carotid artery, embolic material from either the heart or the carotid arteries has a fairly direct route to the eye. Emboli originating from the heart and its valves may be of the following four types:

- *Calcific* emboli from the aortic or mitral valves.

- *Heart valve vegetations* in patients suffering from bacterial endocarditis.

- *Thrombus* originating from the left side of the heart, as a consequence of myocardial infarction (mural thrombi), mitral stenosis associated with atrial fibrillation or mitral valve prolapse.

- *Myxomatous material* from the very rare atrial myxoma.

3. **Carotid emboli**

The bifurcation of the common carotid artery in the neck into external and internal carotid arteries is an extremely vulnerable site for atheromatous ulceration and stenosis. Retinal emboli from the carotid arteries may be of the following types:

- *Cholesterol* emboli (Hollenhorst plaques) appear as intermittent showers of minute, bright, refractile, golden to yellow-orange crystals, often at arteriolar bifurcations

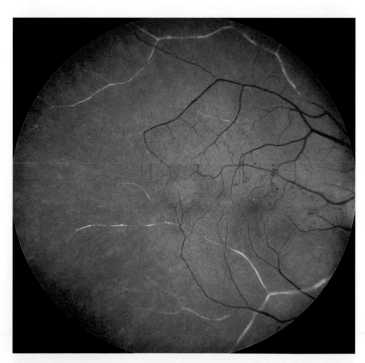

Figure 3.86 Multiple branch retinal artery occlusions associated with polyarteritis nodosa

(Figure 3.87). They rarely cause significant obstruction to the retinal arterioles and are frequently asymptomatic.

- *Fibrinoplatelet* emboli are dull grey, elongated particles which are usually multiple and occasionally fill the entire lumen (Figure 3.88). They may cause a retinal transient ischemic attack (TIA), which is referred to as amaurosis fugax, and occasionally complete obstruction. Amaurosis fugax is characterized by a painless unilateral loss of vision, often described by the patient as a curtain coming down over the eye, usually from top to bottom, but occasionally vice versa. The visual loss, which may be complete, usually lasts a few minutes. Recovery is in the same pattern as the initial loss, although it is usually more gradual. The frequency of attacks may vary from several times a day to one every few months. The attacks may be associated with ipsilateral cerebral TIA with contralateral signs.

- *Calcific* emboli may originate from atheromatous plaques in the ascending aorta or the carotid arteries, as well as from calcified heart valves. They are usually single, white, non-scintillating and often close to the disc (Figure 3.89). When located on the disc itself, they may be easily overlooked because they tend to merge with the disc. Calcific emboli are much more dangerous to the eye than the other two kinds because they may cause a permanent occlusion of the central retinal artery or one of its main branches.

4. **Thrombophilic disorders** such as hyperhomocysteinemia, antiphospholipid antibody syndrome and inherited defects of a natural anticoagulant may be occasionally associated with retinal artery obstruction in young individuals.

Branch retinal artery occlusion

Diagnosis

BRAO is most frequently caused by embolism and occasionally by periarteritis.

1. **Presentation** is with sudden and profound altitudinal or sectorial visual field defect.

2. **Signs**

- Visual acuity may be normal or variable reduced.

- Retinal pallor and opacification corresponding to the area of ischemia (Figure 3.90a).

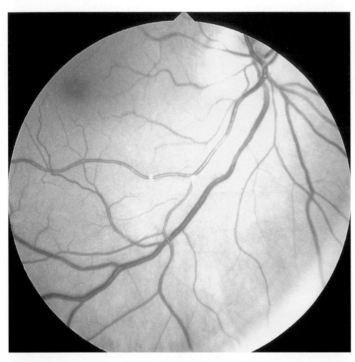

Figure 3.87 Cholesterol retinal emboli (Hollenhorst plaques)

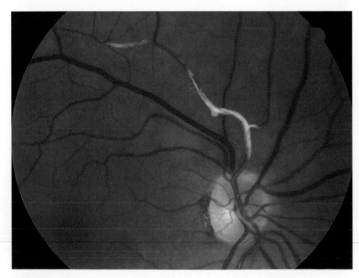

Figure 3.88 Arteriolar occlusion by fibrinoplatelet emboli

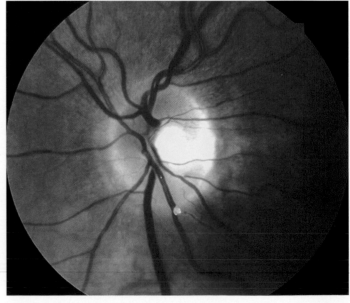

Figure 3.89 Calcific embolus at the inferior edge of the optic disc

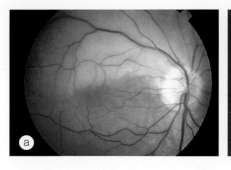

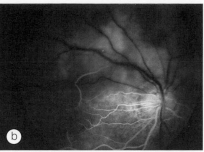

Figure 3.90 Supero-temporal BRAO (see the text)

- Narrowing of arteries and veins with sludging and segmentation of the blood column.

- One or more emboli may be present.

3. **FA** shows great delay in arterial filling and masking of background fluorescence by retinal swelling which is confined to the involved sector (Figure 3.90b).

Prognosis

Unless the obstruction can be relieved within a few hours, the visual field defect becomes permanent and the affected artery remains attenuated. Occasionally, however, recanalization of the obstructed artery may leave only subtle or absent ophthalmoscopic signs.

Central retinal artery occlusion

Diagnosis

Central retinal artery occlusion is most frequently the result of atherosclerosis, although it can also be caused by calcific emboli.

1. **Presentation** is with sudden and profound loss of vision.

2. **Signs**

- Visual acuity is usually reduced to hand movements or light perception. However, in about 20% of individuals, a portion of the papillomacular bundle is supplied by one or more cilioretinal arteries, and in these cases central vision may be preserved.

- Pupillary conduction defect is profound or total (amaurotic pupil).

- Attenuation of arteries and veins with sludging and segmentation of the blood column (Figure 3.91).

- Pallor and opacification, particularly at the posterior pole, resulting from neuronal intracellular swelling.

- The orange reflex from the intact choroidal vessels beneath the foveola stands out in contrast to the surrounding pale retina, giving rise to the 'cherry-red spot' appearance (Figure 3.92).

- In eyes with a cilioretinal artery part of the macula will remain of normal colour (Figure 3.93).

3. **FA** shows great delay in arterial filling and masking of background choroidal fluorescence by retinal swelling. However, a patent cilioretinal artery will fill during the early phase (Figure 3.94).

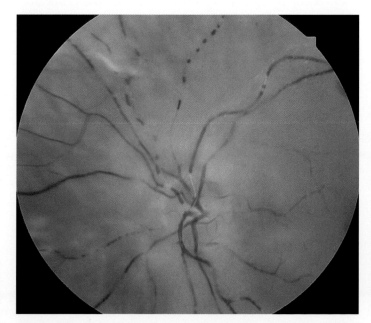

Figure 3.91 Acute CRAO showing vascular attenuation and segmentation of the blood column (cattle-trucking)

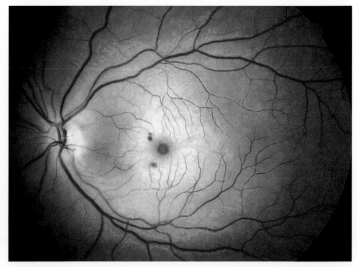

Figure 3.92 Acute CRAO showing pallor of the posterior pole with a cherry-red spot at the fovea

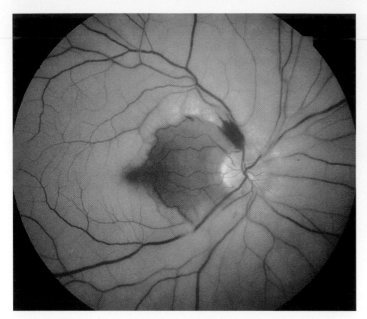

Figure 3.93 Acute CRAO with a patent cilioretinal artery

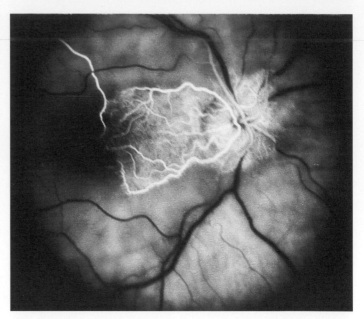

Figure 3.94 FA of a CRAO with a perfused cilioretinal artery

Prognosis

In the vast majority of cases the visual prognosis is extremely poor due to severe retinal ischemia. After a few weeks the retinal whitening and the 'cherry-red spot' disappear although the retinal arteries remain attenuated (Figure 3.95). The inner retinal layers become atrophic and consecutive optic atrophy ensues with permanent loss of all useful vision. Some eyes develop rubeosis iridis which may require laser panretinal photocoagulation, and about 2% develop NVD.

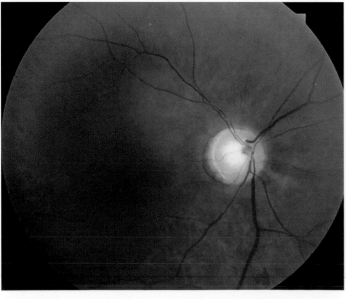

Figure 3.95 Old CRAO showing vascular attenuation and consecutive optic atrophy

Emergency treatment of acute retinal artery occlusion

Although uncommon, retinal artery occlusion is an ocular emergency because it causes irreversible visual loss unless the retinal circulation is re-established prior to the development of ischemic damage. It appears that the prognosis for occlusions caused by calcific emboli is worse than those resulting from either cholesterol or platelet emboli. Theoretically, timely dislodgement of the latter two types of emboli may prevent subsequent visual loss. To this end many mechanical and pharmacological methods have been tried. A recent report by Rumelt and associates suggested that the following aggressive systematic stepwise approach gives the greatest chance of success in patients with occlusions less than 48 hours at presentation.

1. **Initial treatment** is as follows:

   • Ocular massage using a three-mirror contact lens for approximately ten seconds, to obtain retinal artery pulsation or flow cessation, followed by five seconds of release. The aim is to mechanically collapse the arterial lumen and cause prompt changes in arterial flow.

   • During massage the patient is given sublingual isosorbide dinitrate 10 mg to dilate peripheral blood vessels and decrease resistance.

   • Lowering of intraocular pressure by giving a combination of intravenous acetazolamide 500 mg, followed by either intravenous mannitol 20% (1 mg/kg) or oral glycerol 50% (1 mg/kg).

2. **Subsequent treatment**, if the above measures are not successful in re-establishing the circulation after 20 minutes, is as follows:

- Anterior chamber paracentesis.

- Intravenous streptokinase 750,000 units to disintegrate fibrin emboli, combined with intravenous methylprednisolone 500 mg to decrease the risk of streptokinase-related allergy and bleeding.

- Retrobulbar injection of tolazoline 50 mg to decrease retrobulbar resistance to flow.

Cilioretinal artery occlusion

A cilioretinal artery, which is present in 20% of the population, perfuses the retina but is derived from the posterior ciliary circulation.

Diagnosis

1. **Presentation** is with acute onset of severe loss of central vision.

2. **Signs** – pallor and opacification localized to that part of the macula which is normally perfused by the vessel (Figure 3.96a).

3. **FA**

- The arteriovenous early phase shows a corresponding filling defect with masking of choroidal fluorescence (Figure 3.96b).

- The venous phase shows part filling (Figure 3.96c).

- The late phase shows nearly normal filling (Figure 3.96d).

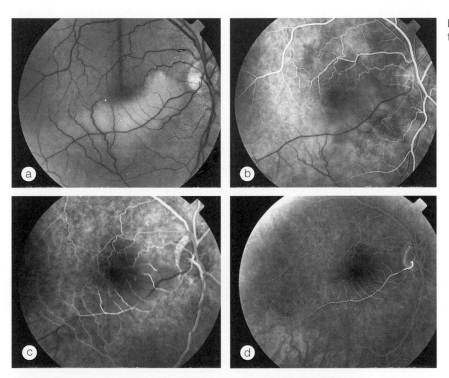

Figure 3.96 Cilioretinal artery occlusion(see the text)

Classification

Cilioretinal artery occlusion occurs in the following three settings:

1. **Isolated** which typically affects patients with an associated systemic vasculitis.

2. **Combined with CRVO** (Figure 3.97), which has a similar prognosis to non-ischemic CRVO.

3. **Combined with anterior ischemic optic neuropathy** (Figure 3.98), which typically affects patients with giant cell arteritis and carries a very poor prognosis.

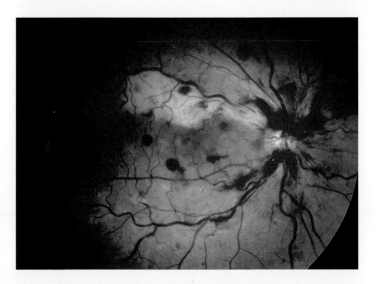

Figure 3.97 Cilioretinal artery occlusion combined with central retinal vein occlusion

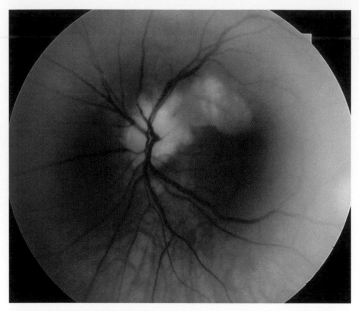

Figure 3.98 Cilioretinal artery occlusion combined with anterior ischemic optic neuropathy

FURTHER READING

Atebara NH, Brown GC, Cater J. Efficacy of anterior chamber paracentesis and carbogen in treating acute nonarteritic central retinal artery occlusion. *Ophthalmology* 1995;102:2029–2035.

Brown GC, Magargal LE, Shields JA, et al. Retinal artery obstruction in children and young adults. *Ophthalmology* 1981;88:18–25.

Dugan JD, Green WR. Ophthalmologic manifestations of carotid artery disease. *Eye* 1991;5:226–238.

Duker JS, Sivalingham A, Brown GC, et al. A prospective study of acute central retinal artery obstruction. *Arch Ophthalmol* 1991;109:339–342.

Glacet-Bernard A, Bayani N, Chretien P, et al. Antiphospholipid antibodies in retinal vascular occlusions. *Arch Ophthalmol* 1994;112:790–795.

Golub BM, Sibony PA, Collier BS, et al. Protein S deficiency associated with central retinal artery occlusion. *Arch Ophthalmol* 1990;108:918–919.

Graham EM. The investigation of patients with retinal vascular occlusion. *Eye* 1990;4:464–468.

Haase CG, Buchner T. Microemboli are not a prerequisite in retinal artery occlusive diseases. *Eye* 1998;12:659–662.

Klein R, Klein BEK, Jensen SC, et al. Retinal emboli and stroke. The Beaver Dam Study. *Arch Ophthalmol* 1999;117:1063–1068.

Mangat HS. Retinal artery occlusion. *Surv Ophthalmol* 1995;40:145–156.

Margo CE, Mack WP. Therapeutic decisions involving disparate clinical outcomes: patient preference survey for treatment of central retinal artery occlusion. *Ophthalmology* 1996;103:691–696.

Martin SC, Rauz S, Marr JE, et al. Plasma total homocysteine and retinal vascular disease. *Eye* 2000;14:590–593.

Sharma S, Brown GC, Pater JL, et al. Does visible retinal embolus increase the likelihood of hemodynamically significant carotid artery stenosis in patients with acute retinal artery occlusions? *Arch Ophthalmol* 1998;116:1602–1606.

Rumelt S, Doremboim Y, Rehany U. Aggressive treatment of central retinal artery occlusion. *Am J Ophthalmol* 1999;128:733–738.

Ocular ischemic syndrome

Pathogenesis

The ocular ischemic syndrome is an uncommon condition which is the result of chronic ocular hypoperfusion secondary to severe ipsilateral atherosclerotic carotid stenosis. It typically affects patients during the seventh decades of life and affects males more frequently than females by a 2:1 ratio. Important systemic associations include diabetes mellitus, hypertension, ischemic heart disease and cerebrovascular disease. The five-year mortality is in the order of 40%, most frequently from cardiac disease. Patients with the ocular ischemic syndrome may also give a history of amaurois fugax due to retinal embolism.

Diagnosis

The ocular ischemic syndrome is unilateral in 80% of cases and affects both anterior and posterior segments. The signs are variable and may be subtle so that the condition may be either missed or misdiagnosed.

1. **Presentation** is usually gradual loss of vision over several weeks or months although occasionally visual loss may be sudden.

2. **Anterior segment signs**

- Diffuse episcleral injection.

- Corneal edema and striae.

- Aqueous flare with few if any cells (ischemic pseudo-inflammatory iritis).

- Mid-dilated and poorly reacting pupil.

- Iris atrophy.

- Rubeosis iridis is common and in about 50% of cases results in the subsequent development of neovascular glaucoma.

- Cataract may be present in very advanced cases.

3. **Fundus signs** (Figure 3.99)

- Venous dilatation with or without mild tortuosity.

- Microaneurysms and dot and blot hemorrhages most frequently in the mid-periphery but may also involve the posterior pole.

- Retinal arteriolar narrowing and occasionally cotton-wool spots.

- Proliferative retinopathy with NVD and occasionally NVE is common.

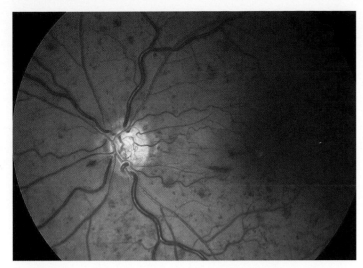

Figure 3.99 Ocular ischemic syndrome showing arteriolar attenuation, venous dilatation, hemorrhages and NVD

- Macular edema.

- Spontaneous arterial pulsation most pronounced near the optic disc is present in most cases or it may be easily induced by exerting gentle pressure on the globe (digital ophthalmodynamometry).

4. **FA** shows delayed and patchy choroidal filling, prolonged arteriovenous transit time, retinal capillary non-perfusion, late leakage and prominent arterial staining.

Management

1. **Anterior segment inflammation** is treated with topical steroids and mydriatics.

2. **Secondary glaucoma** may be treated initially with topical beta-adrenergic antagonists or alpha-adrenergic agonists and oral carbonic anhydrase inhibitors. Advanced cases may require filtration surgery or cyclodestructive procedures.

3. **Proliferative retinopathy** may be treated by laser panretinal photocoagulation although the results are less favorable than in proliferative diabetic retinopathy.

Differential diagnosis

1. **Non-ischemic CRVO**

- *Similarities* – unilateral retinal hemorrhages, venous dilatation and cotton-wool spots.

- *Differences* – normal retinal artery perfusion, veins may be tortuous, hemorrhages are usually more numerous and many are flame-shaped, disc edema is present.

2. **Diabetic retinopathy**

- *Similarities* – dot and blot retinal hemorrhages, venous tortuosity and proliferative retinopathy.

- *Differences* – bilateral and presence of hard exudates.

3. **Hypertensive retinopathy**

- *Similarities* – arteriolar attenuation and focal constriction, hemorrhages and cotton-wool spots.

- *Differences* – invariably bilateral and no venous changes.

Investigations of carotid disease

1. **Palpation** of the patient's cervical carotid arteries should be done gently to avoid dislodging a thrombus. A severe or complete stenosis will be associated with a diminished or absent ipsilateral carotid pulse. Other peripheral pulses may also be abnormal.

2. **Auscultation** over a partial stenosis will give rise to a bruit which is best detected with the bell of the stethoscope. It is important to auscultate along the entire length of the artery and to ask the patient to stop breathing. The most ominous bruit is one that is high-pitched and soft because it indicates a tight stenosis with a low flow of blood. When the lumen is completely obstructed or 90% narrowed, the bruit disappears.

3. **Duplex scanning** involves a combination of high-resolution real-time B-scan ultrasonography with Doppler flow analysis (Figure 3.100). The technique can detect both ulcerative and stenotic lesions and is currently the cheapest available non-invasive test.

4. **Digital intravenous subtraction angiography** involves injection of a contrast medium into the superior vena cava *via* a catheter introduced through the antecubital vein. Images of the carotid arteries are then produced by sophisticated computer-assisted subtraction techniques (Figure 3.101).

5. **Magnetic resonance angiography** is able to visualize the carotids (Figure 3.102) as well as ischemic cerebral lesions.

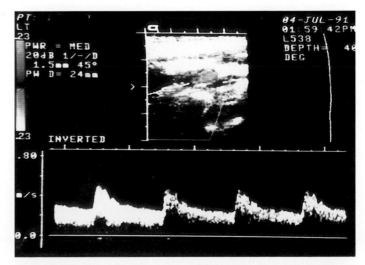

Figure 3.100 Color Doppler scan of the external carotid circulation showing an atheromatous plaque

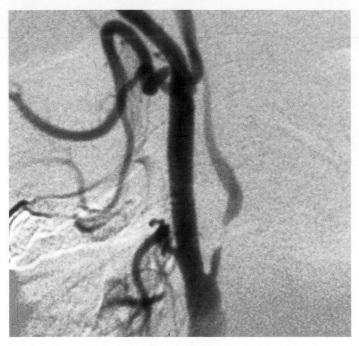

Figure 3.101 Digital subtraction angiogram showing very severe right carotid stenosis

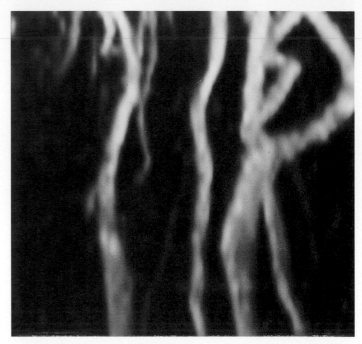

Figure 3.102 MRI angiogram showing severe right carotid stenosis

6. Intra-arterial angiography provides excellent visualization of the carotid system (Figure 3.103) but is associated with potential morbidity.

Management of carotid disease

The aims of management are to prevent stroke and permanent visual impairment. The two current modalities are medical therapy and carotid endarterectomy. The method chosen is dependent on the subsequent risk of stroke and the perioperative morbidity associated with surgical intervention.

1. General measures include screening for associated risk factors such as hypertension, diabetes, hypercholesterolemia, hypercoagulability states and smoking. Risk factors that are identified should be treated appropriately. A cardiological assessment may also be advisable.

2. Antiplatelet therapy with the following agents:

- Aspirin 75–300 mg daily.

- Aspirin combined with dipyridamole (Persantin) 200 mg twice daily if aspirin alone is ineffective.

- Clopidorel (Plavix) 75 mg daily if other measures are inappropriate.

3. Anticoagulants should be considered if antiplatelet therapy is ineffective.

4. Carotid endarterectomy should be considered only in patients who have other risk factors for stroke and symptomatic carotid stenosis greater than 70%.

FURTHER READING

Brown GC, Magargal LE. The ocular ischemic syndrome: clinical, fluorescein angiographic and carotid angiographic features. *Int Ophthalmol* 1988;11:239–251.

Costa VP, Kuzniec S, Molnar LJ, et al. Clinical findings and hemodynamic changes associated with severe occlusive carotid artery disease. *Ophthalmology* 1997;104:1994–2002.

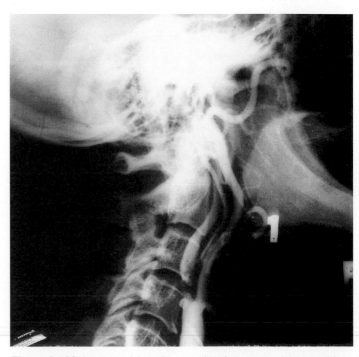

Figure 3.103 Intra-arterial angiogram showing severe right carotid stenosis

Ho AC, Lieb WE, Flaharty PM, et al. Color Doppler imaging of the ocular ischemic syndrome. *Ophthalmology* 1992;99:1453–1462.

Malhotra R, Gregory-Evans K. Management of ocular ischaemic syndrome. Perspectives. *Br J Ophthalmol* 2000;84:1428–1431.

Mizener JB, Podhajsky P, Hayreh SS. Ocular ischaemic syndrome. *Ophthalmology* 1997;104:859–864.

Sivalingham A, Brown GC, Magargal LE, et al. The ocular ischemic syndrome. II. Mortality and systemic morbidity. *Int Ophthalmol* 1990;13:187–191.

Sturrock GD, Mueller HR. Chronic ocular ischaemia. *Br J Ophthalmol* 1984;68:716–723.

Hypertensive retinopathy

Hypertension

Hypertension is a very common condition which, by strict definition, is defined by blood pressure readings on several consecutive occasions of 140/90 or over. In most patients the condition is idiopathic (essential), although it may occasionally be secondary to a renal or metabolic disorder. Presentation is usually in adult life. In the absence of complications, hypertension is asymptomatic. Complications include left ventricular hypertrophy, heart failure, increased risk of atherosclerosis which may result in coronary artery and cerebrovascular disease, and renal disease.

Signs of hypertensive retinopathy

The primary response of the retinal arterioles to systemic hypertension is narrowing. However, the degree of narrowing is dependent on the amount of pre-existing replacement fibrosis (involutional sclerosis). For this reason, hypertensive narrowing is seen in its pure form only in young individuals. In older patients, the rigidity of retinal arterioles caused by involutional sclerosis prevents the same degree of narrowing that is seen in young individuals. In sustained hypertension the blood-retinal barrier is disrupted in small areas, resulting in increased vascular permeability. The fundus picture of hypertensive retinopathy is characterized by the following:

1. **Vasoconstriction** which may be generalized (Figure 3.104) or focal (Figure 3.105). Unfortunately, the ophthalmoscopic diagnosis of generalized narrowing may be difficult, although the presence of focal narrowing makes it highly probable that the blood pressure is raised. Severe hypertension may lead to obstruction of the precapillary arterioles and the development of cotton-wool spots (Figure 3.106).

2. **Leakage**, which is caused by abnormal vascular permeability, leads to the development of flame-shaped retinal hemorrhages and retinal edema (Figure 3.107). Chronic retinal edema may result in the deposition of hard exudates around the fovea in Henle layer and may lead to a macular star configuration (Figure 3.108). Swelling of the optic nerve head is the hallmark of the malignant phase of hypertension (Figure 3.109).

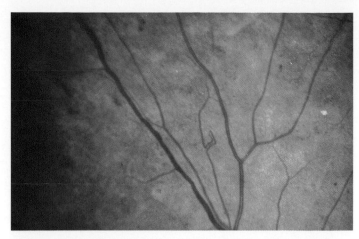

Figure 3.104 Generalized arteriolar attenuation in hypertension

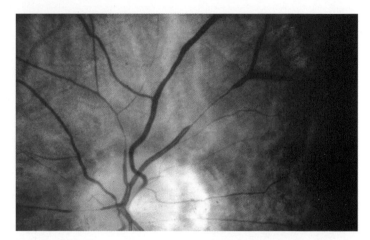

Figure 3.105 Focal arteriolar attenuation in hypertension

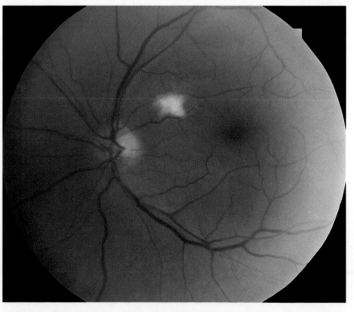

Figure 3.106 Hypertensive retinopathy with one cotton-wool spot

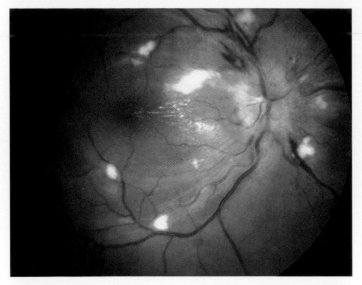

Figure 3.107 Severe hypertensive retinopathy showing cotton-wool spots, flame-shaped hemorrhages, early macular star formation and mild disc swelling

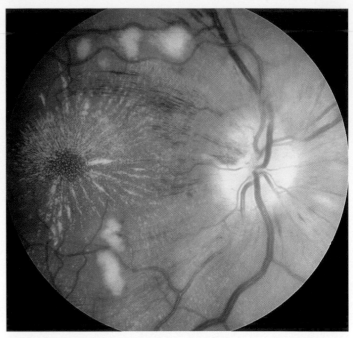

Figure 3.108 Severe hypertensive retinopathy showing a fully-developed macular star, cotton-wool spots, a few flame-shaped hemorrhages and moderate disc swelling

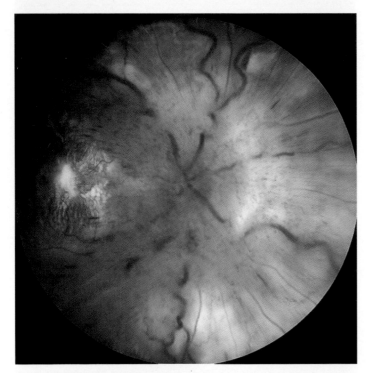

Figure 3.109 Very severe hypertensive retinopathy showing a macular star and very severe disc swelling

with involutional sclerosis in the absence of hypertension. The grading of arteriolosclerosis is shown in Figure 3.112.

4. **Choroidopathy** is rarely of clinical importance and is usually more apparent on FA.

- *Elschnig spots* are small, black spots surrounded by yellow halos which represent focal infarcts (Figure 3.110).

3. **Arteriolosclerosis** is a thickening of the vessel wall, which consists histologically of intimal hyalinization, medial hypertrophy and endothelial hyperplasia. The single most important clinical sign is the presence of changes at arteriovenous crossings (AV nipping). Although this feature alone is not necessarily an indication of the severity of hypertension, its presence makes it probable that hypertension has been present for many years. It is also important to point out that mild changes at arteriovenous crossings are seen in patients

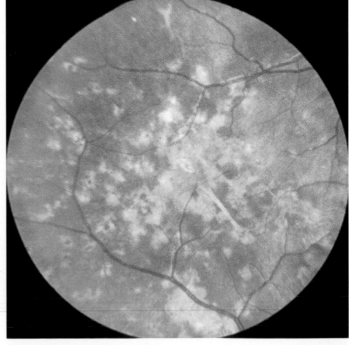

Figure 3.110 Elschnig spots in hypertension

- *Siegrist streaks* are flecks arranged linearly along choroidal vessels (Figure 3.111).

- *Exudative retinal detachment*, which may be bilateral, may occur in patients with severe acute hypertension such as that associated with toxemia of pregnancy.

Grading of arteriolosclerosis

The grading of arteriolosclerosis according to severity is listed below (Figure 3.112).

1. **Grade 1** is characterized by slight broadening of the arteriolar light reflex, mild generalized arteriolar attenuation, particularly of small branches, and vein concealment.

2. **Grade 2** is characterized by obvious broading of the arteriolar light reflex and deflection of veins at arteriovenous crossings (Salus' sign).

3. **Grade 3** is characterized by copper-wiring of arterioles, banking of veins distal to arteriovenous crossings (Bonnet sign), tapering of veins on either side of the crossings (Gunn sign) and right-angled deflection of veins.

4. **Grade 4** is characterized by grade 3 changes and silver-wiring of arterioles.

Ocular associations of hypertension

Patients with hypertension are at increased risk from the following conditions:

- Branch retinal vein occlusion.

- Retinal artery occlusion.

- Retinal artery macroaneurysm.

- Anterior ischemic optic neuropathy.

- Ocular motor nerve palsy.

- Uncontrolled hypertension may adversely effect diabetic retinopathy.

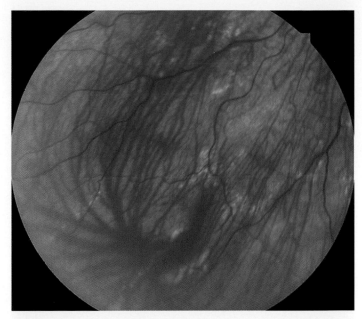

Figure 3.111 Siegrist streaks in hypertension

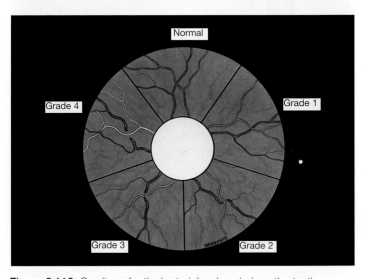

Figure 3.112 Grading of retinal arteriolosclerosis (see the text)

FURTHER READING

Hayreh SS. Classification of hypertensive fundus changes and their order of appearance. *Ophthalmologica* 1989;198:247–260.

Hayreh SS, Servais GE, Virdi PS, et al. Fundus lesions in malignant hypertension. III. Arterial blood pressure, biochemical, and fundus changes. *Ophthalmology* 1986;93:45–59.

Jaffe G, Schatz H. Ocular manifestations of preeclampsia. *Am J Ophthalmol* 1987;103:309–315.

Klein R, Klein BE, Moss SE, et al. Hypertension and retinopathy, arteriolar narrowing, and arteriovenous nicking in a population. *Arch Ophthalmol* 1994;112:92–98.

Scheie HG. Evaluation of ophthalmoscopic changes of hypertension and arteriolar sclerosis. *Arch Ophthalmol* 1953;49:117–138.

Schmidt D, Loffler KU. Elschnig's spots as a sign of severe hypertension. *Ophthalmologica* 1993;206:24–28.

Tso MOM, Jampol LM. Pathophysiology of hyptenive retinopathy. *Ophthalmology* 1982;89:1132–1145.

Walsh JB. Hypertensive retinopathy. Description, classification, and prognosis. *Ophthalmology* 1982;89:1127–1131.

Sickle-cell retinopathy

Introduction

Sickling hemoglobinopathies are caused by one, or a combination, of abnormal hemoglobins which cause the red blood cell to adopt an anomalous shape under conditions of hypoxia and acidosis. As these deformed red blood cells are more rigid than healthy cells, they may become impacted in and obstruct small blood vessels, causing tissue ischemia with a marked local increase in acidosis and hypoxia, and even more sickling. The sickling disorders in which the mutant hemoglobins S and C are inherited as alleles of normal hemoglobin

A have important ocular manifestations. These abnormal hemoglobins may occur in combination with normal hemoglobin A or in association with each other as indicated below:

1. **AS** (sickle-cell trait), which is present in 8% of African-Americans. It is the mildest form and usually requires severe hypoxia or other abnormal conditions to produce sickling.

2. **SS** (sickle-cell disease, sickle-cell anemia), which is present in 0.2% of African-Americans. It causes severe systemic complications, such as painful crises and severe hemolytic anemia. Ocular complications are usually mild and asymptomatic.

3. **SC** (sickle-cell C disease), which is present in 0.4% of African-Americans.

4. **SThal** (sickle-cell thalassemia): both SC and SThal are associated with mild anemia but severe ocular manifestations.

Proliferative retinopathy

Although the most severe forms of retinopathy are associated with SC and SThal diseases, the milder hemoglobinopathies may occasionally also cause retinopathy.

1. **Staging** (Figure 3.113)

- *Stage 1* – peripheral arteriolar occlusion.

- *Stage 2* – peripheral arteriovenous anastomoses which appear to be dilated pre-existent capillary channels. The peripheral retina after the point of vascular occlusion is largely avascular and non-perfused.

- *Stage 3* – sprouting of new vessels from the anastomoses. Initially, the new vessels lie flat on the retina and have a 'sea-fan' configuration and are usually fed by a single arteriole and drained by a single vein (Figure 3.114a). Between 40–50% of 'sea-fans' spontaneously involute as

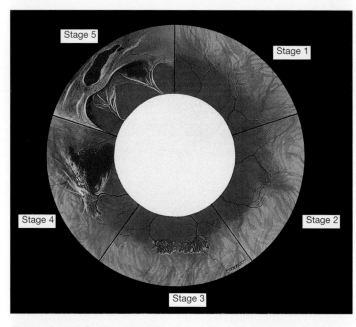

Figure 3.113 Grading of proliferative sickle-cell retinopathy (see the text)

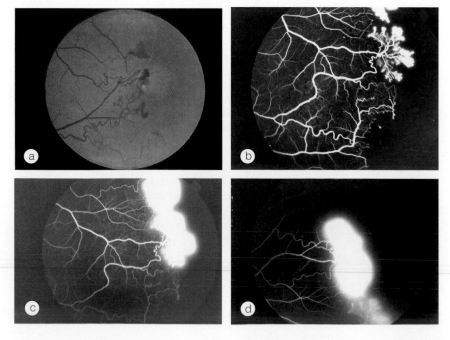

Figure 3.114 Proliferative sickle-cell retinopathy (see the text)

a result of autoinfarction and appear as grayish fibrovascular lesions (Figure 3.115). In other cases the neovascular tufts continue to proliferate, become adherent to the cortical vitreous gel and may bleed as a result of vitreoretinal traction (Figure 3.116).

- *Stage 4* is characterized by varying amounts of vitreous hemorrhage which may be precipitated by relatively trivial ocular trauma.

- *Stage 5* is characterized by extensive fibrovascular proliferation (Figure 3.117) and tractional retinal detachment. Rhegmatogenous retinal detachment may also occur as a result of tear formation adjacent to areas of fibrovascular tissue (Figure 3.118).

2. **FA** shows extensive peripheral capillary non-perfusion (see Figure 3.114b) and massive leakage of dye from sites of neovascularization (see Figure 3.114c and 3.114d).

3. **Treatment** by peripheral retinal scatter photocoagulation to areas of capillary non-perfusion may be required to induce regression in patients with recurrent vitreous haemorrhages. However, unlike DR, the new vessels in sickle cell disease tend to involute spontaneously (autoinfarction) and usually do not require treatment. Pars plana vitrectomy for tractional retinal detachment and/or persistent vitreous hemorrhage usually gives poor results.

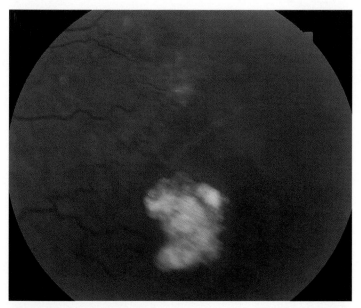

Figure 3.115 Localized fibrovascular lesion in proliferative sickle-cell retinopathy

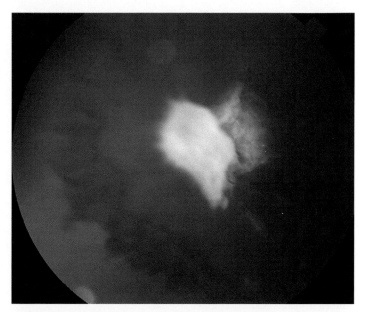

Figure 3.116 Bleeding in proliferative sickle-cell retinopathy

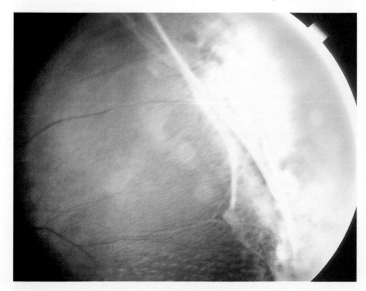

Figure 3.117 Extensive fibrovascular proliferation in sickle-cell retinopathy

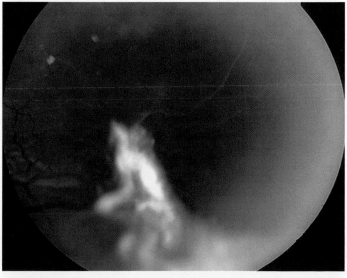

Figure 3.118 Severe fibrovascular proliferation in sickle-cell retinopathy with an adjacent retinal hole which has resulted in retinal detachment

Non-proliferative retinopathy

1. Asymptomatic lesions

- Venous tortuosity is one of the first ophthalmic signs of sickling and is due to peripheral arteriovenous shunts (Figure 3.119).

- 'Silver-wiring' of arterioles in the peripheral retina, which represent previously occluded arterioles.

- 'Salmon patches' are pink, preretinal or superficial intraretinal hemorrhages at the equator which are adjacent to an arteriole (Figure 3.120) which usually resolve without sequelae.

- 'Black sunbursts' are patches of peripheral RPE hyperplasia (Figure 3.121).

- 'Macular depression sign' is an oval depression of the bright central macular reflex due to atrophy and thinning of the sensory retina.

- Peripheral retinal holes and areas of whitening similar to 'white-without-pressure' is an occasional feature (Figure 3.122).

2. Symptomatic lesions

- Chronic macular arteriolar occlusion occurs in about 30% of patients.

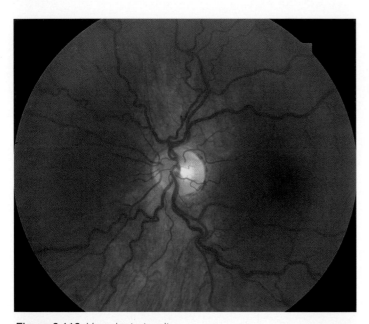

Figure 3.119 Vascular tortuosity

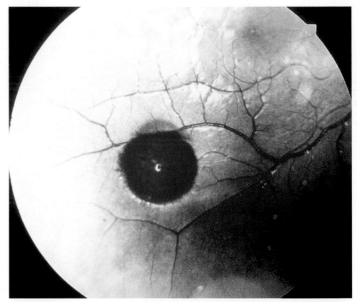

Figure 3.120 Preretinal hemorrhage (salmon patch) in sickle-cell retinopathy

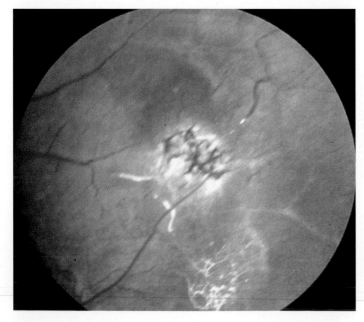

Figure 3.121 Peripheral RPE hyperplasia (black sunburst) in sickle-cell retinopathy

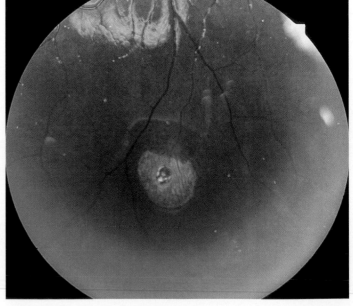

Figure 3.122 Peripheral retinal hole and an area of whitening superiorly in sickle-cell retinopathy

- Acute central retinal artery occlusion is rare.

- Retinal vein occlusion, which may result from hyperviscosity, is uncommon.

- Choroidal vascular occlusion may be seen occasionally, particularly in children.

- Angioid streaks occur in a small minority of patients.

Non-retinal features

1. **Conjunctival lesions** are characterized by isolated dark red vascular anomalies shaped like commas or corkscrews. They involve the small caliber vessels and are most often located inferiorly.

2. **Iris lesions** consist of circumscribed areas of ischemic atrophy, usually at the pupillary edge and extending to the collarette. Rubeosis may be seen occasionally.

FURTHER READING

Condon PI, Serjeant GR. Behaviour of untreated proliferative sickle retinopathy. *Br J Ophthalmol* 1980;64:404–411.

Fox PD, Minninger K, Forshaw ML, et al. Laser photocoagulation for proliferative retinopathy in sickle hemoglobin C disease. *Eye* 1993;7:703–706.

Goldberg MF. Classification and pathogenesis of proliferative sickle retinopathy. *Am J Ophthalmol* 1971;71:649–665.

Jacobson MS, Gargliano DA, Cohen SB, et al. A randomized clinical trial of feeder vessel photocoagulation of sickle cell retinopathy. *Ophthalmology* 1991;98:581–585.

Pulido JS, Flynn HW, Clarkson JG, et al. Pars plana vitrectomy in the management of complications of proliferative sickle retinopathy. *Arch Ophthalmol* 1988;106:1553–1557.

Sanders RJ, Brown GC, Rosenstein RB, et al. Foveal avascular diameter and sickle cell disease. *Arch Ophthalmol* 1991;109:812–815.

van Meurs JC. Evolution of a retinal hemorrhage in patient with sickle cell-hemoglobin C disease. *Arch Ophthalmol* 1995;113:1074–1075.

Retinal artery macroaneurysm

Diagnosis

A retinal artery macroaneurysm is a localized dilatation of a retinal arteriole which usually occurs in the first three orders of the arterial tree. It has a predilection for elderly hypertensive women and involves one eye in 90% of cases.

1. **Presentation** may be in one of the following ways:

- Some patients may have no symptoms and the condition is detected by chance.

- Insidious impairment of central vision due to macular edema and hard exudate formation.

- Sudden visual loss resulting from vitreous hemorrhage is uncommon.

2. **Signs**

- Saccular or fusiform dilatation of the arterial wall, which in some cases may be enlarged several times the size of the artery, most frequently at bifurcations or arteriovenous crossings of a branch of the superior or inferior temporal arterioles (Figures 3.123a).

Figure 3.123 Retinal artery macroaneurysm (see the text)

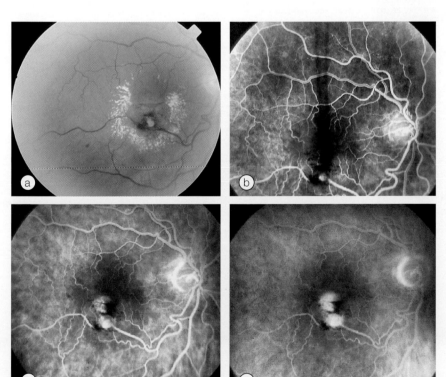

123

- Associated retinal hemorrhage is present in 50% of cases.

- Multiple macroaneurysms along the same or different arteriole are present in 20% of cases.

3. **FA** findings are dependent on the patency of the lesion and the presence or absence of associated hemorrhage. The typical appearance is that of immediate uniform filling of the macroaneurysm (Figure 3.123b) with late leakage (Figure 3.123c and 3.123d). Incomplete filling is the result of partial or complete obliteration of the lumen by thrombosis.

Prognosis

1. **Spontaneous involution** following thrombosis and fibrosis is very common. This may occur either prior to, or after the development of leakage or hemorrhage (Figure 3.124).

2. **Chronic leakage** resulting in edema which may give rise to accumulation of hard exudates at the fovea is common (see Figure 3.126a) and may result in permanent loss of central vision.

3. **Rupture** resulting in bleeding, which may be vitreous, preretinal, intraretinal or subretinal is less common. In these cases the underlying lesion may be overlooked and the diagnosis missed (Figure 3.125).

Management

1. **Observation** is indicated in the following situations:

- Eyes with good visual acuity in which the macula is not threatened should be observed in anticipation of spontaneous involution.

- Eyes with retinal hemorrhage without significant edema or exudation.

2. **Argon laser photocoagulation** should be considered if edema or hard exudates threaten or involve the fovea (Figure 3.126a), particularly if there is documented visual deterioration. The burns may be applied to the lesion itself, the surrounding area, or both (Figure 3.126b). It may take several months for the edema and hard exudates to absorb.

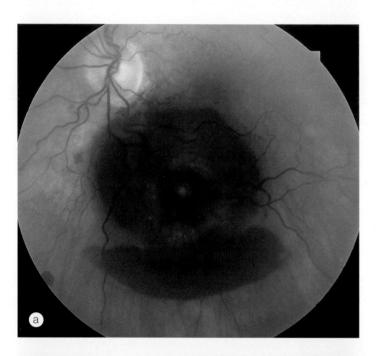

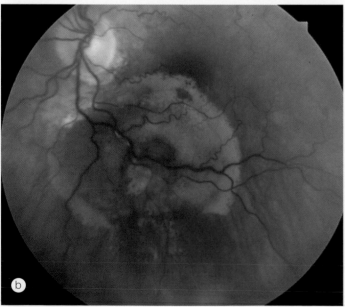

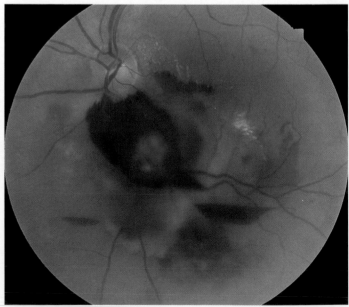

Figure 3.124 (a) Retinal artery macroaneurysms associated with a large subretinal haemorrhage; (b) following spontaneous absorption of blood

Figure 3.125 Retinal artery macroaneurysm resulting in retinal, preretinal and vitreous hemorrhage

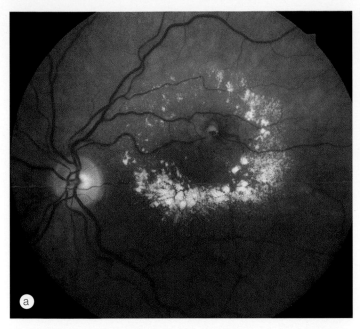

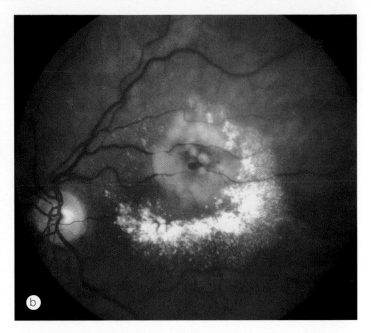

Figure 3.126 (a) Chronic leakage from a retinal artery macroaneurysm resulting in hard exudate formation involving the fovea; (b) immediately following laser photocoagulation

3. **YAG-laser photodestruction** may be considered in eyes with large non-absorbing preretinal hemorrahages overlying the macula (Figure 3.127) in order to disperse the blood into the vitreous cavity from where it may be absorbed more quickly.

Differential diagnosis

Retinal artery macroaneurysm should be considered in the differential diagnosis of the following conditions.

1. **Hard exudates at the posterior pole**

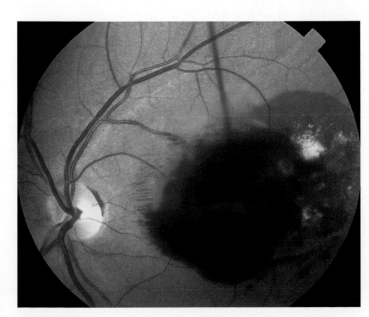

Figure 3.127 Large preretinal hemorrhage arising from a retinal artery macroaneurysm

- Background diabetic retinopathy.
- Exudative age-related macular degeneration.
- Old retinal branch vein occlusion.
- Retinal telangiectasia.
- Small retinal capillary hemangioma.
- Radiation retinopathy.

2. **Deep retinal or subretinal hemorrhages at the posterior pole**

- Choroidal neovascularization.
- Valsalva retinopathy which follows a sudden strain or cough.
- Idiopathic polypoidal choroidal vasculopathy.
- Blunt ocular trauma.
- Choroidal melanomas.
- Terson syndrome is characterized by a preretinal hemorrhage which typically occurs in association with a subarachnoid hemorrhage.

FURTHER READING

Abdel-Khalek MN, Richardson J. Retinal macroaneurysms: natural history and guidelines for treatment. *Br J Ophthalmol* 1986;70:2–11.

Brown DM, Sobol WM, Folk JC et al. Retinal arteriolar macroaneurysms: long-term visual outcome. *Br J Ophthalmol* 1994;78:534–538.

Homayun M, Lewis H, Flynn HW Jr, et al. Management of submacular hemorrhage associated with retinal artery macroaneurysm. *Am J Ophthalmol* 1998;126:358–361.

Iijima H, Satoh S, Tsukahara S. Nd:YAG laser photodisruption of preretinal hemorrhage due to retinal macroaneurysm. *Retina* 1998;18:430–434.

Lavin MJ, Marsh RJ, Peart S, et al. Retinal artery macroaneurysms. A retrospective study of 40 patients. *Br J Ophthalmol* 1987;71:817–825.

McCabe CM, Flynn HW Jr, McLean WC, et al. Nonsurgical management of macular hemorrhage secondary to retinal artery macroaneurysms. *Arch Ophthalmol* 2000;118:78–85.

Panton RW, Goldberg MF, Faber MD. Retinal artery macroaneurysms; risk factors and natural history. *Br J Ophthalmol* 1990;74:595–600.

Rabb MF, Gagliano DA, Teske MP. Retinal artery macroaneurysms. *Surv Ophthalmol* 1988;33:73–96.

Primary retinal telangiectasias

The primary retinal telangiectasias are a group of rare, idiopathic, congenital or acquired, retinal vascular anomalies characterized by dilatation and tortuosity of retinal vessels, formation of multiple aneurysms, varying degrees of leakage and deposition of lipid exudates. Retinal telangiectasias always involves the capillary bed, although arterioles and venules may also be affected. The vascular malformations frequently progress and may become symptomatic later in life as a result of hemorrhage, edema or lipid exudation. Because the condition is not associated with any other systemic or ocular disease, it should be distinguished from secondary telangiectasias. According to severity primary retinal telangiectasias can be divided into three main types: (a) *idiopathic juxtafoveolar retinal telangiectasia*, (b) *Leber miliary aneurysms* and (c) *Coats disease*. Some authorities consider Leber miliary aneurysms to be a localized and milder form of Coats disease.

Idiopathic juxtafoveolar retinal telangiectasia

Idiopathic juxtafoveolar telangiectasia is a rare, congenital or acquired, condition which can be divided into the following types.

1. **Group 1A – unilateral parafoveal telangiectasia** typically affects men during the fifth decade of life.

- *Presentation* is with mild to moderate blurring of vision.

- *Signs* – telangiectasia, 1.5–2 discs in diameter, located temporal to the fovea and frequently associated with hard exudates (Figure 3.128a). Figure 3.128d shows the leakage and hard exudate deposition within the middle retinal layers.

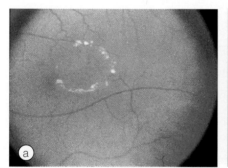
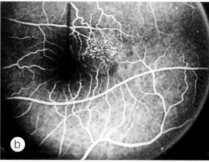
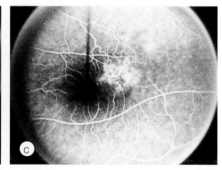

Figure 3.128 Idiopathic juxtafoveolar retinal telangiectasia – group 1A (see the text)

- *FA* – shows capillary dilatation (Figure 3.128b), and the late phase shows leakage (Figure 3.128c)

- *Prognosis* is guarded although laser photocoagulation to areas of leakage may be beneficial in preventing visual loss.

2. **Group 1B – unilateral parafoveal telangiectasia** typically affects men during the sixth decade of life.

- *Presentation* is with mild blurring of vision.

- *Signs* – telangiectasia confined to one clock hour at the edge of FAZ (Figure 3.129a). Figure 3.129d shows the telangiectatic capillaries within the middle retinal layers.

- *FA* shows focal capillary telangiectasia (Figure 3.129b) and absence of leakage (Figure 3.129c).

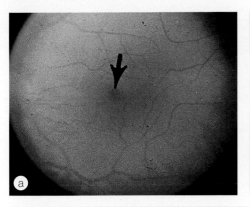
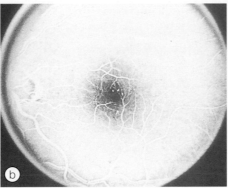
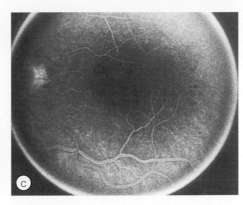

Figure 3.129 Idiopathic juxtafoveolar retinal telangiectasia – group 1B (see the text)

photocoagulation may be of benefit in patients with CNV but not otherwise.

4. **Group 3 – bilateral perifoveal telangiectsia and capillary occlusion** is the most severe type and typically affects patients during the sixth decade of life.

- *Presentation* is with slowly-progressive loss of central vision.

- *Signs* – marked aneurysmal dilatation of terminal capillaries and progressive occlusion of parafoveal capillaries. Optic atrophy may also be present.

- *FA* shows widening of FAZ but absence of leakage.

- *Prognosis* is usually poor.

- *Prognosis* is good and laser photocoagulation is not appropriate.

3. **Group 2 – bilateral parafoveolar telangiectasia** typically affects patients during the fifth and sixth decades of life.

- *Presentation* is with mild, slowly progressive disturbance of central vision.

- *Signs* – symmetrical telangiectasia, one disc or less in diameter, involving all or a part of the parafoveolar retina without hard exudates (Figure 3.130a and 3.130b) but frequently associated with stellate plaques of RPE hyperplasia. Occasional associations include many glistening white juxtafoveolar dots and solitary small yellow central deposits.

- *FA* shows dilated capillaries outside the FAZ (Figure 3.130b) and late leakage (Figure 3.130d).

- *Prognosis* is guarded because of the development of secondary foveal atrophy and occasionally CNV. Laser

Leber miliary aneurysms

1. **Presentation** is in adult life with unilateral impairment of central vision.

2. **Signs**

- Fusiform and saccular dilatation of venules and arterioles, most commonly involving the temporal retinal periphery (Figure 3.131 and see Figure 3.133a).

- Chronic leakage results in intraretinal hard exudate formation which may involve the macula (Figure 3.132).

3. **FA** during the early phase highlights the vascular anomalies and shows areas of retinal non-perfusion (Figure 3.133b and 1.133c). The late phase shows leakage (Figure 3.133d).

4. **Prognosis** is variable and is dependent on the extent of fovea involvement by hard exudates at the time of diagnosis.

5. **Treatment**, to ablate the vascular anomalies by photocoagulation may be beneficial if applied early.

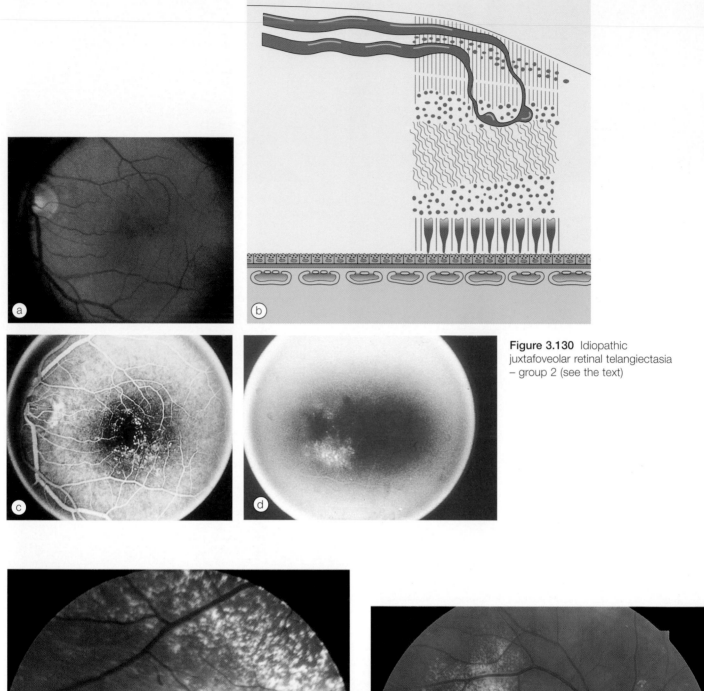

Figure 3.130 Idiopathic juxtafoveolar retinal telangiectasia – group 2 (see the text)

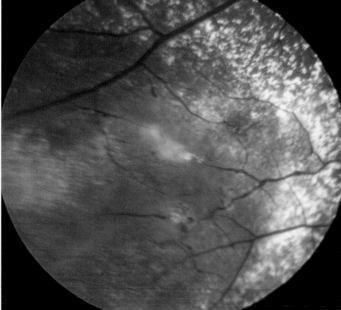

Figure 3.131 Peripheral lesions in Leber miliary aneurysms

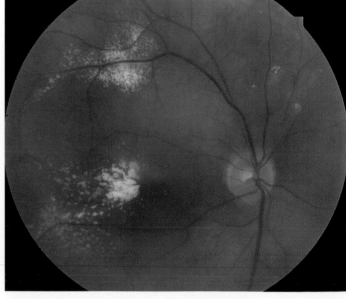

Figure 3.132 Hard exudates in Leber miliary aneurysms

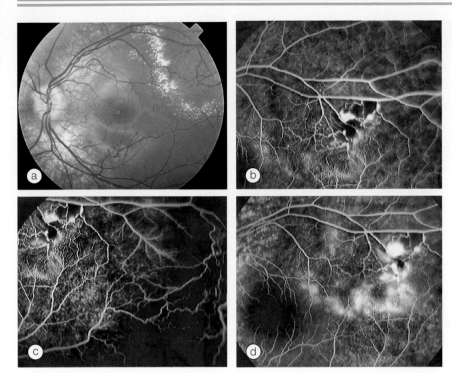

Figure 3.133 Leber miliary aneurysms (see the text)

Coats disease

Coats disease is the most severe form of retinal telangiectasia. It is invariably unilateral and more common in boys than girls.

1. **Presentation** is typically in the first decade of life (average age eight years) with visual loss, strabismus or a white fundus reflex (leukocoria) (Figure 3.134). In the differential diagnosis it is important to exclude retinoblastoma although this usually presents earlier.

2. **Signs** in chronological order:

- Areas of intraretinal and subretinal yellowish exudation associated with overlying dilated and tortuous retinal blood vessels (Figure 3.135).

- Increasing subretinal exudation (Figures 3.136, 3.137 and 3.138a).

- Exudative retinal detachment and a retrolental mass which gives rise to leukocoria.

3. **FA** highlights the underlying vascular malformations consisting of tortuosity, telangiectasia, aneurysm formation, non-perfusion and anomalous vascular communications with variable blockage by hard exudation (Figure 3.138b–3.138d).

4. **Prognosis** is frequently poor once the retina has detached due to the subsequent development of cataract, uveitis, neovascular glaucoma and phthisis bulbi.

5. **Treatment** with photocoagulation or cryotherapy, if applied early, may prevent progression and occasionally improve vision.

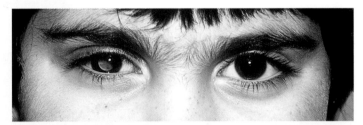

Figure 3.134 White pupil (leukocoria) in advanced Coats disease

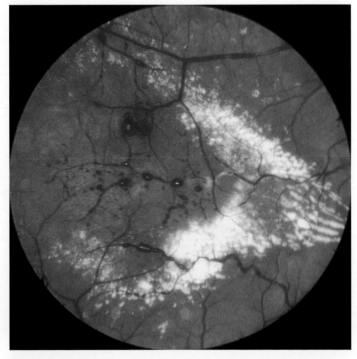

Figure 3.135 Early Coats disease showing vascular changes and retinal exudates

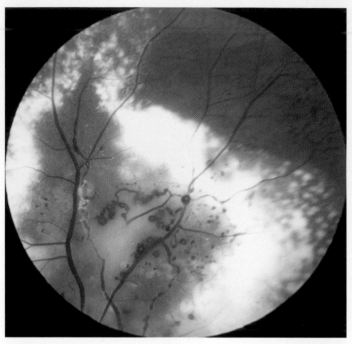

Figure 3.136 More extensive involvement in Coats disease

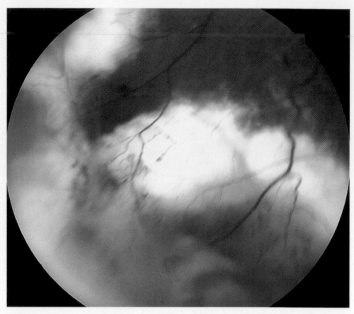

Figure 3.137 Very extensive hard exudate formation and early exudative retinal detachment in Coats disease

Figure 3.138 Coats disease (see the text)

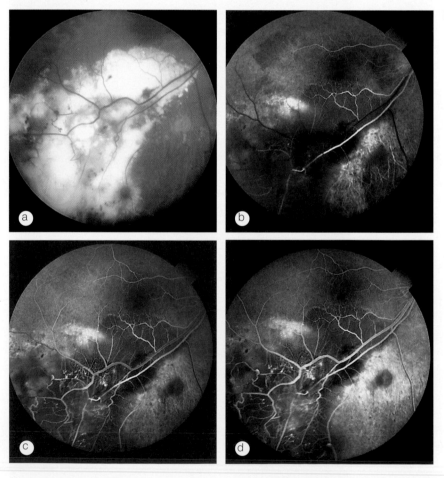

6. Differential diagnosis includes other causes of unilateral leukocoria and retinal detachment in children such as: late-onset retinoblastoma, toxocariasia, incontinentia pigmenti and retinal capillary hemangioma.

FURTHER READING

Egerer I, Tasman W, Tomer TL. Coats disease. *Arch Ophthalmol* 1974;92:109–112.

Gass JDW, Oyakawa RT. Idiopathic juxtafoveal retinal telangiectasis. *Arch Ophthalmol* 1982;100:769–780.

Morales AG. Coats' disease. Natural history and results of treatment. *Am J Ophthalmol* 1965;60:855–865.

Ridley ME, Shields JA, Brown GC, et al. Coats' disease. Evaluation of management. *Ophthalmology* 1982;89:1381–1387.

Shields JA, Shields CL, Honovar SG, et al. Classification and management of Coats disease: The 2000 Proctor Lecture. *Am J Ophthalmol* 2001; 131:572–583.

Siliodor SW, Augsburger JJ, Shields JA, et al. Natural history and management of advanced Coats' disease. *Ophthalmol Surg* 1988;19:89–93.

Tarkkanen A, Laatikainen L. Coats' disease: clinical angiographic, histopathological findings and clinical management. *Br J Ophthalmol* 1983;67:766–776.

Radiation retinopathy

Radiation retinopathy may develop following treatment of intraocular tumours by plaque therapy (brachytherapy) or external beam radiation of sinus, orbital or nasopharyngeal malignancies.

1. Presentation The time interval is highly variable and unpredictable. The most usual latent interval is between 6 months and 3 years.

2. Signs in order of severity are as follows:

- Discrete foci of capillary occlusion with irregular dilatation of capillary collateral channels and microaneurysms best seen on FA (Figure 3.139).

- Macular edema, hard exudates and flame-shaped retinal hemorrhages (see Figure 3.143a).

- Severe retinal telangiectasia with increase in hard exudate formation (Figure 3.140).

- Ischemic retinal necrosis characterized by widespread arteriolar occlusion, cotton-wool spots, and superficial and deep retinal haemorrhages, involving both central and peripheral retina.

3. FA is useful in showing the early microvascular changes, extent of capillary non-perfusion and leakage (see Figure 3.143b and 3.143c).

4. Prognosis depends on the severity of involvement. Poor prognostic features are the presence of papillopathy and proliferative retinopathy which may result in vitreous hemorrhage and tractional retinal detachment.

5. Treatment by laser photocoagulation may be beneficial for macular edema and proliferative retinopathy. Papillopathy is treated with systemic steroids.

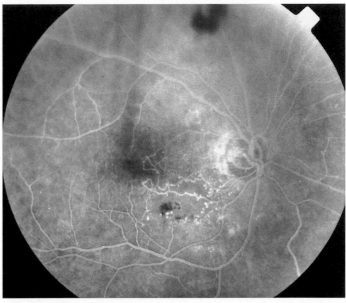

Figure 3.139 FA of early radiation retinopathy showing an area of retinal capillary non-perfusion associated with microvascular changes

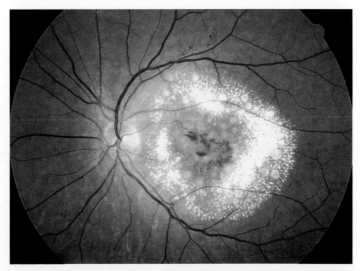

Figure 3.140 Severe radiation retinopathy with hard exudates involving the macula

Case study

1. History
A 61-year-old woman presented with a three week history of photopsia involving the right visual field.

2. Examination right eye

- Visual acuity was 6/6.

- Fundus examination showed a large choroidal melanoma involving the infero-nasal quadrant with a surrounding rim of subretinal fluid (Figure 3.141a).

3. FA

- *Early phase* showed hypofluorescence of the mass with spotty surface hyperfluorescence (Figure 3.142b).

- *Later phases* showed more diffuse hyperfluorescence (Figure 3.142c and 3.142d).

4. Ultrasonography

- Strong border echo, internal hollowing with shadowing of the orbital fat pattern (Figure 3.142). The dimensions of the mass were 10.5 mm × 11 mm × 4 mm.

5. Systemic investigations

- Liver function tests and chest radiographs were normal.

6. Treatment

- A 15 mm diameter radioactive plaque was sutured over the tumor base and left in place for 96 hours.

7. Course

- After six months visual acuity was 6/12.

- Fundus examination showed regression of the tumor with necrotic atrophy.

- A new finding was the presence of hard exudates and flame-shaped between the optic disc and fovea (Figure 3.143a).

- FA during the early phase showed small areas of hypofluorescence due to capillary non-perfusion and blockage by hemorrhages (Figure 3.143b). The late phase showed diffuse hyperfluorescence due to leakage (see Figure 3.143c).

8. Diagnosis

- Early radiation retinopathy secondary to plaque radiotherapy.

9. Treatment

- Grid laser photocoagulation was applied to the sites of leakage in the papillomacular bundle between the fovea and optic disc.

10. Outcome
Six months later visual acuity was 6/12 with reduction in edema and number of hard exudates.

11. Comment
This patient had an excellent response to laser photocoagulation for early radiation retinopathy. If the condition had not been diagnosed early then the outlook would have been very much less favorable.

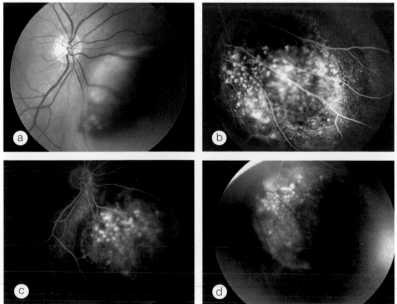

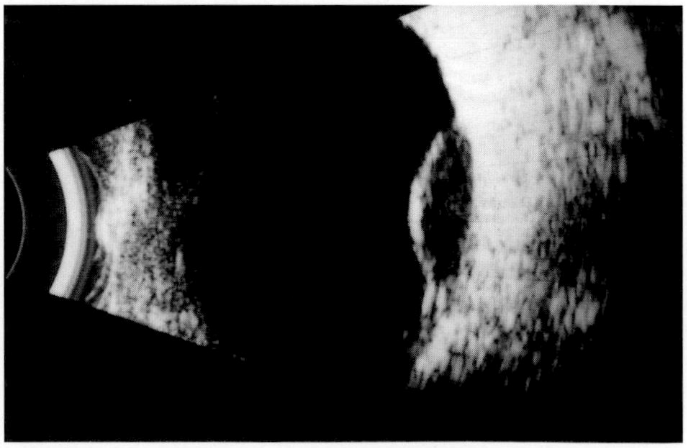

Figure 3.142 B-scan of a choroidal melanoma showing strong border echo, internal hollowing and shadowing of the orbital fat pattern

Figure 3.141 Choroidal melanoma (see the text)

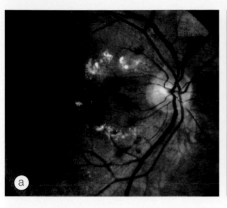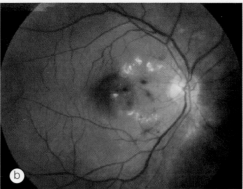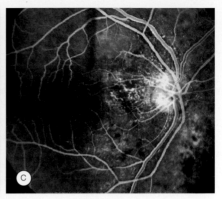

Figure 3.143 Radiation retinopathy (see the text)

FURTHER READING

Amoaku WMK, Archer DB. Fluorescein angiographic features, natural history and treatment for radiation retinopathy. *Eye* 1990;4:757–667.

Archer DB. Doyne Lecture; responses of retinal and choroidal vessels to ionising radiation. *Eye* 1993;7:1–13.

Gragoudas ES, Li W, Lane AM, et al. Risk factors for radiation retinopathy and papillopathy after intraocular irradiation. *Ophthalmology* 1999;106:1571–1578.

Gunduz K, Shields CL, Shields JA, et al. Radiation retinopathy following plaque radiotherapy for posterior uveal melanomas. *Arch Ophthalmol* 1999;117:609–614.

Hykin PG, Shields CL, Shields JA, et al. The efficacy of focal laser therapy in radiation-induced macular edema. *Ophthalmology* 1998;105:1425–1429.

Purtscher retinopathy

1. **Pathogenesis** of this uncommon condition is uncertain. It has been postulated that there is an underlying microvascular damage resulting in occlusion and ischemia.

2. **Associations**, which are wide and varied, include the following:

- *Severe trauma* to the head or a chest compression injury.

- *Embolism* which may consist of fat, air or amniotic fluid.

- *Systemic diseases* which include acute pancreatitis, pancreatic carcinoma, connective tissue diseases, lymphomas, thrombotic thrombocytopenic purpura and following bone marrow transplantation.

3. **Signs** – multiple, superficial, white retinal patches, resembling large cotton-wool spots (Figure 3.144 and 3.145a) which may be associated with superficial peripapillary hemorrhages.

4. **FA** shows variable early capillary non-perfusion and blockage by hemorrhages and edema (Figure 3.145b) and late staining of blood vessels (Figure 3.145c).

5. **Treatment** of the underlying cause is desirable but not always possible.

6. **Prognosis** is guarded. Although the acute fundus changes usually resolve within a few weeks permanent visual impairment occurs in approximately 50% of cases as a result of macular or optic nerve damage.

FURTHER READING

Chuang EL, Miller FS, Kalina RE. Retinal lesions following long bone fractures. *Ophthalmology* 1985;92:370–374.

Power MH, Regillo CD, Custis PH. Thrombotic thrombocytopenic purpura associated with Purtscher retinopathy. *Arch Ophthalmol* 1997;115:128–129.

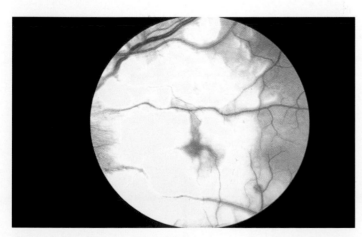

Figure 3.144 Purtscher retinopathy

Case study

1. History

A 42-year-old man was involved in a road traffic accident the previous evening. He suffered a compression type injury against the steering wheel. The right side of his face was struck but he did not recall any loss of consciousness or immediate change in vision. However, shortly thereafter he noticed that his vision was becoming blurred, particularly in his left eye.

2. Examination

Right eye

- Visual acuity was 6/9.

- There was a large subconjunctival hemorrhage.

- Fundus examination several patches of retinal whitening along the supero-temporal arcade and the nasal aspect of the macula.

Left eye

- Visual acuity was CF at one metre.

- Fundus examination showed many large patches of retinal whitening at the posterior pole and around the optic disc (see Figure 3.145a).

3. FA left eye

- *Arteriovenous phase* showed slow choroidal filling and relative block of fluorescence within the macula (see Figure 3.145b).

- *Later phases* showed capillary non-perfusion at the fovea and staining of retinal vessels (see Figure 3.135c).

4. Diagnosis

Bilateral Purtscher retinopathy secondary to chest compression injury.

5. Outcome

- Eight months later visual acuity was 6/6-1 right and CF left.

- The right fundus showed subtle irregularities temporal to the macula.

- The left fundus showed severe optic atrophy.

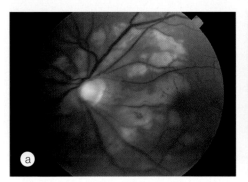
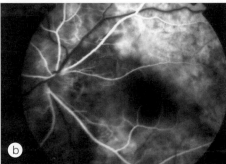
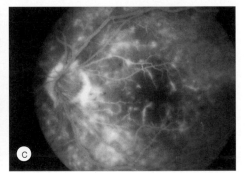

Figure 3.145 Purtscher retinopathy (see the text)

Chapter 4

Inflammatory fundus disorders

Toxoplasmosis

Pathogenesis

Toxoplasma gondii is an obligate intracellular protozoan. The cat is the definitive host and other animals, such as mice, livestock and humans, are intermediate hosts (Figure 4.1).

1. Forms of the parasite

- *Sporocyst* (oocyst) which is excreted in cat feces.

- *Bradyzoite* which is encysted in tissues.

- *Tachyzoite* (trophozoite) which is the proliferating active form responsible for tissue destruction and inflammation.

2. Ways of human infection

- *Ingestion of undercooked* meat (lamb, pork, beef) containing bradyzoites of an intermediate host.

- *Ingestion of sporocysts* following accidental contamination of hands when disposing of cat litter trays and then subsequent transfer on to food. Infants may also become infested by eating dirt (pica) containing sporocysts.

- *Transplacental spread* of the parasite (tachyzoite) can occur to the fetus if a pregnant woman becomes infected (infested).

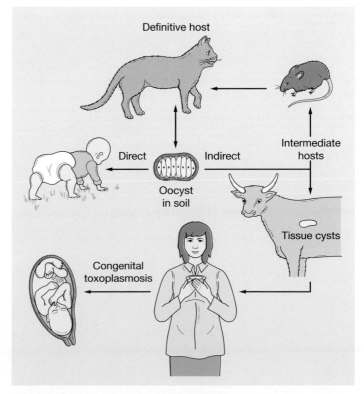

Figure 4.1 Life cycle of *Toxoplasma gondii*

Diagnostic tests

The diagnosis of retinitis caused by toxoplasmosis is based on a compatible fundus lesion and positive serology for toxoplasma antibodies. Any antibody titre is significant because in recurrent ocular toxoplasmosis no correlation exists between the titre and the activity of retinitis.

1. **Indirect immunofluorescent antibody** tests utilize dead organisms that are exposed to the patient's serum and antihuman globulin labelled with fluorescein. The results are read using a fluorescent microscope.

2. **Hemagglutination** tests involve coating of lysed organisms on to red blood cells which are then exposed to the patient's serum. Positive sera cause the red cells to agglutinate.

3. **Enzyme-linked immunosorbent assay** involves binding of the patient's antibodies to an excess of solid phase antigen. This complex is then incubated with an enzyme-linked second antibody. Assessment of enzyme activity provides measurement of specific antibody concentration. The test can also be used to detect antibodies in the aqueous which are more specific than those in the serum.

Congenital systemic toxoplasmosis

Toxoplasmosis is transmitted to the fetus through the placenta when a pregnant woman becomes infected. If the mother is infected before pregnancy, the fetus will be unscathed. The severity of involvement of the fetus is dependent on the duration of gestation at the time of maternal infection. For example, infection during early pregnancy may result in stillbirth, whereas if it occurs during late pregnancy it may result in convulsions, paralysis, hydrocephalus and visceral involvement. Intracranial calcification may be seen on plain skull radiographs or CT (Figure 4.2). However, just as in the acquired form, most cases of congenital systemic toxoplasmosis are subclinical. In these children, bilateral healed chorioretinal scars (Figure 4.3) may be discovered later in life, either by chance or when the child is found to have defective vision.

Acquired systemic toxoplasmosis

1. **In immunocompetent patients** it may take one of the following forms:

- *Subclinical*, which has no symptoms, is the most frequent.

- *Lymphadenopathic syndrome*, which is uncommon and self-limiting. It is characterized by cervical lymphadenopathy, fever, malaise and pharyngitis.

- *Meningoencephalitis*, which is characterized by convulsions and altered consciousness occurs in a minority of patients.

- The *exanthematous form*, resembling a rickettsial infection, is the rarest.

2. **In immunocompromised patients**, such as AIDS patients or organ graft recipients, systemic infection may be life-threatening. The most common manifestation in AIDS patients is an intracerebral space occupying lesion which resembles a cerebral abscess on MRI.

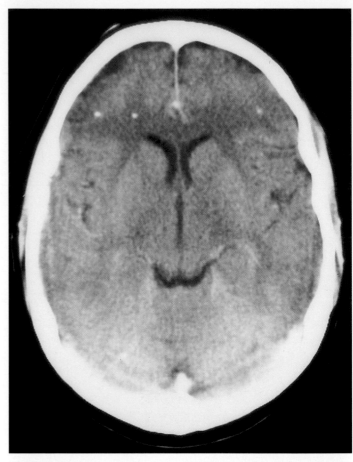

Figure 4.2 CT scan the head showing intracerebral calcification due to congenital toxoplasmosis

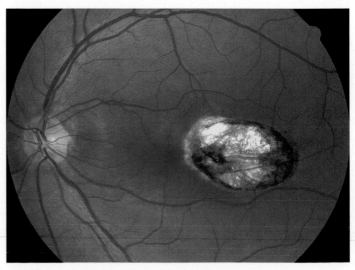

Figure 4.3 Macular scar due to congenital toxoplasmosis

Clinical features of toxoplasma retinitis

Toxoplasma is the most frequent cause of infectious retinitis in immunocompetent individuals. Although most cases are thought to occur as a reactivation of prenatal infection, it has been suggested that postnatally acquired toxoplasma retinitis may be more frequent than previously realized. Recurrent episodes of inflammation are common and occur when the cysts rupture and release hundreds of tachyzoites into normal retinal cells. This usually takes place between the ages of 10 and 35 years (average age 25 years). The scars from which recurrences arise may be the residua of previous congenital infection or, less frequently, remote acquired involvement. Active retinitis is usually associated with anterior uveitis which may be non-granulomatous or granulomatous (Figure 4.4). It is therefore very important to examine the fundus in all patients with anterior uveitis. The signs are as follows:

1. Unifocal superficial necrotizing retinitis

- A solitary inflammatory focus near an old pigmented scar ('satellite lesion') is by far the most common finding (Figure 4.5).

- The inflammatory focus may be small (Figure 4.6) or large (Figure 4.7) and is associated with an overlying vitreous haze.

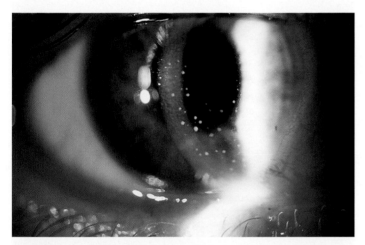

Figure 4.4 Granulomatous anterior uveitis associated with toxoplasma retinitis

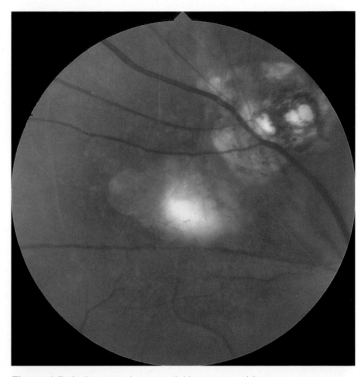

Figure 4.5 Active toxoplasma retinitis near an old scar

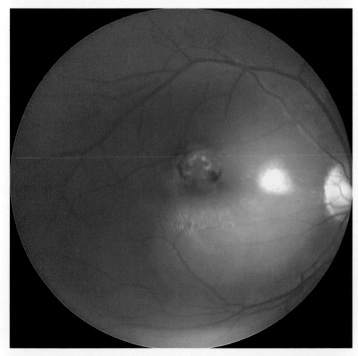

Figure 4.6 Small active focus of toxoplasma retinitis involving the papillomacular bundle and a larger old scar near the fovea

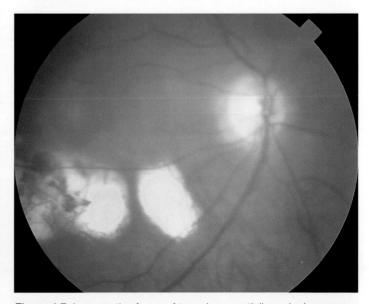

Figure 4.7 Large active focus of toxoplasma retiniis and a large scar

- Very severe vitritis may greatly impair visualization of the fundus, although the inflammatory focus may still be discernible ('headlight in the fog' appearance) (Figure 4.8).

- Associated features include vasculitis and, in some cases, the detached posterior hyaloid face becomes covered by inflammatory precipitates.

2. **Papillitis** (inflammation of the optic nerve head) may be secondary to active retinitis located in the juxtapapillary area (Jensen choroiditis) (Figure 4.9). Very occasionally, the optic nerve head itself is the primary site of involvement.

Course and complications of toxoplasma retinitis

The rate of healing is dependent on the virulence of the organism, the competence of the host's immune system, the size of the lesion and the use of antimicrobial drugs. In uncompromised hosts, the retinitis heals within one to four months. The vitreous haze gradually clears, although some vitreous condensation may remain. The inflammatory focus is replaced by a sharply demarcated atrophic scar surrounded by a hyperpigmented border (Figure 4.10a). On FA the scar is

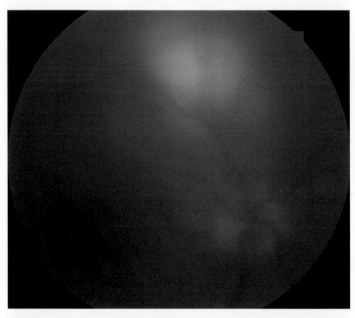

Figure 4.8 Active toxoplasma retinitis and severe vitritis giving rise to a 'headlight in the fog' appearance

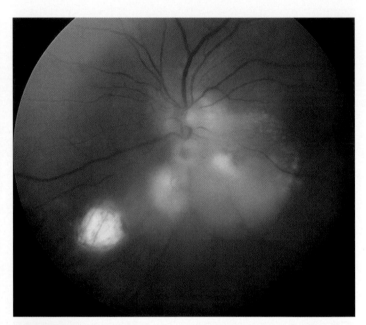

Figure 4.9 Active juxtapapillary toxoplasma retinitis

Figure 4.10 Inactive toxoplasma retinitis (see the text)

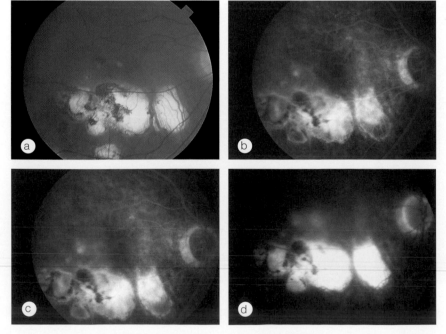

characterized by a RPE window defect (Figure 4.10b and 4.10c) and late staining (Figure 4.10d). Resolution of anterior uveitis is a reliable sign of posterior segment healing. After the first attack, the mean recurrence rate within three years is about 50%, and the average number of recurrent attacks per patient is 2.7. Eyes with toxoplasmosis may lose vision from various direct or indirect causes:

- *Direct involvement* by an inflammatory focus of the fovea (Figure 4.11), papillomacular bundle (see Figure 4.6), optic nerve head or a major blood vessel.

- *Indirect involvement* by epiretinal or vitreoretinal traction may result in macular pucker or tractional retinal detachment.

Management of toxoplasma retinitis

1. Indications for treatment
In the immunocompetent patient not all active lesions require treatment because small peripheral foci are frequently self-limiting and innocuous. The following are the main indications for treatment:

- A lesion threatening or involving the macula, papillomacular bundle, optic nerve head or a major blood vessel.

- A very severe vitritis because it may subsequently lead to vitreous fibrosis and tractional retinal detachment.

- In AIDS patients all lesions should be treated irrespective of location or severity.

2. Therapeutic regimen
Currently there is no universally agreed therapeutic regimen of active lesions. It has been shown that treatment does not reduce either the duration of inflammation nor the incidence of recurrences although it appears to reduce the ultimate size of the chorioretinal scar. The following drugs may be used:

- *Systemic steroids* are recommended in eyes with vision-threatening lesions, particularly if associated with severe vitritis. Steroids are, however, contraindicated in AIDS patients.

- *Clindamycin* 300 mg four times daily is given orally for three weeks. However, if used alone in some patients, it may cause a pseudomembranous colitis secondary to clostridial overgrowth. Treatment of colitis is with oral vancomycin 500 mg six-hourly for ten days. The risk of colitis is reduced when clindamycin is used together with a sulphonamide that inhibits clostridial overgrowth.

- *Sulphonamide* therapy is with either sulphadiazine or the mixed sulphonamide Sulphatriad (if available). The loading oral dose is 2 g followed by 1 g four times daily for three to four weeks. Side-effects of sulphonamides include renal stones, allergic reactions and Stevens-Johnson syndrome.

- *Pyrimethamine* (Daraprim) is a strong anti-toxoplasma agent which may cause thrombocytopenia, leucopenia, and folate deficiency. For this reason, weekly blood counts should be performed and the drug used only in combination with oral folinic acid 4 mg three times a week (mixed with orange juice), because this counteracts the side-effects. The loading dose is 50 mg followed by 25–50 mg daily for four weeks. Pyrimethamine should not be used in patients with AIDS.

- *Co-trimoxazole* (Septrin) consists of a combination of trimethoprim 160 mg and sulphamethoxazole 800 mg. When used in oral doses of 960 mg twice daily for four to six weeks, it may be effective alone or in combination with clindamycin. Side-effects are similar to those of the sulphonamides.

- *Atovaquone* 750 mg three times daily has been used mainly in the treatment of pneumocystosis and toxoplasmosis in AIDS but it is also effective in the treatment of toxoplasma retinitis in immunocompetent individuals. The drug is relatively free of serious side-effects but is expensive.

- *Azithromycin* 500 mg daily on three successive days may be an effective alternative for patients who cannot tolerate other drugs.

FURTHER READING

Bosch-Griessen EH, Rothova A. Recurrent ocular disease in postnatally acquired toxoplasmosis. *Am J Ophthalmol* 1999;128:421–425.

Bosch-Griessen EH, Rothova A. Sense and nonsense of corticosteroid administration in the treatment of ocular toxoplasmosis. *Br J Ophthalmol* 1998;82:858–860.

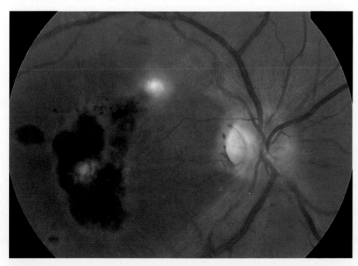

Figure 4.11 Foveal involvement by an old scar with a small active focus at its superior edge

Bosch-Grierson EH, Karimi S, Slima JS, et al. Retinal detachment in ocular toxoplasmosis. *Ophthalmology* 2000;107:36–40.

Gilbert RE, Stanford MR. Is ocular toxoplasmosis caused by prenatal or postnatal infection? Perspective. *Br J Ophthalmol* 2000;84:224–226.

Holland GN. Reconsidering the pathogenesis of ocular toxoplasmosis. *Am J Ophthalmol* 1999;128:502–505.

Klaren VNA, van Doornik CEM, Ongkosuwito JV, et al. Differences between intraocular and serum antibody responses in patients with ocular toxoplasmosis. *Am J Ophthalmol* 1998;126:698–706.

Mets MB, Holfels E, Boyer KM, et al. Eye manifestation of congenital toxoplasmosis. *Am J Ophthalmol* 1997;123:1–16.

Pavesio CE, Lightman S. *Toxoplasma gondii* and ocular toxoplasmosis: pathogenesis. *Br J Ophthalmol* 1996;80:1099–1107.

Pearson PA, Piracha AR, Sen HA, et al. Atovaquone for treatment of toxoplasma retinochoroiditis in immunocompetent patients. *Ophthalmology* 1999;106:148–153.

Rothova A, Bosch-Driersen EH, van Loon NH, et al. Azithromycin for ocular toxoplasmosis. *Br J Ophthalmol* 1998;82:1306–1308.

Rothova A, Meeken C, Buitenhuis HJ, et al. Therapy for ocular toxoplasmosis. *Am J Ophthalmol* 1993;115:517–523.

Histoplasmosis

Systemic histoplasmosis

Histoplasmosis is a fungal infection caused by *Histoplasma capsulatum*. The disease is acquired by inhalation and the organisms pass *via* the bloodstream to the spleen, liver and, on occasion, the choroid, setting up multiple foci of granulomatous inflammation. In the vast majority of patients, the fungemia is innocuous and asymptomatic, because the organisms disappear after a few weeks. A small minority of patients develop severe, disseminated systemic histoplasmosis. Although ocular histoplasmosis has never been reported in patients with active, systemic histoplasmosis, eye disease has an increased prevalence in areas where histoplasmosis is endemic, such as the Mississippi – Missouri river valley.

Diagnostic tests

1. **Histoplasma skin testing**, although positive in about 90% of patients with ocular involvement, it is now seldom performed.

2. **Complement fixation tests** are of limited value because they usually become negative several years after the original infection.

3. **Radiographs** may occasionally show old calcified granulomata in the lungs and spleen.

4. **Tissue typing** of patients with ocular disease, particularly if associated with maculopathy, shows an increased prevalence of HLA-B7.

Ocular histoplasmosis

Ocular histoplasmosis is asymptomatic unless it causes a maculopathy. The earliest symptom of macular involvement is metamorphopsia. The following types of fundus lesion are seen which are bilateral in 60% of cases:

1. **Atrophic 'histo' spots** consist of roundish, slightly irregular, yellowish-white lesions about 200 μm in diameter. Small pigment clumps may be present within or at the margins of the scars although some spots are not associated with pigmentation. The lesions are scattered in the mid-retinal periphery (Figure 4.12a and 4.12b, and Figure 4.13) and the posterior pole (Figure 4.12c and Figure 4.14).

2. **Peripapillary atrophy** may be diffuse or focal, or a combination of both.

- *Diffuse*, circumferential, choroidal atrophy extends up to half a disc diameter beyond the disc margin (Figure 4.15).

- *Focal* peripapillary lesions are less common and are irregular and punched out, resembling the peripheral spots (Figure 4.16).

3. **Linear streaks** of chorioretinal atrophy may be seen in the fundus periphery (Figure 4.17).

4. **Absence of intraocular inflammation**.

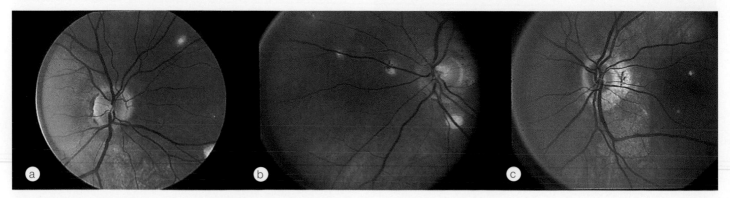

Figure 4.12 'Histo' spots in ocular histoplasmosis

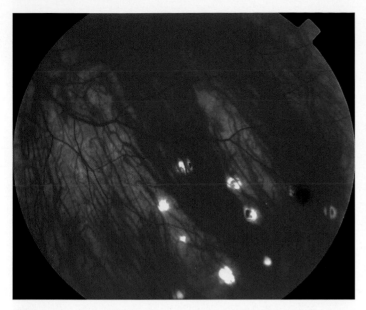

Figure 4.13 Peripheral 'histo' spots in ocular histoplasmosis

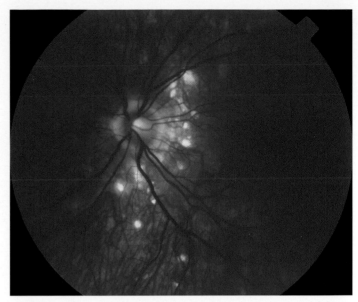

Figure 4.14 Central 'histo' spots in ocular histoplasmosis

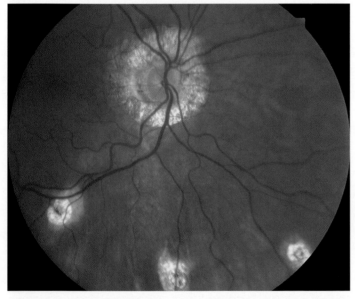

Figure 4.15 Circumferential peripapillary atrophy and peripheral 'histo' spots in ocular histoplasmosis

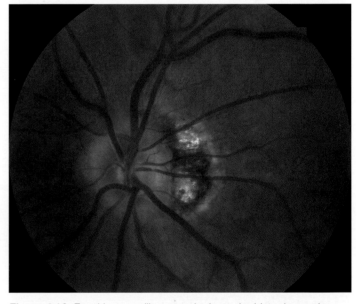

Figure 4.16 Focal juxtapapillary atrophy in ocular histoplasmosis

Exudative maculopathy

1. **Choroidal neovascularization** (CNV) is a late manifestation which usually develops between the ages of 20 and 45 years in about 5% of eyes. In most cases, CNV is associated with an old macular 'histo spot', although occasionally they develop within a peripapillary lesion. Very rarely, the CNV occurs in the absence of a pre-existing scar.

2. **The clinical course** of maculopathy is variable and follows one of the following patterns:

- The CNV may initially leak fluid and give rise to metamorphopsia, blurring of central vision and a

scotoma. Careful slitlamp biomicroscopy with a fundus contact lens shows that the macula is elevated by serous fluid and an underlying focal yellow-white or grey lesion. In 12% of eyes the subretinal fluid absorbs spontaneously and visual symptoms regress.

- A dark green-black ring frequently develops on the surface of the yellow-white lesion and bleeding occurs into the sub-sensory retinal space causing a marked drop in visual acuity. In a few eyes, the subretinal hemorrhage resolves and visual acuity improves.

- In some eyes, the initial CNV remains active for about 2 years giving rise to repeated hemorrhages. This finally causes a profound and permanent impairment of central

141

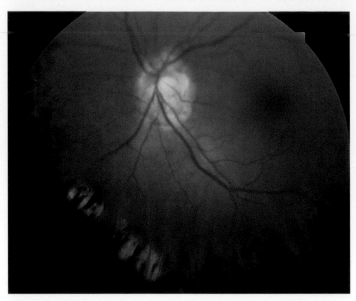

Figure 4.17 Linear streaks of chorioretinal atrophy in ocular histoplasmosis

vision resulting from the development of a fibrous disciform scar at the fovea. Patients with maculopathy in one eye and an asymptomatic atrophic macular scar in the other are likely to develop a disciform lesion in the second eye. They should therefore test themselves every day with an Amsler grid to detect early metamorphopsia because without treatment 60% of eyes with CNV have a final visual acuity of less than 6/60.

3. Treatment of CNV

- *Laser photocoagulation* is at present the treatment of choice. Pre-treatment FA is vital in evaluating the extent and location of CNV (see below).

- *Surgical removal* of subfoveal CMV may be indicated in selected cases.

FURTHER READING

Fine SL, Wood WJ, Singerman LJ, et al. Laser treatment for subfoveal neovascular membranes in ocular histoplasmosis syndrome: results of a pilot randomized clinical trial. *Arch Ophthalmol* 1993;111:19–20.

Jost BF, Olk RJ, Burgess DB. Factors related to spontaneous visual recovery in the ocular histoplasmosis syndrome. *Retina* 1987;7:1–8.

Macular Photocoagulation Study Group. Five-year follow-up of fellow eyes in individuals with ocular histoplasmosis and unilateral extrafoveal or juxtafoveal choroidal neovascularization. *Arch Ophthalmol* 1996;114:677–688.

Olk RJ, Burgess, DB, McCormick PA. Subfoveal and juxtafoveal subretinal neovascularization in the presumed ocular histoplasmosis syndrome. Visual prognosis. *Ophthalmology* 1984;91:1592–1602.

Case study

1. History

A 42-year-old female presented with a three week history of mild metamorphopsia and blurred vision in her left eye.

2. Examination left eye

- Visual acuity was 6/12–1.

- Slitlamp examination showed absence of intraocular inflammation.

- Fundus examination showed numerous peripheral punched-out atrophic chorioretinal scars and a small solitary atrophic lesion in the temporal macula. The fovea showed an area of edema associated with a few small hemorrhages (Figure 4.18a).

3. FA left eye

- *Arterial phase* showed the following three abnormalities (Figure 4.18b): (a) a lesion just above the centre of the fovea which showed a lacy filling pattern of hyperfluorescence typical of CNV; (b) a very small hyperfluorescent spot temporal to the CNV which remained the same throughout the angiogram due to a RPE window defect which had not been apparent at fundus examination, and (c) a larger area of focal hypofluorescence in the temporal macula which later became hyperfluorescent.

- *Venous phase* showed increase in hyperfluorescence but not in size of the CNV (Figure 4.18c).

- *Late phase* showed intense hyperfluorescence of the CNV due to leakage (Figure 4.18d).

4. Diagnosis

- Ocular histoplasmosis associated with juxtafoveal CNV and an adjacent 'histo spot'.

5. Treatment

- Laser photocoagulation to CNV.

6. Outcome

- Two months later visual acuity was 6/9 with resolution of edema and hemorrhages.

7. Comment

This patient had a favorable outcome of treatment of CNV associated with histoplasmosis which carries a far better prognosis than a similar juxtafoveal lesion in patients with age-related macular degeneration. However, close follow-up is indicated because of the possibility of recurrence not only from the treated site but also from the other scar in the temporal macula.

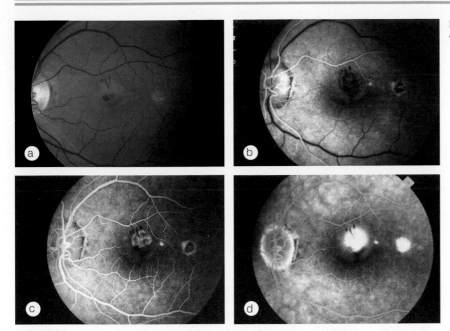

Figure 4.18 Treatment of CNV associated with ocular histoplasmosis (see the text)

Acquired immune deficiency syndrome

Systemic features

Acquired immune deficiency syndrome (AIDS) is caused by the human immunodeficiency virus (HIV) which is predominantly transmitted by sexual intercourse. In some cases it is transmitted through contaminated blood or syringes. The majority (70%) of patients with AIDS in the Western world are homosexual males, and 20% are intravenous drug abusers. The remainder consists of heterosexual partners of persons with AIDS, recipients of contaminated blood and newborn infants of high risk mothers. AIDS was initially defined as the occurrence of opportunistic infections, Kaposi sarcoma or lymphoma, or both, in patients who are not immunosuppressed from other causes. The definition was subsequently expanded to include HIV-infected patients with severe immunosuppression in the absence of opportunistic infections. Patients can be HIV positive some years before they develop the clinical manifestations of AIDS. One of the hallmarks of progressive immune deficiency is a steady decline in the absolute number of CD4+ T-lymphocytes. The life expectancy of AIDS patients has been significantly improved with the introduction of new drugs. Current treatment is with highly active antiretroviral therapy (HAART) which consists of triple therapy with a combination of two nucleoside analogues and one protease inhibitor.

1. **Opportunistic infections in AIDS**

* *Protozoa*: toxoplasmosis, *Pneumocystis carinii* and microsporidium.

* *Viruses*: cytomegalovirus, herpes simplex virus, varicella zoster virus, molluscum contagiosum and Epstein-Barr virus.

* *Fungi*: cryptococcus neoformans, histoplasmosis and candida.

* *Bacteria*: tuberculosis and atypical myobacteria.

* *Spirocheates*: syphilis.

2. **Malignancies** – Kaposi sarcoma, lymphoma and carcinoma.

HIV retinal microangiopathy

Retinal microangiopathy develops in 60% of patients with AIDS. It is characterized by cotton-wool spots (Figure 4.19)

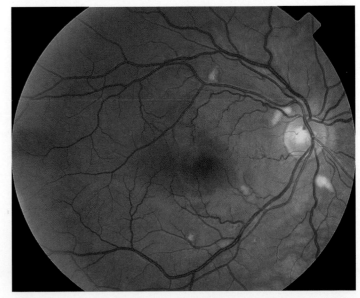

Figure 4.19 Cotton wool spots associated with HIV retinal microangiopathy

which may be associated with retinal hemorrhages and microaneurysms. The lesions may be mistaken for early CMV retinitis. However, in contrast to CMV retinitis, the cotton-wool spots are usually asymptomatic and almost invariably disappear spontaneously after several weeks. Possible causes of the microangiopathy include immune complex deposition and HIV infection of the retinal vascular endothelium.

Cytomegalovirus retinitis

CMV retinitis eventually affects 25% of patients with AIDS and its appearance usually signifies severe systemic involvement, although on rare occasions it is the initial manifestation of the disease.

1. Signs

- *Indolent CMV retinitis* frequently starts in the periphery and progresses slowly. It is characterized by a mild granular opacification which may be associated with a few punctate hemorrhages but there is no vasculitis (Figure 4.20).

- *Fulminating retinitis* is characterized by a dense, white, well-demarcated, geographical area of confluent opacification (Figure 4.21). Retinal hemorrhages may develop either within the area of retinitis or along its leading edge (Figure 4.22). Vitritis is mild. The infective process spreads slowly but relentlessly as a 'brushfire-like' extension along the course of the retinal blood vessels and may involve the optic nerve head (Figure 4.23). Retinal

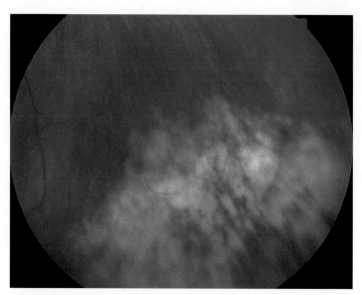

Figure 4.20 Indolent cytomegalovirus retinitis

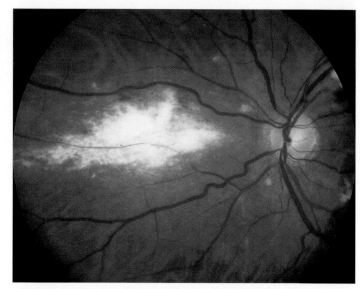

Figure 4.21 Confluent retinal opacification in fulminating cytomegalovirus retinitis

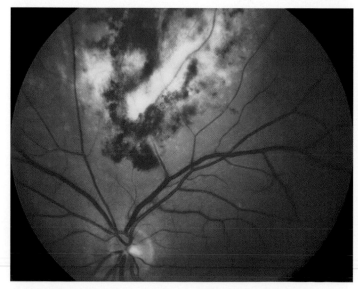

Figure 4.22 Retinal hemorrhages associated with fulminating cytomegalovirus retinitis

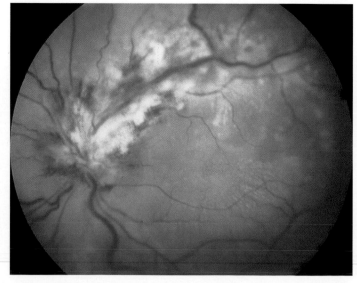

Figure 4.23 Fulminating cytomegalovirus retinitis involving the optic disc

vasculitis characterized by perivascular sheathing is a prominent feature (Figure 4.24). Retinal detachment may occur in eyes with severe involvement.

2. **Regression** is characterized by fewer hemorrhages, less opacification, and diffuse atrophic and pigmentary changes (Figure 4.25).

3. **Complications**

- *Macular complications* include necrosis, cystoid edema, epiretinal membranes, and hard exudate formation (Figure 4.26).

- *Other complications* include retinal detachment and consecutive optic atrophy.

4. **Treatment** with the following drugs may be used as monotherapy or in combination.

- *Ganciclovir* is initially given intravenously (induction) 10 mg/kg every 12 hours for two to three weeks, then 5 mg/kg every 24 hours. Patients with stable retinitis may be treated with oral ganciclovir 300 mg daily for prophylaxis and maintenance. Ganciclovir is effective in 80% of patients but 50% subsequently relapse and require reinduction of therapy. The drug carries a high risk of bone marrow suppression which often forces interruption of treatment.

- *Intravenous foscarnet*, is initially given as 60 mg/kg every eight hours for two to three weeks and then every 24 hours. Its side-effects include nephrotoxicity, electrolyte disturbances and seizures. Foscarnet can also be given intravitreally.

- *Intravitreal ganciclovir*, in the form of either injections or slow-release devices (Vitrasert), appears to be as effective as intravenous therapy. The duration of the implant is eight months. However, it fails to protect the fellow eye from retinitis. Intravitreal injections may also cause serious complications such as vitreous hemorrhage, retinal detachment and endophthalmitis.

- *Intravenous cidofovir*, 5 mg/kg once weekly for two weeks and then every two weeks may be used where other agents are unsuitable. It must be administered in combination with probenecid. Side-effects include nephrotoxicity and neutropenia. Cidofovir can also be given intravitreally.

5. **Prognosis**

- Without treatment the eye becomes blind within six weeks to six months.

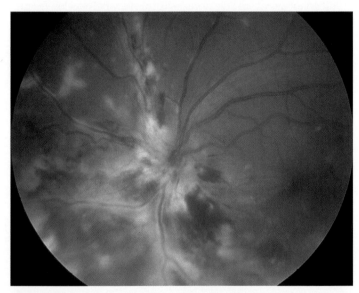

Figure 4.24 Vascular sheathing associated with fulminating cytomegalovirus retinitis

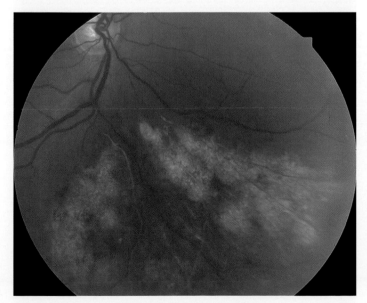

Figure 4.25 Regressing cytomegalovirus retinitis

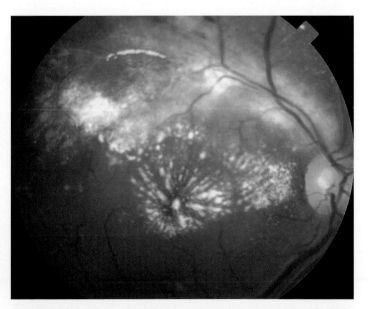

Figure 4.26 Hard exudates forming a macular star associated with fulminating cytomegalovirus retinitis

- With treatment there is a 95% response with decrease in size of the lesions. However, there is a 100% relapse within two weeks when treatment is discontinued and a 50% relapse rate within six months in patients on maintenance therapy.

Choroidal pneumocystosis

Pneumocystis carinii, an opportunistic protozoan parasite, is a major cause of morbidity and mortality in AIDS. The presence of choroidal involvement can be an important sign of extrapulmonary systemic dissemination. Most patients with choroiditis have received inhaled pentamidine as prophylaxis against *P. carinii* pneumonia because systemic prophylaxis protects against choroiditis, while aerosolized pentamidine protects only the lungs, allowing the organisms to disseminate throughout the body. The presence of choroiditis implies a grave prognosis for life.

1. **Signs**

- Variable number of flat, yellow, round, choroidal lesions which are frequently bilateral and not associated with vitritis (Figure 4.27).

- Even when the fovea is involved there is little, if any, impairment of visual acuity.

2. **Treatment** with intravenous trimethoprim, sulphamethoxazole or parenteral pentamidine causes resolution of the lesions within several weeks (Figure 4.28).

Progressive outer retinal necrosis

Progressive outer retinal necrosis (PORN) is caused by varicella-zoster virus and only affects patients with AIDS. It may be anteceded by herpes zoster ophthalmicus in some patients.

1. **Presentation** rapidly progressive visual loss which is initially unilateral in 75% of cases.

2. **Signs** in chronological order:

- Peripheral, circumferential, multifocal, deep outer retinal opacification with minimal associated vitritis (Figure 4.29).

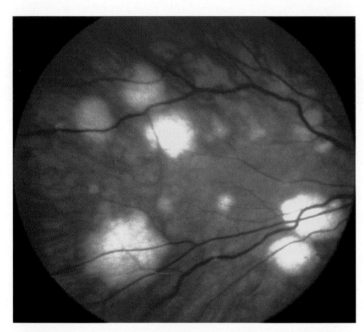

Figure 4.27 Choroidal pneumocystosis

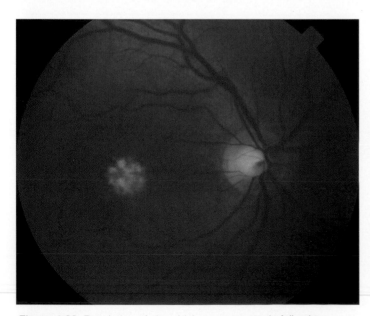

Figure 4.28 Resolution of choroidal pneumocystosis following treatment

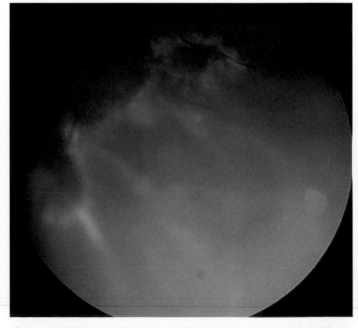

Figure 4.29 Progressive outer retinal necrosis involving the periphery

- Subsequent full-thickness retinal necrosis and spread to involve the macula (Figure 4.30).

3. **Prognosis** is extremely poor, because the condition responds poorly to antiviral therapy and most patients become blind in both eyes within a few weeks as a result of macular necrosis or retinal detachment. In addition 50% are dead five months after the diagnosis.

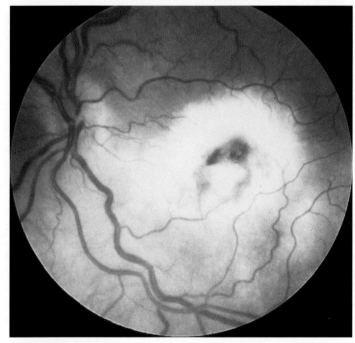

Figure 4.30 Macular involvement by progressive outer retinal necrosis

Other fundus lesions

1. **Toxoplasma retinitis** in AIDS is different from the condition in immunocompetent patients and may need lifelong treatment. It tends to be more severe, bilateral, multifocal, not adjacent to old scars, and is often associated with central nervous system involvement.

2. **Cryptococcus choroiditis** is usually associated with meningitis and is characterized by asymptomatic creamy choroidal lesions which are not associated with vitritis. Small white spheres at the vitreoretinal interface may also occur. Some patients with cryptococcosis may lose vision from coexisting cryptococcal involvement of the optic nerves which manifests as either disc swelling or retrobulbar neuritis. Other fungal infections that may involve the posterior segment in AIDS patients are candidiasis and, rarely, histoplasmosis.

4. **Large-cell intraocular lymphoma** which may mimic uveitis.

FURTHER READING

Belfort R Jr. The ophthalmologist and the global impact of the AIDS epidemic. LV Edward Jackson Memorial Lecture. *Am J Ophthalmol* 2000;129:1–8.

Cassoux N, Lumbroso L, Bogaghi B, et al. Cystoid macular oedema and cytomegalovirus retinitis in patients with HIV disease treated with highly active antiretroviral therapy. *Br J Ophthalmol* 1999;83:47–49.

Holland GN. Treatment options for cytomagalovirus retinitis. A time for reassessment. *Arch Ophthalmol* 1999;117:1549–1550.

Holland GN. New issues in the management of patients with AIDS-related cytomegalovirus retinitis. Commentary. *Arch Ophthalmol* 2000;118:704–706.

Jabs DA, Bartlett JG. AIDS and ophthalmology: a period of transition. *Am J Ophthalmol* 1997;124:227–233.

Jabs DA, Bolton SG, Dunn JP, et al. Discontinuing anticyclomegalovirus therapy in patients with immune reconstitution after combination antiretroviral therapy. *Am J Ophthalmol* 1998;126:817–822.

Lee V, Subak-Sharpe I, Shah S, et al. Changing trends in cytomegalovirus retinitis triple therapy. *Eye* 1999;13:59–64.

Macdonald JC, Karavellas MP, Torriani FJ, et al. High active antiretroviral therapy-related immune recovery in AIDS patients with cytomegalovirus retinitis. *Ophthalmology* 2000;107:877–883.

Maguire AM, Nichols CW, Crooks GW. Visual loss in cytomegalovirus retinitis caused by cystoid macular edema in patients without acquired immune deficiency syndrome. *Ophthalmology* 1996;103:601–605.

Mitchell SM, Membrey WL, Youle MS, et al. Cytomegalovirus retinitis after initiation of highly active antiretroviral therapy: a 2 year prospective study. *Br J Ophthalmol* 1999;83:652–655.

Raina J, Bainbridge JWB, Shah SM. Decreased visual acuity in patients with cytomegalovirus retinitis and AIDS. *Eye* 2000;14:8–12.

Reed JB, Schwab IR, Gordon J, et al. Regression of CMV retinitis associated with protease inhibitor treatment of AIDS. *Am J Ophthalmol* 1997;124:199–205.

Roth DB, Feuer WJ, Blenke AJ, et al. Treatment of cytomegalovirus retinitis with the ganciclovir implant. *Am J Ophthalmol* 1999;127:276–282.

Sarcoidosis
Systemic features

Sarcoidosis is an idiopathic, multisystem, granulomatous disease with frequent ocular manifestations. Eye problems may occur in patients with few, if any, constitutional symptoms, as well as those with inactive systemic disease. The posterior segment is involved in about 25% of patients with ocular sarcoid and is usually associated with anterior uveitis.

1. **Presentation**

- *Acute-onset* sarcoid typically occurs in the third decade in one of the following ways:
  a. Lofren syndrome which is characterized by fever, erythema nodosum, hilar lymphadenopathy and frequently arthralgia.

b. Heerfordt syndrome (uveoparotid fever) which is characterized by fever, parotid gland enlargement and uveitis.

c. Seventh nerve palsy which may be associated with other neurological features.

• *Insidious-onset* sarcoid typically presents during the fifth decade with fatigue, dyspnoea and arthralgia.

2. Signs

• *Pulmonary involvement* varies in severity from asymptomatic hilar lymphadenopathy (Figure 4.31) to progressive pulmonary fibrosis with formation of bullae and bronchiectasis (Figure 4.32).

• *Skin lesions* include erythema nodosum (Figure 4.33), lupus pernio (Figure 4.34) and granulomas.

• *Neurological involvement* includes cranial nerve palsies, most frequently facial (Figure 4.34), meningeal

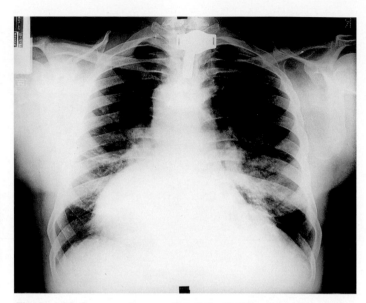

Figure 4.32 Severe pulmonary fibrosis in chronic sarcoidosis

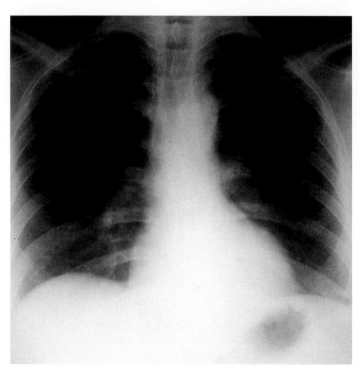

Figure 4.31 Hilar lymphadenopathy in acute sarcoidosis

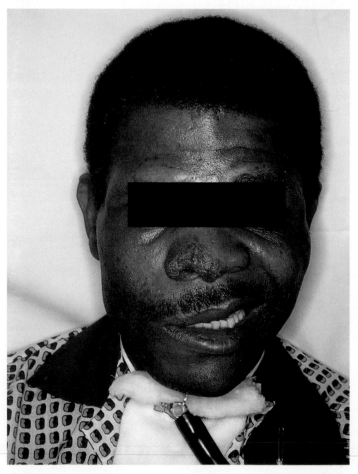

Figure 4.34 Lupus pernio involving the nose and facial nerve palsy in sarcoidosis

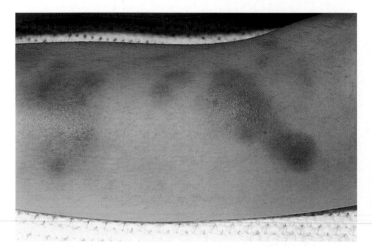

Figure 4.33 Erythema nodosum in acute sarcoidosis

148

infiltration as well as intracranial and intraspinal granulomas.

- *Miscellaneous lesions* may involve the reticuloendothelial system, liver, kidneys, bones and the heart.

Diagnostic tests

Although the diagnosis of sarcoidosis is usually relatively straightforward, in some patients many of the above features may be absent and the following special investigations may be useful.

1. **Chest radiographs** show abnormalities in approximately 90% of patients with sarcoidosis.

2. **Biopsy**

- *Lung* biopsy is accurate in diagnosing sarcoidosis in about 90% of cases.

- *Conjunctival* biopsy is positive in about 70% of patients irrespective of the presence of intraocular involvement.

- *Lacrimal gland* biopsy by a transconjunctival route may be considered in patients with suspected sarcoidosis, particularly if the lacrimal glands are enlarged or if they demonstrate increased gallium uptake. Biopsies are positive in 25% of patients with non-enlarged glands and in 75% with enlarged glands.

3. **Kvein-Slitzbach skin test** is positive in 85–90% of patients with early or active systemic disease, but sensitivity decreases with time. Because it is difficult to obtain the antigen required to perform this test it is seldom used.

4. **Serum angiotensin-converting enzyme** (ACE) is a useful test which is elevated in patients with active sarcoidosis and normal during remission. The normal level for adults is 32.1 +/– 8.5 IU. In patients with suspected neurosarcoid, ACE should be measured in the cerebrospinal fluid.

5. **Calcium assay** may be useful because calcium metabolism is abnormal in patients with sarcoidosis. Hypercalciuria is common but hypercalcemia is unusual.

6. **Gallium-67 scans** of the head, neck and thorax frequently show increased uptake.

7. **Bronchoalveolar lavage** shows a raised proportion of activated T-helper lymphocytes.

Anterior uveitis

1. **Acute anterior uveitis** typically affects patients with acute-onset sarcoid. It can usually be controlled by topical treatment with steroids and mydriatics.

2. **Chronic granulomatous anterior uveitis** typically affects older patients with chronic lung disease. The inflammation is characterized by mutton fat keratic precipitates and iris nodules. Treatment is initially topical but frequently periocular or systemic steroid administration is required. If severe and longstanding it may lead to secondary cataract, glaucoma, band keratopathy and CME.

Intermediate uveitis

Intermediate uveitis is relatively uncommon. It is characterized by vitreous inflammation and snowball opacities (Figure 4.35). Treatment is initially with posterior sub-tendon injection of steroids. The main complication is chronic CME. Because some patients with sarcoidosis may not have systemic symptoms it is important to rule out the possibility in patients with presumed idiopathic intermediate uveitis.

Posterior uveitis

The posterior segment is involved in about 25% of patients with ocular sarcoid and may take the following forms:

1. **Retinal periphlebitis** may be subclinical and only visible on FA (Figure 4.36) or more extensive sheathing (Figure 4.37) which, if severe, may be associated with perivenous exudates referred to as 'candlewax drippings' (Figure 4.38). Occasionally severe periphlebitis may result in branch retinal vein occlusion. Although acute lesions may resolve spontaneously or with the use of systemic steroids, vascular sheathing, once established, usually persists.

2. **Choroidal granulomas** are relatively uncommon and vary in appearance:

- Multiple, small, pale-yellow, infiltrates, usually most numerous inferiorly are the most common type (Figure 4.39).

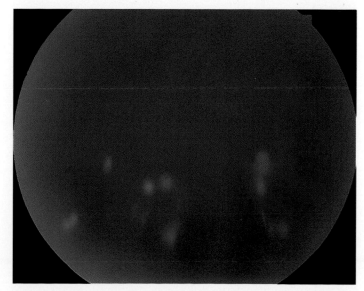

Figure 4.35 Snowball vitreous opacities associated intermediate sarcoid uveitis

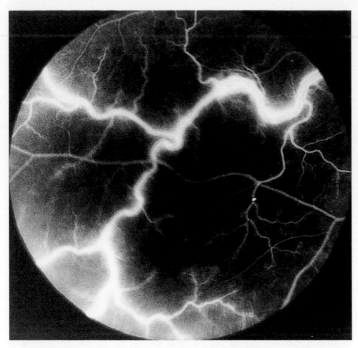

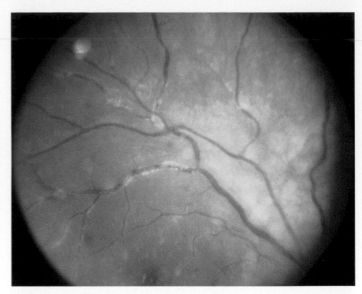

Figure 4.37 Retinal periphlebitis in sarcoidosis

Figure 4.36 FA of retinal periphlebitis in sarcoidosis

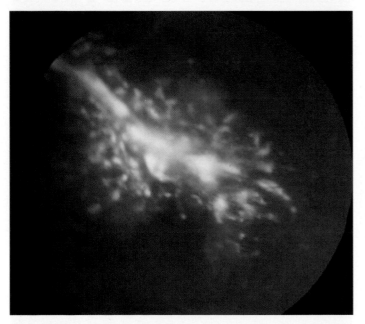

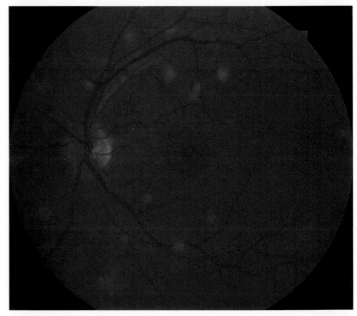

Figure 4.38 Severe retinal periphlebitis with 'candlewax drippings' in sarcoidosis

Figure 4.39 Multiple, small, choroidal granulomas in sarcoidosis

- Multiple, large, confluent, infiltrates which may have ameboid margins are less common (Figure 4.40).

- Large solitary choroidal granuloma (Figure 4.41) is the least common and may be mistaken for an amelanotic choroidal melanoma.

3. **Retinal granulomas** are characterized by small, discrete, yellow lesions (Figure 4.42).

4. **Preretinal granulomas** are also uncommon and are typically located inferiorly anterior to the equator (Landers sign) (Figure 4.43).

5. **Peripheral retinal neovascularization** (Figure 4.44) may occur in association with retinal capillary dropout seen on FA. In black patients neovascularization may be mistaken for that associated with sickle-cell retinopathy (see Chapter 3).

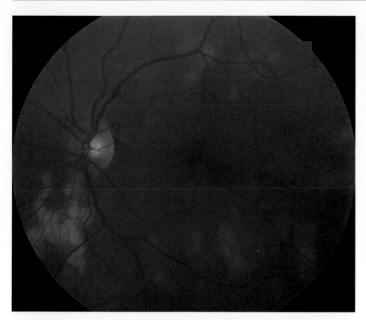

Figure 4.40 Multiple, large confluent choroidal granulomas in sarcoidosis

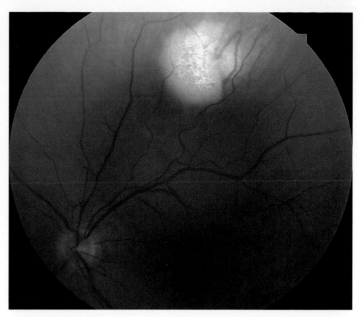

Figure 4.41 Solitary, large choroidal granuloma in sarcoidosis

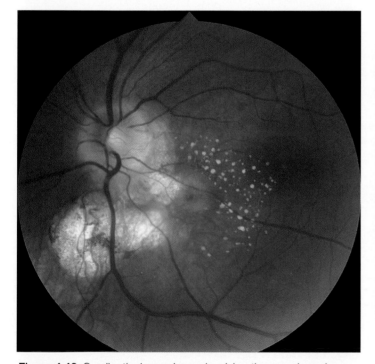

Figure 4.42 Small retinal granulomas involving the macula and a juxtapapillary scar in sarcoidosis

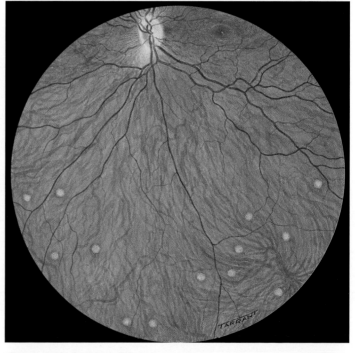

Figure 4.43 Small, peripheral pre-retinal granuloma in sarcoidosis

Optic nerve lesions

The optic nerve may be involved by one of the following:

1. **Focal granulomas** which do not usually affect vision (Figure 4.45).

2. **Papilledema**, which is usually secondary to involvement of the central nervous system, may occur in the absence of other eye lesions (Figure 4.46).

3. **Persistent disc edema** of unknown cause is a frequent finding in patients with retinal or vitreous involvement.

Differential diagnosis

1. **Intermediate uveitis**

- Idiopathic.

- Lyme disease.

151

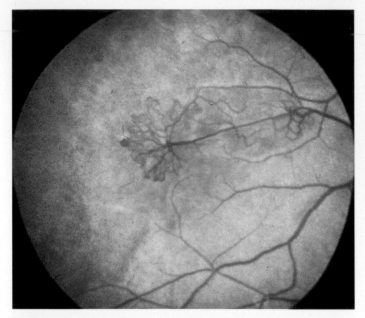

Figure 4.44 Peripheral retinal neovascularization in sarcoidosis

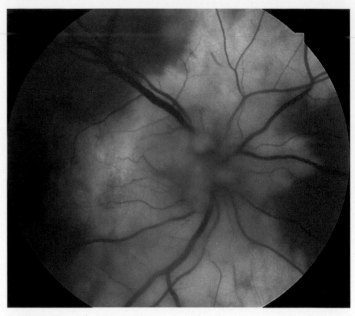

Figure 4.45 Optic nerve head and peripapillary involvement in sarcoidosis

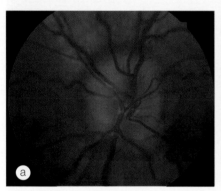

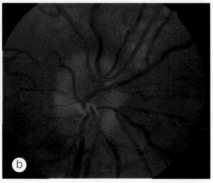

Figure 4.46 Papilledema

- Multiple sclerosis.
- Non-Hodgkin large B-cell lymphoma.
- Whipple disease.

2. Small choroidal lesions

- Multifocal choroiditis with panuveitis.
- Birdshot chorioretinopathy.
- Tuberculosis.

3. Large choroidal infiltrates

- Metastatic tumour.
- Large cell lymphoma.
- Harada disease.
- Serpiginous choroidopathy.

4. Periphlebitis

- Tuberculosis.
- Behçet disease.

- Cytomegalovirus retinitis.
- Cat-scratch fever.
- Crohn disease.

FURTHER READING

Brod RD. Presumed sarcoid choroidopathy mimicking birdshot retinochoroidopathy. *Am J Ophthalmol* 1990;109:357–358.

Dana M-R, Merayo-Lloves J, Schaumberg DA, et al. Prognosticators for visual outcome in sarcoid uveitis. *Ophthalmology* 1999;103:1846–1853.

Dev S, McCallum RM, Jaffe GJ. Methotrexate treatment for sarcoid-associated panuveitis. *Ophthalmol* 1999;106:111–118.

Edelsten C, Pearson A, Joyles E, et al. The ocular and systemic prognosis of patients presenting with sarcoid uveitis. *Eye* 1999;13:748–753.

Jabs DA, Johns CJ. Ocular involvement in chronic sarcoidosis. *Am J Ophthalmol* 1986;102:297–301.

Karma A, Huhti E, Poukkula A. Course and outcome of ocular sarcoidosis. *Am J Ophthalmol* 1988;106:467–472.

Power WJ, Neves RA, Rodriguez A, et al. The value of combined serum angiotensin-conversion enzyme and gallium scan in the diagnosis of ocular sarcoidosis. *Ophthalmology* 1995;102:2007–2011.

Rothova A. Ocular involvement in sarcoidosis. Perspectives. *Br J Ophthalmol* 2000;84:110–116.

Stavrou P, Linton S, Young DW, et al. Clinical diagnosis of ocular sarcoid. *Eye* 1997;11:365–370.

Thorne JE, Brucker AJ. Choroidal white lesions as early manifestations of sarcoidosis. *Retina* 2000;20:8–15.

Behçet disease

Systemic features

Behçet disease is an uncommon, idiopathic, multisystem disease which typically affects young men from the eastern Mediterranean region and Japan. It is associated with an increased incidence of HLA-B51.

1. **Presentation** is usually in the third and fourth decades of life, with localized lesions such as aphthous stomatitis. As there are no definitive diagnostic laboratory tests, the diagnostic criteria can be divided into major and minor as follows:

2. **Major diagnostic criteria**

- *Recurrent aphthous stomatitis* is a universal finding and a very common presenting feature. The ulcers are painful and shallow with a yellowish necrotic base. They tend to occur in crops, which may involve the tongue (Figure 4.47), gums, lips and buccal mucosa.

- *Skin lesions* – erythema nodosum-like lesions on the shins (Figure 4.48), acneiform lesions, vasculitis (Figure 4.49) and hypersensitivity (dermatographism) (Figure 4.50).

- *Recurrent genital ulceration* of the penis (Figure 4.51) and scrotum in males, and of the labia and vagina in females is present in about 90% of patients.

- *Uveitis.*

3. **Minor diagnostic criteria**

- *Arthritis* involving the knees, ankles and occasionally sarcoiliitis.

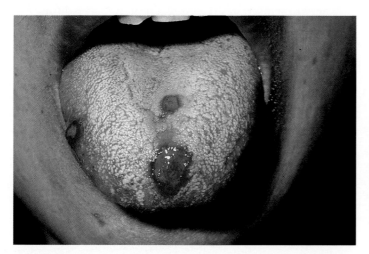

Figure 4.47 Aphthous ulceration of the tongue in Behçet disease

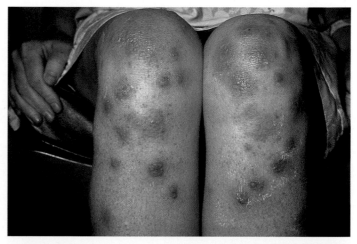

Figure 4.48 Erythema nodosum-like skin lesions in Behçet disease

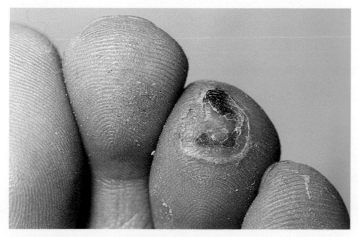

Figure 4.49 Vasculitis in Behçet disease

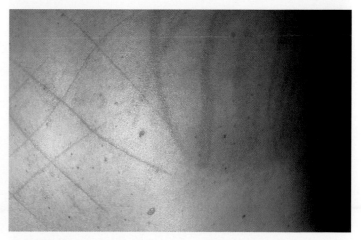

Figure 4.50 Dermatographism associated with skin hypersensitivity in Behçet disease

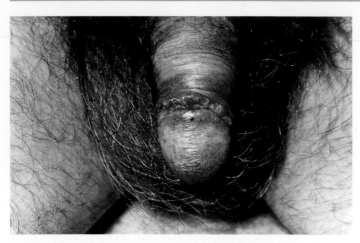

Figure 4.51 Genital ulceration in Behçet disease

- *Epididymitis* in males.
- *Intestinal ulceration* involving the ileocecal region.
- *Vascular* – obliterative thrombophlebitis of superficial and deep veins (Figure 4.52), large vessel arterial occlusion and aneurysm formation.
- *Central nervous system* brain stem syndromes and meningoencephalitis.

According to the presence or absence of the above criteria Behçet disease can be divided into complete and incomplete types as follows:

4. **Complete type** is characterized by four major criteria occurring either simultaneously or at different times during the course of the disease.

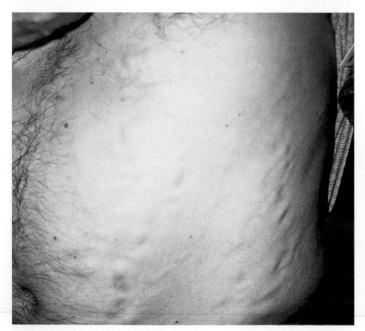

Figure 4.52 Dilated superficial veins secondary to deep obliterative thrombophlebitis in Behçet disease

5. **Incomplete type** is characterized by one of the following:

- Three major criteria.
- Two major criteria plus two minor criteria.
- Uveitis plus another major criterion.
- Uveitis plus two minor criteria.

Ocular features

The following ocular complications occur in up to 95% of men and 70% of women with Behçet disease. They are frequently bilateral and usually follow the systemic manifestations of the disease, although occasionally they may be the presenting feature. It is unusual for the systemic and ocular manifestations to develop simultaneously.

1. **Acute recurrent anterior uveitis** which may be simultaneously bilateral and frequently associated with a transient mobile hypopyon (Figure 4.53). Initially it responds well to treatment with topical steroids, but it may subsequently become chronic and eventually lead to phthisis bulbi.

2. **Retinitis** characterized by scattered, white, necrotic superficial infiltrates (Figure 4.54) may be seen during the acute stage of the systemic disease. The lesions are usually transient and heal without scarring.

3. **Retinal vasculitis** may involve both veins (periphlebitis) (Figure 4.55) and arteries (periarteritis) and is a serious problem because it may result in vascular occlusions and macular ischemia (Figure 4.56).

4. **Vascular leakage** may give rise to diffuse retinal edema, CME and disc edema.

5. **Vitritis**, which may be severe and persistent, is universally present in eyes with uveitis.

6. **Prognosis** is guarded, and between 5–10% of patients become blind despite treatment. The end stage of

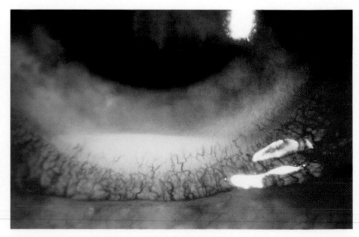

Figure 4.53 Hypopyon in Behçet disease

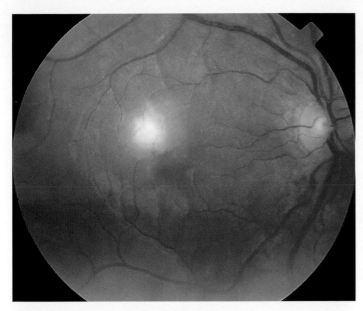

Figure 4.54 Retinitis in Behçet disease

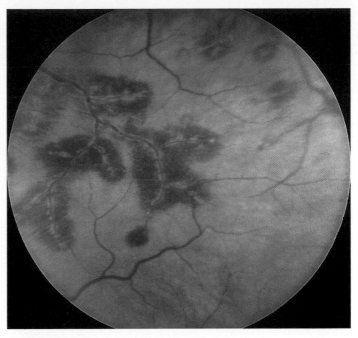

Figure 4.55 Retinal periphlebitis in Behçet disease

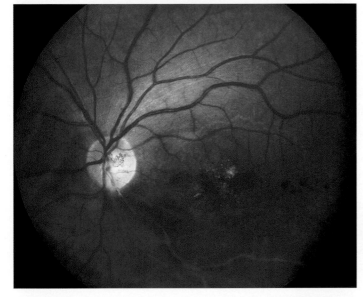

Figure 4.56 Vasculitis resulting in branch retinal vein occlusion in Behçet disease

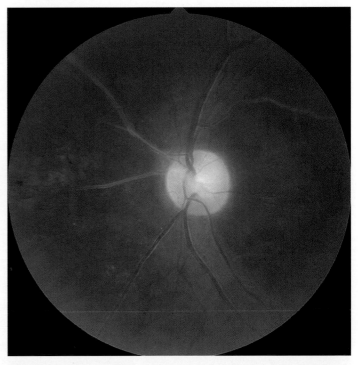

Figure 4.57 Old vascular occlusion and consecutive optic atrophy in Behçet disease

posterior segment involvement is characterized by optic atrophy, vascular attenuation and sheathing, variable chorioretinal scarring (Figure 4.57), and macular ischemia.

Treatment

1. **Anterior uveitis** is treated with topical steroids and mydriatics.

2. **Posterior uveitis** is treated with high doses of systemic steroids. Unfortunately, the inflammation frequently becomes steroid-resistant and requires alternative

Case study

1. History

A 35-year-old woman developed an upper respiratory tract infection associated with a sore throat, tongue ulcers, headache, malaise, episodic diarrhea, swelling of the left knee and wrists, and erythematous lesions on the arms and genitalia. She also noticed mildly blurred vision in both eyes. She was treated by her family doctor with antibiotics with little benefit and was referred to an ophthalmologist because of her eye problems.

2. Examination

Right eye

- Visual acuity was 6/9.

- Slitlamp biomicroscopy showed mild anterior uveitis (cells +2) and vitritis (cells +2).

- Fundus examination showed optic disc swelling, several superficial white retinal infiltrates, small hemorrhages and vasculitis (Figure 4.58a).

Left eye

- Similar to the right (Figure 4.58b).

3. FA

- Late hyperfluorescence of the optic discs, more marked in the left, due to leakage (Figure 4.58c and d).

4. Diagnosis

- Bilateral panuveitis and retinitis; and Behçet disease on the basis of four major criteria.

5. Treatment

- Topical treatment of anterior uveitis was with steroids and mydriatics.

- Systemic treatment was with oral prednisolone 80 mg daily and azathioprine 100 mg daily.

6. Course

- After a few days there was a dramatic improvement with disappearance of joint swelling and skin lesions.

- Systemic treatment was gradually tapered and discontinued after two months.

7. Outcome

- Three months later the uveitis was inactive and visual acuity in both eyes was 6/6.

8. Comment

Despite the very favorable response to treatment of both the ocular and systemic manifestations, it is important to realize that Behçet disease is frequently a recurrent disease.

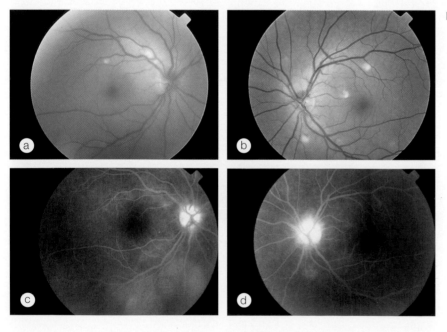

Figure 4.58 Behçet disease (see the text)

therapy with drugs also used to treat the systemic manifestations of the disease such as cyclosporine, colchicine, azathioprine, chlorambucil and levamisole.

Differential diagnosis

In patients with incomplete forms of Behçet disease, the systemic diagnosis may be uncertain because there are no definitive laboratory tests. It is therefore important to consider the following conditions:

1. **Recurrent anterior uveitis with hypopyon** may be associated with spondyloarthropathies. However, the uveitis is not usually simultaneously bilateral and the hypopyon is not mobile because it is frequently associated with a fibrinous exudate. In Behçet disease the uveitis is frequently simultaneously bilateral and the hypopyon shifts with gravity as the patient changes head positions.

2. **Retinal vasculitis** may be associated with sarcoidosis. However, sarcoid vasculitis involves only veins in a segmental manner and is rarely occlusive. In contrast, Behçet disease usually involves both arteries and veins, is diffuse and frequently occlusive.

3. **Retinal infiltrates** similar to those in Behçet disease may be seen in viral retinitis such as the acute retinal necrosis syndrome. However, in viral retinitis the infiltrates eventually coalesce. Multiple retinal infiltrates also occur in idiopathic acute multifocal retinitis. In contrast to Behçet disease the clinical course is favourable with return to normal vision within two to four months of onset.

FURTHER READING

BenEzra D, Cohen E. Treatment and visual prognosis in Behçet's disease. *Br J Ophthalmol* 1986;70:589–592.

Demiroglu H, Barista I, Dundar S. Risk factor assessment and prognosis of eye involvement in Behçet disease in Turkey. *Ophthalmology* 1997;104:701–705.

el-Asar AM, al-Momen AK, Alamro SA, et al. Bilateral central retinal vein occlusion in Behçet disease. *Clin Rheumatol* 1996;15:511–513.

International Behçet's study group. Criteria for diagnosis of Behçet's disease. *Lancet* 1990;335:1078–1080.

Michelson JB, Chisari FV. Behçet's disease. *Surv Ophthalmol* 1982;26:190–203.

Mochizuki M, Akduman L, Nussenblatt RB. Behçet disease. In: Pepose JS, Holland GN, Wilhelmus KR, editors. *Ocular immunology and inflammation*. St Louis: Mosby, 1996:663–675.

Sakamoto M, Akazawa K, Nishioka Y, et al. Prognostic factors of vision in patients with Behçet's disease. *Ophthalmology* 1995;102:317–321.

Tabbara KF. Chlorambucil in Behçet's disease: a reappraisal. *Ophthalmology* 1983;90:906–908.

Vogt-Koyanagi-Harada disease

The Vogt-Koyanagi-Harada (V-K-H) disease is an idiopathic, multisystem disorder which typically affects Hispanic, Japanese and pigmented individuals. Japanese patients have an increased prevalence of HLA-DR4 and Dw15. In practice, V-K-H can be sub-divided into Vogt-Koyanagi syndrome, characterized mainly by skin changes and anterior uveitis, and Harada disease, in which neurological features and exudative retinal detachment predominate.

Systemic features

1. **Localized alopecia** occurs in about 60% of patients.

2. **Poliosis**, a premature localized whitening of hair, involving the lashes and eyebrows is also common and usually develops several weeks after the onset of the disease. It may sometimes surround areas of alopecia.

3. **Vitiligo**, which consists of patches of skin hypopigmentation (Figure 4.59), usually follows the onset of visual symptoms by several weeks.

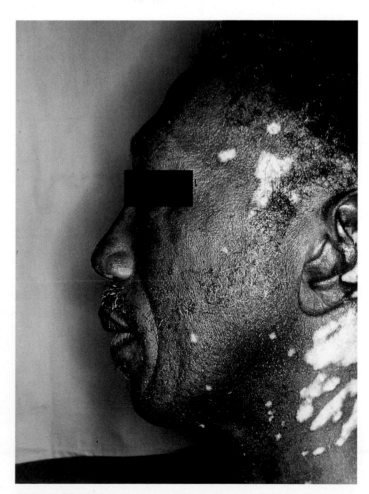

Figure 4.59 Vitiligo

4. Neurological

- *Meningitis*, which causes headache and neck stiffness, develops simultaneously with uveitis.

- *Encephalopathy* is less frequent than meningitis. It may be manifest as convulsions, cranial nerve palsies and paresis.

- *Auditory* features include tinnitus, vertigo and deafness.

- *CSF lymphocytosis* is present during the acute phase of the disease.

Ocular features

1. **Chronic granulomatous anterior uveitis** is characterized by mutton fat keratic precipitates and iris nodules. It runs a protracted course and frequently leads to the formation of posterior synechiae and cataract. Severe anterior uveitis typically occurs in patients with Vogt-Koyanagi syndrome, but mild anterior uveitis may also be seen in patients with Harada disease.

2. **Posterior segment** involvement occurs in patients with Harada disease and is frequently bilateral. In chronological order the findings are as follows:

- Multifocal choroiditis.

- Multifocal detachments of the sensory retina (Figure 4.60).

- Exudative retinal detachment (Figure 4.61).

- Residual lesions consist of atrophy and proliferation of the RPE.

3. **Treatment** of posterior segment involvement is with systemic steroids. Steroid-resistant patients may require systemic cyclosporine.

4. **Prognosis** is guarded and only 50% of patients have a final visual acuity better than 6/12.

5. **Differential diagnosis** of bilateral exudative retinal detachments

- Metastatic carcinoma to the choroid.

- Uveal effusion syndrome.

- Posterior scleritis.

- Toxemia of pregnancy.

- Bullous central serous retinopathy.

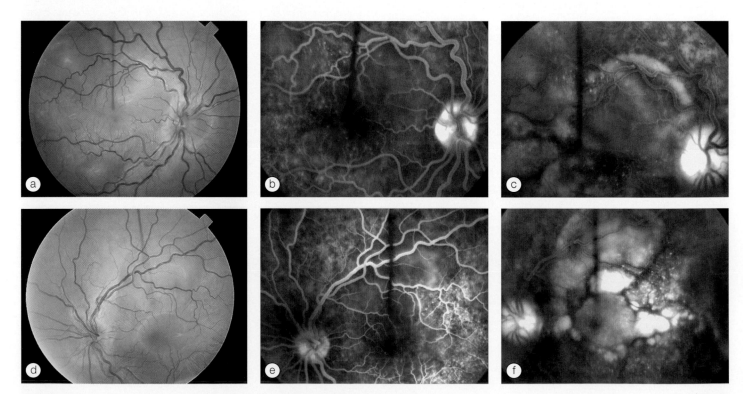

Figure 4.60 Multifocal detachments of the sensory retina in Harada disease (see the text)

Case study

1. History

An 18-year-old Hispanic woman presented with a week's history of subacute-onset of bilateral blurring of vision and headaches.

2. Examination

Right eye

- Visual acuity was 6/24.

- Slitlamp biomicroscopy showed mild anterior uveitis (cells +1) and mild vitritis (cells +2).

- Fundus examination showed optic disc hyperemia and retinal vascular tortuosity. There were also numerous deep yellow lesions and exudative macular detachments (see Figure 4.60a).

Left eye

- Visual acuity was CF at one meter.

- Slitlamp and fundus findings were similar to the right eye (see Figure 4.60d).

3. FA

Right eye

- *Early phase* showed numerous pinpoints of hyperfluorescence (see Figure 4.60b).

- *Later phase* showed large hyperfluorescent areas due to pooling of dye under the exudative retinal detachments (see Figure 4.60c).

Left eye

- Similar to the right eye (see Figure 4.60e and 4.60f).

4. Diagnosis

- Bilateral macular exudative retinal detachments: and Harada disease.

5. Treatment

- Oral prednisone 100 mg daily with gradual tapering every four days.

6. Course

- Within four weeks the retinal detachments resolved and the optic discs and retinal vessels returned to normal.

7. Outcome

Two months later visual acuity in both eyes was 6/9. Fundus examination showed residual pigmentary changes involving the perimacular areas and mid-periphery.

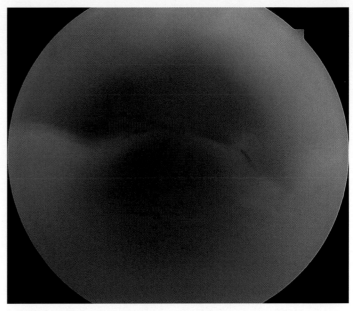

Figure 4.61 Inferior exudative retinal detachment in Harada disease

FURTHER READING

Beniz J, Forster DJ, Lean JS. Variations in clinical features of Vogt-Koyanagi-Harada syndrome. *Retina* 1991;11:275–280.

Kahn M, Pepose JS, Green WR et al. Immunocytologic findings in a case of Vogt-Koyanagi-Harada syndrome. *Ophthalmology* 1993;100:1191–1198.

Moorthy RS, Inomata H, Rao NA. Vogt-Koyanagi-Harada syndrome. *Surv Ophthalmol* 1995;39:265–292.

Perry HD, Font RL. Clinical and histopathologic observations in severe Vogt-Koyanagi-Harada syndrome. *Am J Ophthalmol* 1997;83:242–254.

Rao N. Mechanisms of inflammatory response in sympathetic ophthalmia and VKH syndrome. *Eye* 1997;11:213–216.

Rathinam SR, Namperumalsamy P, Nozik RA, et al. Vogt-Koyanagi-Harada syndrome after cutaneous injury. *Ophthalmology* 1999;106:635–638.

Rubasamen PE, Gass JDM. Vogt-Koyanagi-Harada syndrome; clinical course, therapy, and long-term outcome. *Arch Ophthalmol* 1991;109:682–687.

Acquired syphilis

Systemic features

Acquired syphilis is a sexually transmitted infection caused by the spirochaete *Treponema pallidum*. It is a systemic disease which, when untreated, has overt and covert stages:

1. The **primary stage** typically develops 9–90 days after exposure and is characterized by a painless ulcer (chancre) at the site of infection with associated regional lymphadenopathy.

2. The **secondary stage** usually appears by the eighth week of infection, although there may be considerable delay. Mucocutaneous involvement is usually the presenting feature. A macular, papular or mixed skin rash which may involve the trunk (Figure 4.62) or the palms and soles, is common. Systemic involvement may cause malaise, fever, generalized lymphadenopathy, meningitis, nephritis and hepatitis. The latent stage follows resolution of secondary syphilis and can be detected only by serological tests.

3. The **tertiary stage** occurs in about 30% of untreated patients within 5–30 years. The main lesions of tertiary syphilis are:

- Aortitis.

- Neurosyphilis which causes tabes dorsalis or general paralysis of the insane.

- Benign late syphilis characterized by gummata in tissues other than the cardiovascular system and CNS.

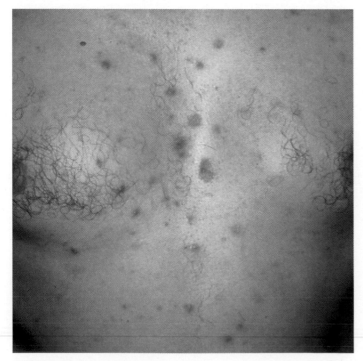

Figure 4.62 Rash in secondary syphilis

Syphilis and AIDS

Patients at risk from AIDS are also at increased risk from other sexually transmitted diseases, such as syphilis, so that the two conditions can coexist. It appears that concomitant HIV infection may alter the natural course of syphilis, rendering the disease more aggressive with unusual manifestations. All patients with AIDS should therefore also be tested for syphilis and *vice versa*.

Diagnostic tests

One or both of the following tests should be ordered when screening patients with uveitis for syphilis.

1. **FTA-ABS** (fluorescent treponemal antibody absorption) test is specific for treponemal antibodies. Once positive, it remains positive throughout the patient's life despite treatment. However, the test is not titratable and is read as: reactive, weakly reactive or non-reactive.

2. **MHA-TP** (microhemagglutination assay with *Treponema pallidum* antigen) is specific for treponemal antibodies but it may be negative in early primary syphilis.

Ocular features

Ocular syphilis is uncommon and there are no pathognomonic signs. Eye involvement typically occurs during the secondary and tertiary stages although occasionally it may also be seen during the primary stage. The ability of syphilis to mimic many different ocular disorders can lead to misdiagnosis and delay of appropriate therapy. The disease must therefore be suspected in any case of intraocular inflammation that is resistant to conventional therapy. External features include madarosis, scleritis, keratitis and iridocyclitis. Posterior segment disease may take one of the following forms.

1. **Vitritis** is the most common finding.

2. **Multifocal chorioretinitis** is the next most common finding. Healed lesions appear as focal areas of chorioretinal atrophy associated with hyperpigmentation (Figure 4.63). Occasionally extensive pigmentary changes with perivascular bone spicules, similar to those seen in retinitis pigmentosa, may be associated with night blindness and a ring scotoma.

3. **Unifocal chorioretinitis** is less common and frequently bilateral. It is characterized by an inflammatory focus near the disc (juxtapapillary choroiditis) or at the macula (central choroiditis).

4. **Neuroretinitis** primarily involves the retina and optic nerve head, and is independent of choroidal inflammation. The fundus shows disc edema and a macular star (Figure 4.64). The retinal veins may be engorged, and peripapillary cotton-wool spots or flame-shaped hemorrhages may appear. Unless treated with antisyphilitic drugs, neuroretinitis is progressive. The

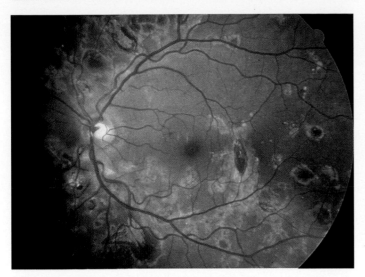

Figure 4.63 Old syphilitic multifocal chorioretinitis

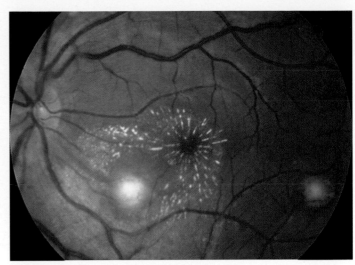

Figure 4.64 Active syphilitic neuroretinitis

retinal blood vessels eventually become replaced by white strands and optic atrophy ensues (Figure 4.65).

Treatment

Conventional doses of penicillin are inadequate in ocular syphilis and the therapeutic regimen is the same as for neurosyphilis which should be ruled out. One of the following three regimen may be used:

1. 12–24 mega units (MU) of aqueous penicillin G intravenously daily for 10–15 days.

2. Alternative treatment is with either Procaine penicillin intramuscularly 2.4 MU daily supplemented with oral probenecid (2 g daily), or oral amoxycillin 3 g twice daily, for 28 days.

3. Patients allergic to penicillin can be treated with oral tetracycline 500 mg four times daily for 30 days or oral erythromycin 500 mg four times daily for 30 days.

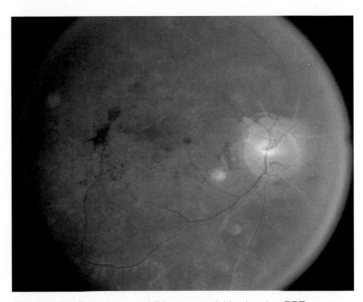

Figure 4.65 End-stage syphilitic neuroretinitis showing RPE changes, vascular sheathing and attenuation, and consecutive optic atrophy

FURTHER READING

Barile GR, Flynn TE. Syphilis exposure in patients with uveitis. *Ophthalmology* 1997;104:1605–1609.

Browning DJ. Posterior segment manifestations of active ocular syphilis. Their response to a neurosyphilis regimen of penicillin therapy, and the influence of human immunodeficiency virus status on response. *Ophthalmology* 2000;107:2015–2023.

Friberg TR. Syphilitic chorioretinitis. *Arch Ophthalmol* 1989;107:1676–1677.

Halpern LS, Berger AS, Grand MG. Syphilitic disc edema and periphlebitis. *Retina* 1990;10:223–225.

Kuo IC, Kapusta MA, Rao N. Vitritis as the primary manifestation of ocular syphilis in patients with HIV infection. *Am J Ophthalmol* 1998;125:306–311.

Margo CE, Hamed LM. Ocular syphilis. *Surv Ophthalmol* 1992;37:203–220.

Shalaby IA, Dunn JP, Semba RD, et al. Syphilitic uveitis in human immunodeficiency virus-infected patients. *Arch Ophthalmol* 1997;115:469–473.

Tamesis RR, Foster CS. Ocular syphilis. *Ophthalmology* 1990;97:1281–1287.

Toxocariasis

Pathogenesis

Toxocariasis is caused by infection (infestation) with a common intestinal ascarid (roundworm) of dogs called *Toxocara canis*. About 80% of puppies between the ages of two and six months are infested with this worm. Human infection is by accidental ingestion of soil or food contaminated with ova shed in dog feces. Very young children who eat dirt (pica) or are in close contact with puppies are at particular risk of acquiring the disease. In the human intestine, the ova develop into larvae which penetrate the intestinal wall and travel to various organs, such as the liver, lungs, skin, brain and eyes. When the larvae die, they disintegrate and cause an inflammatory reaction followed by granulation. Clinically, human infection can take one of the following forms:

1. **Visceral larva migrans** (VLM) is caused by severe systemic infection which usually occurs at about the age of two years. The clinical features, which vary in severity, include a low-grade fever, hepatosplenomegaly, pneumonitis, convulsions and, rarely, death. The blood shows a leucocytosis and marked eosinophilia.

2. **Ocular toxocariasis** differs markedly from VLM. Patients with ocular involvement are otherwise healthy and they have a normal white cell count with absence of eosinophilia. A history of pica is less common, and the average age at presentation is considerably older (7.5 years) compared with VLM (2 years). The three most common ocular lesions are:

* *Chronic endophthalmitis-like picture.*

* *Posterior pole granuloma.*

* *Peripheral granuloma.*

Other less common manifestations include: anterior uveitis, optic disc granuloma, optic papillitis, a localized vitreous abscess and retinal tracks. Only the three most common lesions will be described; all affect only one eye.

Diagnostic tests

1. **Enzyme-linked immunosorbent assay** (ELISA) can be used to determine the level of serum antibodies to *Toxocara canis*. When ocular toxocariasis is suspected, exact ELISA titers should be requested, including testing of undiluted serum. Any positive titer is consistent with, but not necessarily diagnostic of, toxocariasis. It must therefore be interpreted in conjunction with the clinical findings. A positive titer does not therefore exclude the possibility of retinoblastoma.

2. **Ultrasonography** may be useful both in establishing the diagnosis in eyes with hazy media and in excluding other causes of leukocoria.

Chronic endophthalmitis

1. **Presentation** is between the ages of two and nine years with leukocoria, strabismus or unilateral visual loss.

2. **Signs**

* Anterior uveitis and vitritis.

* In some cases, there may be a peripheral granuloma.

* In other cases the peripheral retina and pars plana are covered by a dense greyish-white exudate, similar to the 'snowbanking' seen in pars planitis (Figure 4.66).

3. **Treatment**

* Systemic or periocular steroids may be helpful in some cases.

* Vitreoretinal surgery may be beneficial in some eyes with tractional retinal detachment.

4. **Prognosis** in most cases is very poor and some eyes eventually require enucleation. The main causes of visual loss are:

* Tractional retinal detachment secondary to contraction of vitreoretinal membranes.

* Ocular hypotony and phthisis bulbi caused by separation of the ciliary body from the sclera brought about by contraction of a cyclitic membrane.

* Cataract.

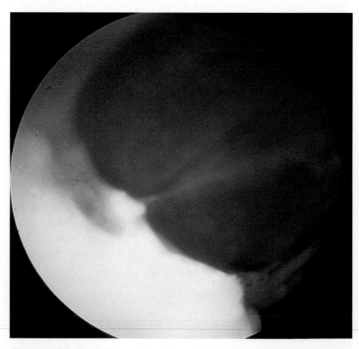

Figure 4.66 Extensive peripheral exudation in chronic toxocara endophthalmitis

Posterior pole granuloma

1. **Presentation** is typically with unilateral visual impairment between the ages of 6 and 14 years.

2. **Signs**

• Anterior uveitis and vitritis are absent.

• Round, yellow-white, solid granuloma which varies between one to two disc-diameters in diameter.

• Usually the granuloma is located either at the macula (Figure 4.67) or between the macula and the optic disc.

• Occasionally the granuloma involves the optic nerve head.

• Associated findings include retinal stress lines, distortion of blood vessels, and occasionally the lesion is surrounded by yellow hard exudates.

• Once formed, the granuloma is usually stationary and the extent of visual loss is dependent on its location.

3. **Complications**, which are rare, include retinal detachment and subretinal hemorrhage.

Peripheral granuloma

1. **Presentation** is usually during adolescence or adult life as a result of visual impairment from distortion of the macula or retinal detachment. In uncomplicated cases, the lesion may remain undetected throughout life.

2. **Signs**

• Anterior uveitis and vitritis are absent.

• A white hemispherical granuloma located at or anterior to the equator in any quadrant of the fundus (Figure 4.68).

• Vitreous bands frequently extend from the lesion to the posterior fundus and on contracting may give rise to 'dragging' of the disc and straightening of blood vessels (Figure 4.69).

3. **Complications** in severe cases are the following:

• *Macular heterotopia* caused by contraction of the bands connecting the granuloma with the optic nerve head.

• *Retinal detachment* caused by contraction of vitreoretinal bands. In some cases vitreoretinal surgery may be successful in reattaching the retina.

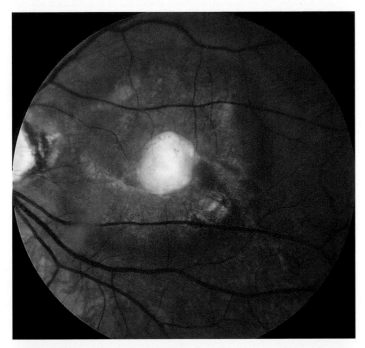

Figure 4.67 Posterior toxocara granuloma

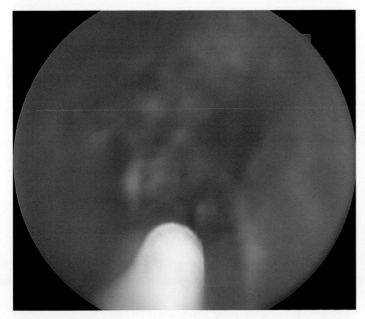

Figure 4.68 Peripheral toxocara granuloma

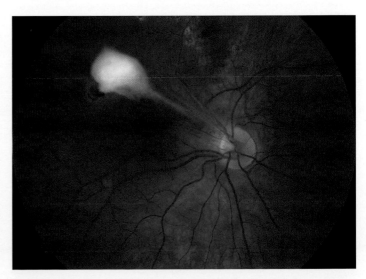

Figure 4.69 Vitreous bands between the optic disc and a toxocara granuloma

FURTHER READING

Dinning WJ, Gillespie SH, Cooling RJ, et al. Toxocariasis: a practical approach to management of ocular disease. *Eye* 1988;2:580–582.

Sharkey JA, McKay PS. Ocular toxocariasis in a patient with repeatedly negative ELISA titre to *Toxoplasma canis*. *Br J Ophthalmol* 1993;77:253–254.

Shields JA. Ocular toxocariasis: a review. *Surv Ophthalmol* 1984;28:361–381.

Small KW, McCuen BW, deJuan E, et al. Surgical management of retinal traction caused by toxocariasis. *Am J Ophthalmol* 1989;108:10–14.

Sorr EM. Meandering ocular toxocariasis. *Retina* 1984;4:90–96.

Wan WL, Cano MR, Pince KJ, et al. Echographic characteristics of ocular toxocariasis. *Ophthalmology* 1991;98:28–32.

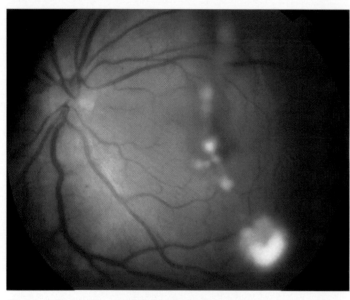

Figure 4.70 Multifocal candida retinitis with early vitreous involvement

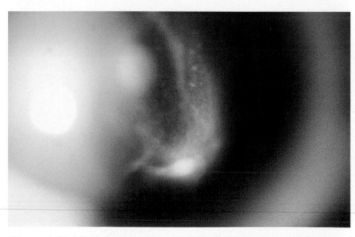

Figure 4.71 Vitritis and a 'cotton-ball' filtrate in ocular candidiasis

Candidiasis

Systemic risk factors

Candida albicans, a yeast-like fungus, is a frequent commensal of the human skin, mouth, gastrointestinal tract and vagina. Candidiasis is an opportunist infection in which the organism acquires pathogenic properties. Candidemia, which may result in ocular involvement, occurs in three main groups of patients.

1. **Drug addicts** may become infected through the use of non-sterile needles and syringes. Not infrequently, they have no obvious evidence of disseminated candidiasis, and negative blood and urine cultures for *Candida* sp. In this group, the diagnosis may be missed unless the skin is carefully examined for evidence of injection site scars.

2. **Patients with long-term indwelling catheters** used for hemodialysis or intravenous nutrition following extensive bowel surgery, are at increased risk.

3. **Compromised hosts** are severely debilitated patients with decreased immunity either from an underlying systemic disease (AIDS, malignancies) or from long-term treatment with drugs, such as antibiotics, steroids and cytotoxic agents.

Diagnosis

1. **Presentation** is with gradual unilateral blurring of vision and floaters.

2. **Signs** in chronological order are as follows:

• The initial focus is in the choroid.

• The organisms then invade the retina and give rise to a multifocal retinitis manifest as small, round, white, slightly elevated lesions with indistinct borders (Figure 4.70).

• The retinal lesions enlarge and extend into the vitreous gel, giving rise to floating white 'cotton-ball' colonies (Figure 4.71).

• Chronic endophthalmitis characterized by severe vitreous infiltration (Figure 4.72).

3. **Course** is relatively chronic and may result in the development of retinal necrosis and retinal detachment.

4. **Vitreous biopsy** and culture may be required to confirm the diagnosis (see below).

Treatment

1. **Medical treatment** is with a combination of oral flucytosine 150 mg/kg daily and fluconazole 200–400 mg daily for three weeks.

2. **Pars plana vitrectomy** is indicated for moderate to severe vitreous involvement (endophthalmitis). At the time of vitrectomy, smears and cultures should be taken to

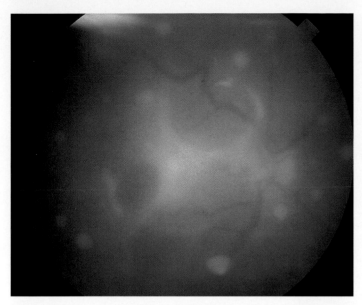

Figure 4.72 Chronic candida endophthalmitis with many 'cotton-balls'

confirm the diagnosis and test the sensitivity of the organisms to antifungal agents and an injection of 5 mg of amphotericin B is given into the central vitreous cavity.

Differential diagnosis

1. Multifocal retinitis

• Behçet syndrome.

• Cytomegalovirus retinitis.

• Idiopathic acute multifocal retinitis.

2. Vitreous cotton-balls

• Idiopathic intermediate uveitis.

• Sarcoidosis.

FURTHER READING

Chignell AH. Endogenous candidiasis. *J Royal Soc Med* 1992;85:721–724.

Donahue SP, Greven CM, Zuravleff JJ, et al. Intraocular candidiasis in patients with candidemia. Clinical implications derived from a prospective multicenter study. *Ophthalmology* 1994;101:1302–1309.

Luttrull JK, Wan WL, Kubak BM, et al. Treatment of ocular fungal infections with oral fluconazole. *Am J Ophthalmol* 1995;119:477–481.

Congenital rubella
Systemic features

Rubella (German measles) is usually a benign febrile exanthema. Congenital rubella results from transplacental transmission of virus to the fetus from an infected mother, usually during the first trimester of pregnancy. This may lead to serious chronic fetal infection and malformations. It appears that the risk to the fetus is closely related to the stage of gestation at the time of maternal infection. Fetal infection is about 50% during the first eight weeks, 33% between weeks 9 and 12, and about 10% between weeks 13 and 24. Each of the various organs affected has its own period of susceptibility to the infection, after which no gross malformations are produced. Systemic complications of maternal rubella include: spontaneous abortion, stillbirth, congenital heart malformations, deafness, microcephaly, mental handicap, hypotonia, hepatosplenomegaly, thrombocytopenic purpura, pneumonitis, myocarditis and metaphyseal bone lesions.

Retinopathy

Retinal involvement is the most common ocular complication, but the exact incidence is unknown because cataracts frequently impair visualization of the fundus. Retinopathy may involve one or both eyes.

1. Signs

• 'Salt-and-pepper' pigmentary disturbance, most often involving the posterior pole and most marked at the macula (Figure 4.73a).

• The optic nerve head and retinal blood vessels are usually normal, although the foveal reflex may be absent.

2. FA

• *Venous phase* – oval areas of hypofluorescence within which retinal and choroidal blood vessels are normal (Figure 4.73b).

• *Late phase* – the hypofluorescent spots are surrounded by a ring of hyperfluorescence from leakage from the surrounding choroid and diffuse mottled hyperfluorescence caused by irregular loss of the RPE (Figure 4.73c and 4.73d).

3. Prognosis is usually good and visual acuity may be normal or slightly impaired. A small percentage of eyes may later develop CNV (Figure 4.74).

Other ocular manifestations

1. Cataract is the second most common complication, affecting about 15% of infants. The pearly nuclear cataract may be bilateral or unilateral, and is frequently associated with microphthalmos.

2. Microphthalmos affects 10–20% of infants and is associated with cataracts, optic nerve abnormalities and glaucoma.

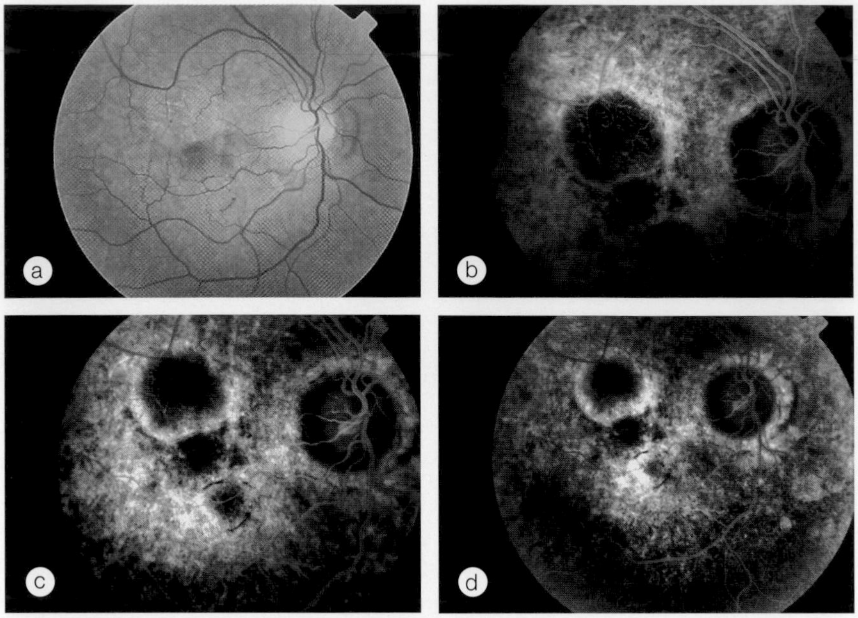

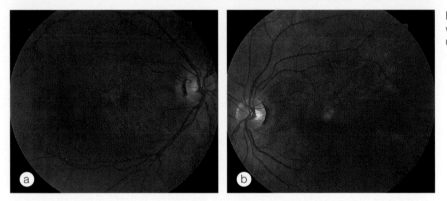

Figure 4.73 Rubella retinopathy (see the text)

Figure 4.74 Bilateral old rubella retinopathy with left macular scarring due to previous CNV

3. **Glaucoma** develops in about 10% of eyes, usually during the neonatal period. It may or may not be associated with cataract. When occurring in a microphthalmic eye, the raised intraocular pressure could enlarge the cornea to normal size. When occurring in a normal-size eye the cornea may become larger than normal (buphthalmos). Corneal haze resulting from corneal edema is also an important feature of glaucoma.

4. **Miscellaneous manifestations**, which are less common, are corneal haze, iritis, iris atrophy and extreme refractive errors. Pendular nystagmus and strabismus may develop as a consequence of the various ocular abnormalities.

FURTHER READING

Givens KT, Lee DA, Jones T, et al. Congenital rubella syndrome: ophthalmic manifestations and associated systemic disorders. *Br J Ophthalmol* 1993;77:358–363.

Krill AE. The retinal disease of rubella. *Arch Ophthalmol* 1967;77:445–449.

Wolff SM. The ocular manifestations of congenital rubella. *Trans Am Ophthalmol Soc* 1972;70:577–614.

Acute retinal necrosis

Acute retinal necrosis (ARN) is a rare but devastating necrotizing retinitis. It typically affects otherwise healthy individuals of all ages. ARN is a biphasic disease which tends to be caused by herpes simplex in younger patients and herpes zoster in older individuals. Males are more frequently affected than females by a 2:1 ratio. The disease is unilateral in two-thirds of cases.

Diagnosis

1. **Presentation** is initially unilateral and varies according to severity. Some patients develop severe visual impairment over a few days associated with pain whereas others have an insidious onset with mild visual symptoms such as floaters.

2. **Signs**, in chronological order, are as follows:

   - Anterior granulomatous uveitis is universal and unless the fundus is examined the diagnosis may be missed.

   - Moderate to severe vitritis is universal.

   - Peripheral retinal periarteritis is universal.

   - Multifocal, deep, yellow-white, retinal infiltrates (Figure 4.75).

   - The lesions gradually become confluent and represent a full-thickness necrotizing retinitis (Figure 4.76).

   - The posterior pole is usually spared until late so that visual acuity may remain fairly good despite severe necrosis of the surrounding retina.

   - Other signs include disc edema, choroidal thickening and retinal hemorrhages.

3. **Course** lasts 6–12 weeks with resolution of the acute lesions, leaving behind a transparent and necrotic retina with hyperpigmented borders (Figure 4.77). Unless the patient received appropriate treatment the second eye becomes involved in 30% of patients, usually within two months, although in some patients the interval may be much longer.

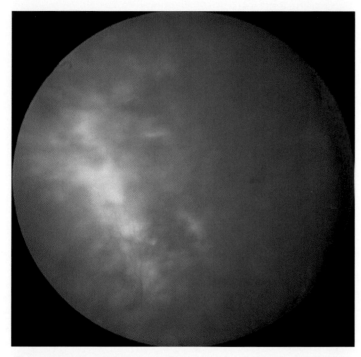

Figure 4.75 Peripheral retinal infiltrates in acute retinal necrosis

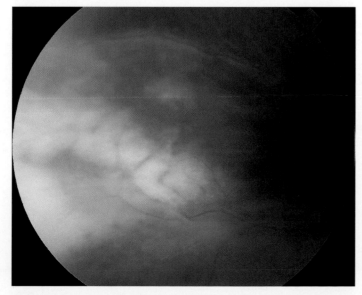

Figure 4.76 Confluent retinal infiltration in acute retinal necrosis

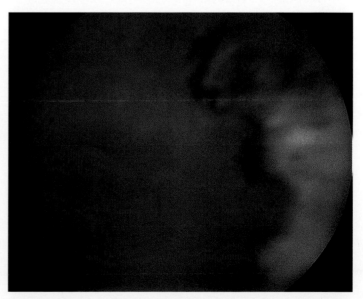

Figure 4.77 Resolved acute retinal necrosis with a hyperpigmented border

Prognosis

The prognosis is relatively poor, with 60% of patients having a final visual acuity of less than 6/60. The following are the main vision-threatening complications:

1. **Rhegmatogenous retinal detachment** which develops as a result of the formation of retinal holes at the margin of uninvolved and involved zones. The results of treatment by vitrectomy are good.

2. **Tractional retinal detachment** which is less common and caused by secondary condensation and fibrosis of the vitreous base.

3. **Ischemic optic neuropathy** caused by thrombotic arteriolar occlusion and infiltration of the optic nerve by inflammatory cells.

4. **Retinal vein occlusion** secondary to periphlebitis.

Treatment

1. **Systemic aciclovir** initially given intravenously for ten days and then orally for four to six weeks may hasten resolution of the acute retinal lesions but does not prevent retinal detachment. Long-term therapy may be required in some patients to prevent recurrences.

2. **Systemic steroids** are started a few days after the initiation of antiviral therapy.

3. **Aspirin** may be used in an effort to prevent vascular obstructive complications.

4. **Prophylactic peripheral laser photocoagulation**, which creates a chorioretinal adhesion in areas of potential retinal break formation, may be effective in preventing retinal detachment if applied early.

5. **Vitreoretinal surgery**, including silicone injection, may be successful in treating complicated retinal detachments.

Differential diagnosis

1. **Behçet disease**

- *Similarities* – panuveitis, retinitis and necrotizing periarteritis.

- *Differences* – onset and course are more chronic, presence of systemic features and non-granulomatous anterior uveitis.

2. **Cytomegalovirus retinitis**

- *Similarities* – retinitis and vasculitis.

- *Differences* – onset and course are more chronic, mild or absent vitritis and anterior uveitis.

3. **Progressive outer retinal necrosis**

- *Similarities* – progressive retinal necrosis with a poor prognosis.

- *Differences* – only occurs in AIDS, more rapid course and absence of intraocular inflammation.

FURTHER READING

Blumenkranz MS, Culbertson WW, Clarkson JG, et al. Treatment of the acute retinal necrosis syndrome with intravenous acyclovir. *Ophthalmology* 1986;93:296–300.

Blumenkratz MS, Clarkson JG, Culbertson WW, et al. Visual results and complications after retinal reattachment in the acute retinal necrosis syndrome. *Retina* 1989;9:170–174.

Crapotta JA, Freeman WR, Feldman RM, et al. Visual outcome in acute retinal necrosis. *Retina* 1993;13:208–213.

Culbertson WW, Blumenkranz MS, Pepose JS, et al. Varicella zoster virus is a cause of the acute retinal necrosis syndrome. *Ophthalmology* 1986;93:559–569.

Duker JS, Blumenkranz MS. Diagnosis and management of the acute retinal necrosis (ARN) syndrome. *Surv Ophthalmol* 1991;35:327–343.

Duker JS, Nielsen JC, Eagle RC Jr, et al. Rapidly progressive acute retinal necrosis secondary to herpes simplex virus type 1. *Ophthalmology* 1990;97:1638–1643.

Holland GN. Standard diagnostic criteria for the acute retinal nerosis syndrome. *Am J Ophthalmol* 1994;117:663–666.

Acute posterior multifocal placoid pigment epitheliopathy

Diagnosis

Acute posterior multifocal placoid pigment epitheliopathy (APMPPE) is an uncommon, idiopathic, bilateral, self-limiting condition which typically affects healthy young adults. In about one-third of patients APMPPE follows a flu-like illness, and a few may also develop erythema nodosum. It is thought that in some cases APMPPE may be the initial manifestation of a central nervous system angiitis. The condition affects both sexes equally and there is an association with HLA-B7 and HLA-DR2.

1. **Presentation** is with subacute visual impairment and paracentral scotomas. Within a few days the fellow eye also becomes affected.

2. **Signs**

- Multiple, large, cream-colored or grayish-white, subretinal plaque-like lesions of variable size (Figure 4.78).

- The lesions typically begin at the posterior pole and then extend to involve the post-equatorial fundus.

- Vitritis in 50% of cases.

- Occasionaly findings include anterior uveitis, disc edema and retinal periphlebitis.

3. **Course** – after a few weeks during which the fundus lesions fade leaving variable residual multifocal areas of depigmentation and clumping of the RPE (Figure 4.79).

4. **FA** of active lesions shows early dense hypofluorescence due to blockage (Figure 4.80b and 4.80d) and late

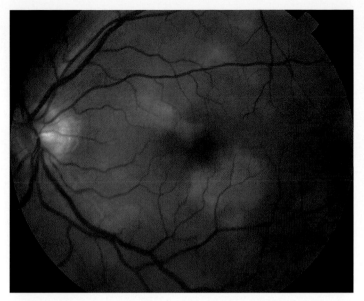

Figure 4.78 Fresh lesions in acute posterior multifocal placoid pigment epitheliopathy

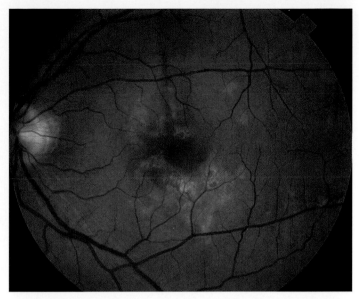

Figure 4.79 Residual lesions in posterior multifocal placoid pigment epitheliopathy

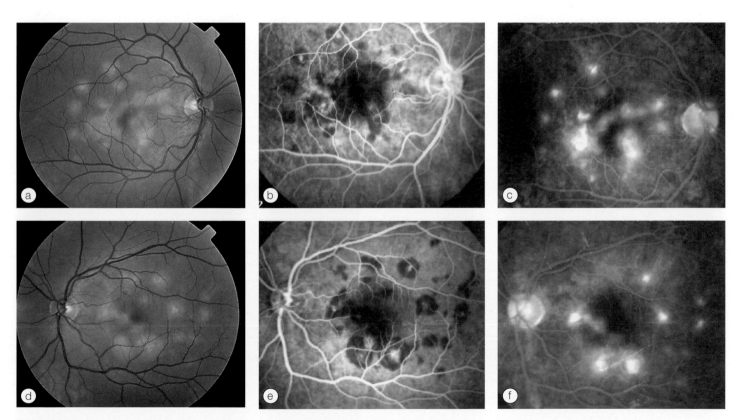

Figure 4.80 Acute posterior multifocal placoid pigment epitheliopathy (see the text)

hyperfluorescence due to staining (Figure 4.80c and 4.80f). These findings can be explained by occlusion of the choriocapillaris which leads to swelling of the RPE.

Prognosis

Despite the lack of treatment the prognosis is good in the vast majority of cases with a slow recovery to normal or near normal vision which may take up to six months. Some patients complain of residual paracentral scotomas. CNV is a very rare late complication.

Differential diagnosis

1. Serpiginous choroidopathy

- *Similarities* – early lesions may resemble APMPPE.

- *Differences* – older age group, chronic and poor prognosis.

2. MEWDS

- *Similarities* – causes subacute visual loss in healthy young adults and has a good prognosis.

- *Differences* – fundus lesions are smaller and unilateral.

3. Harada disease

- *Similarities* – diffuse choroidal infiltrates during acute stage and similar residual RPE changes during the inactive stage.

- *Differences* – typically affects specific ethnic groups, exudative retinal detachment.

FURTHER READING

Damato BE, Nanjiani M, Foulds WS. Acute posterior multifocal placoid pigment epitheliopathy. A follow-up study. *Trans Ophthalmol Soc UK* 1983;103:517–522.

Gass JMD. Acute posterior multifocal placoid pigment epitheliopathy. *Arch Ophthalmol* 1968;80:177–185.

Isashiki M, Koide H, Yamashita T, et al. Acute posterior multifocal placoid pigment epitheliopathy associated with diffuse retinal vasculitis and late haemorrhagic macular detachment. *Br J Ophthalmol* 1986;70:255–259.

Kersten DH, Lessell S, Carlow TJ. Acute posterior multifocal placoid pigment epitheliopathy and late-onset meningoencephalitis. *Ophthalmology* 1987;94:393–396.

Laatikainen LT, Immonen IJR. Acute posterior multifocal placoid pigment epitheliopathy in connection with acute nephritis. *Retina* 1988;8:122–124.

Ryan SJ, Maumenee AE. Acute posterior multifocal placoid pigment epitheliopathy. *Am J Ophthalmol* 1972;81:1066–1077.

Savino PJ, Weinberg RJ, Yasin JC, et al. Diverse manifestations of acute posterior multifocal placoid pigment epitheliopathy. *Am J Ophthalmol* 1974;77:679–662.

Serpiginous choroidopathy

Diagnosis

Serpiginous choroidopathy is a rare, idiopathic, progressive inflammatory chorioretinopathy which typically affects patients between the fourth and sixth decades of life. The disease is usually bilateral, but the extent of involvement is frequently asymmetrical. Both sexes are equally affected.

1. **Presentation** is with unilateral blurring of central vision or metamorphopsia as a result of macular involvement. After a variable period of time the fellow eye is also affected although it is not uncommon to find evidence of inactive asymptomatic disease in the fellow eye at the time of presentation.

2. **Signs**

- Active lesions consist of gray-white to yellow-white subretinal lesions with hazy borders.

- The lesions typically start around the optic disc and then gradually spread outwards in a snake-like manner along the major vascular arcades and towards the macula (Figure 4.81).

- Rarely the initial lesion involves the macula.

- Vitritis is present in about 30% of eyes and a mild anterior uveitis may also be present in some cases.

3. **Course**

- The course lasts many years in an episodic and recurrent fashion and it is not uncommon for disease activity to recur after several months of remission.

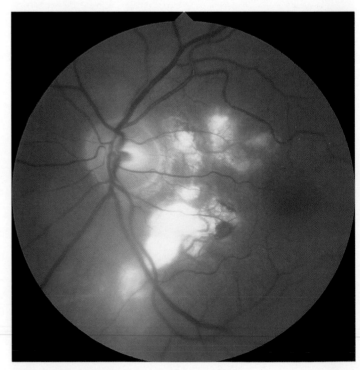

Figure 4.81 Active serpiginous choroidopathy

- Recurrences are characterized by yellow-gray extensions at the level of the choriocapillaris, contiguous or as satellites to existing areas of chorioretinal atrophy.

- Inactive lesions are characterized by scalloped, atrophic, 'punched-out' areas of choroidal atrophy associated with RPE changes (Figure 4.82).

4. **FA** of active lesions shows early hypofluorescence due to blockage and late hyperfluorescence due to staining.

5. **EOG** is decreased.

Prognosis

The prognosis is generally poor. Visual loss caused by involvement of the fovea occurs in about 50% of cases. It is usually profound and permanent. Some eyes develop CNV associated with an old scar which may be amenable to laser photocoagulation. Subretinal fibrosis is a rare late complication.

Treatment

Currently there is no definitive treatment strategy for serpiginous choroidopathy. Treatment options include triple therapy with a combination of systemic corticosteroids, azathioprine and cyclosporine although a recent report has suggested that early monotherapy with cyclosporine may be adequate.

FURTHER READING

Araujo AAQ, Wells AP, Dick AD, et al. Early treatment with cyclosporin in serpiginous choroidopathy maintains remission and good visual outcome. *Br J Ophthalmol* 2000;84:979–982.

Hardy RA, Schatz H. Macular geographic helicoid choroidopathy. *Arch Ophthalmol* 1987;105:1237–1242.

Hooper PL, Kaplan HJ. Triple agent immunosuppression in serpiginous choroiditis. *Ophthalmology* 1991;98:944–952.

Jampol LM, Orth D, Daily MJ. Subretinal neovascularization with geographic (serpiginous) choroiditis. *Am J Ophthalmol* 1979;88:683–689.

Mansour AM, Jampol LM, Packo KH, et al. Macular serpiginous choroidopathy. *Retina* 1988;8:125–131.

Secchi AG, Tognon MS, Maselli C. Cyclosporine-A in the treatment of serpiginous choroiditis. *Int Ophthalmol* 1990;14:395–399.

Wu JS, Lewis H, Fine SL, et al. Clinicopathologic findings in a patient with serpiginous choroidopathy and treated choroidal neovascularization. *Retina* 1989;9:292–301.

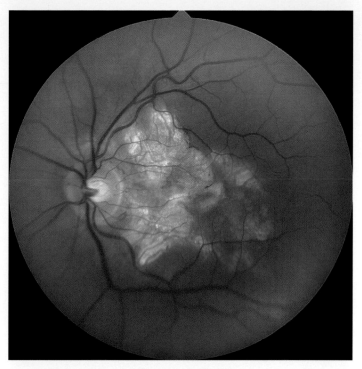

Figure 4.82 Inactive serpiginous choroidopathy

Birdshot retinochoroidopathy

Diagnosis

Birdshot retinochoroidopathy is an uncommon, bilateral, probably autoimmune, chronic inflammatory disease of the retina and choroid which typically affects middle-aged individuals. About 90% of patients are positive for HLA-A29.

1. **Presentation** is with painless impairment of central vision associated with nyctalopia, and with vitreous floaters. Disturbances of color vision are also common. The severity of visual disturbance is frequently out of proportion to the measured visual acuity, indicating diffuse retinal dysfunction.

2. **Signs** are usually bilateral but may be asymmetrical.

- Minimal if any anterior uveitis.

- Diffuse vitritis without snowbanking.

- Acute lesions consist of distinctive, subretinal, poorly defined, cream-coloured, small (100–300 μm) ovoid spots distributed in one of the following four patterns:
   a. Involving the macula (Figure 4.83) and mid-periphery (Figure 4.84).
   b. With relative macular sparing (Figure 4.85).
   c. With macular predominance.
   d. Asymmetric with predominance of lesions in the inferonasal fundus with relative macular sparing.

3. **Course** is characterized by exacerbations and remissions over several years. With time some of the lesions may become confluent. Inactive lesions consist of well delineated, white atrophic spots (Figure 4.86).

4. FA during the active stage may be useful in demonstrating the presence of CME and CNV. Initially, the lesions may remain silent throughout the angiogram if they do not affect the RPE. Thus more lesions may be seen clinically than angiographically. Later there may be staining of the lesions as the RPE becomes affected (Figure 4.87b).

5. ERG is decreased.

Prognosis

The prognosis is guarded. About 20% of patients have a self limited course and maintain normal visual acuity. The remainder have variable impairment of visual acuity in one or both eyes as a result of one or more of the following complications:

- CME which is eventually present in over 50% of cases.

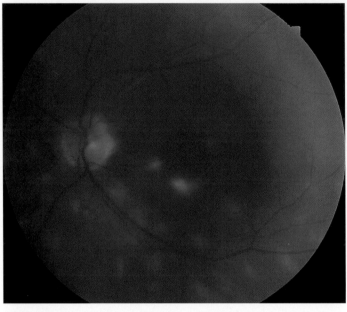

Figure 4.83 Active birdshot retinochoroidopathy with macula involvement

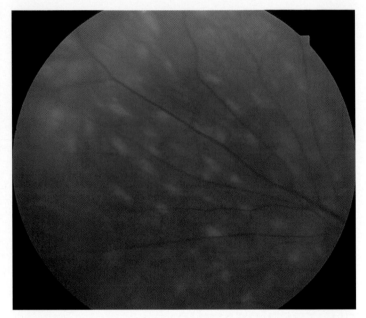

Figure 4.84 Mid-peripheral lesions in birdshot retinochoroidopathy

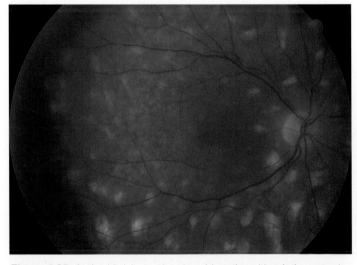

Figure 4.85 Active birdshot retinochoroidopathy with relative macular scaring

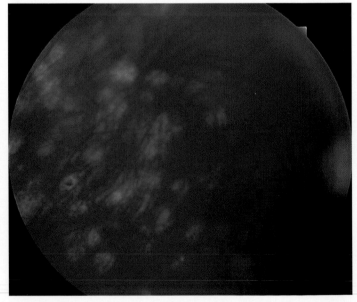

Figure 4.86 Inactive birdshot retinochoroidopathy

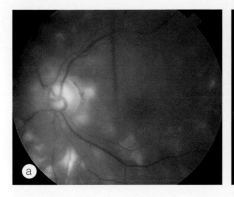
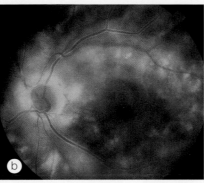

Figure 4.87 Active birdshot chorioretinopathy (see the text)

- Epiretinal membrane formation which may progress to macular pucker is the next most common affecting about 10% of patients.

- CNV which eventually occurs in 6% of patients.

Treatment

Although there is currently no definitive treatment strategy for birdshot retinochoroidopathy, the following should be considered:

1. **Steroids** administered either by periocular injection or systemically give inconsistent results. Because of the chronicity of the disease the complications of longterm systemic steroids therapy are frequently significant and may be unacceptable.

2. **Cyclosporin**, in uncontrolled studies, has been shown to be superior to steroid therapy and may prove to be the treatment of choice.

Differential diagnosis

1. **Sarcoidosis** may occasionally mimic birdshot particularly in patients without systemic manifestations.

2. **Multifocal choroiditis and panuveitis**

- *Similarities* – multifocal choroidal lesions and vitritis, chronic course.

- *Differences* – lesions are smaller, better delineated and frequently hyperpigmented.

FURTHER READING

Brod RD. Presumed sarcoid choroidopathy mimicking birdshot retinochoroidopathy. *Am J Ophthalmol* 1990;109:357–358.

Howe, LH, Stanford MR, Graham EM, et al. Choroidal abnormalities in birdshot chorioretinopathy: an indocyanine green angiography study. *Eye* 1997;11:554–559.

Fuerst DJ, Tessler HH, Fishman GA, et al. Birdshot retinochoroidopathy. *Arch Ophthalmol* 1994;102:214–219.

Gasch AT, Smith JA, Whitcup SM. Birdshot retinochoroidopathy. Perspectives. *Br J Ophthalmol* 1999;83:241–249.

Gass JDM. Vitiliginous chorioretinitis. *Arch Ophthalmol* 1981;99:1778–1787.

LeHoang P, Ozdemir N, Benhamou A, et al. HLA-A29.2 subtype associated with birdshot retinochoroidopathy. *Am J Ophthalmol* 1992;113:33–35.

Ryan SJ, Maumenee AE. Birdshot retinochoroidopathy. *Am J Ophthalmol* 1980;89:31–45.

Soubrane G, Bokobza R, Coscas G. Late developing lesions in birdshot retinochoroidopathy. *Am J Ophthalmol* 1990;109:204–210.

Vitale AT, Rodriguez A, Foster CS. Low-dose cyclosporine therapy in the treatment of birdshot retinochoroidopathy. *Ophthalmology* 1994;101:822–831.

Multifocal choroiditis with panuveitis

Diagnosis

Multifocal choroiditis with panuveitis is an uncommon, usually bilateral, recurrent choroidal inflammatory disease. Although the exact etiology is unknown, it has been suggested that Epstein-Barr virus infection may be responsible. The disease typically occurs during the fourth decade of life and affects females more commonly than males by a 3:1 ratio.

1. **Presentation** is usually with blurring of central vision which may be associated with vitreous floaters and photopsia.

2. **Signs**

- A variable number of discrete, round or ovoid, yellowish-gray lesions located at the level of the RPE and choriocapillaris. The lesions range in diameter from 50–350 μm and involve the posterior pole (Figure 4.88) and periphery.

- Occasionally, in older patients, the lesions are confined to the periphery.

- Vitritis of variable severity is universal and anterior uveitis is present in 50% of cases.

- Mild disc edema may occasionally be present.

- The blind spot may be enlarged.

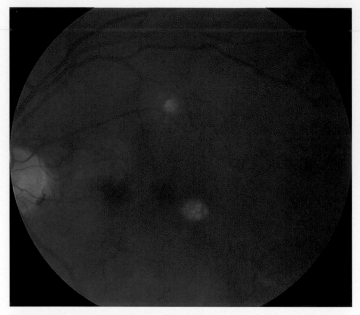

Figure 4.88 Active multifocal choroiditis

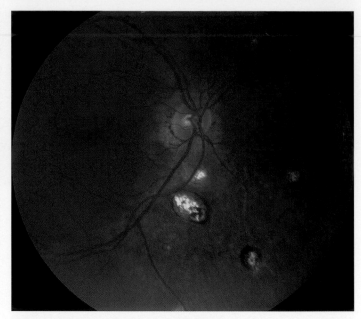

Figure 4.89 Healed multifocal choroiditis

3. **Course** is prolonged and may last many months with the development of new lesions and recurrent inflammatory episodes. Inactive lesions have sharp 'punched-out' margins and pigmented borders (Figure 4.89).

4. **FA** of active lesions shows early blockage and late staining. Old inactive lesions show early hyperfluorescence which subsequently fades during the late phase.

5. **ERG** is normal or mildly reduced.

Prognosis

The prognosis is guarded because of the high rate of visual loss due to one or more of the following:

- Direct involvement of the fovea.

- CNV which may develop in association with old macular lesions.

- Diffuse subretinal fibrosis which is uncommon but serious.

- CME.

Treatment

There is currently no definitive treatment strategy. Conventional therapy with steroids, mainly systemic, is moderately effective with response rates of 50% or more. In order to reduce the complications of long-term systemic steroid therapy other immunosuppressive agents frequently have to be administered. Eyes with CNV may require laser photocoagulation.

Differential diagnosis

1. **Sarcoidosis**

- *Similarities* – multifocal choroiditis with vitritis and anterior uveitis.

- *Differences* – lesions are usually more numerous in the inferior fundus and absence of CNV.

2. **Ocular histoplasmosis**.

- *Similarities* – multifocal punched out chorioretinal scars and CNV.

- *Differences* – absence of intraocular inflammation and fresh lesions do not develop.

3. **Punctate inner choroidopathy**

- *Similarities* – multifocal choroidal lesions affecting the posterior pole and CNV.

- *Differences* – absence of intraocular inflammation and preponderance for young myopic females.

FURTHER READING

Ben Ezra D, Forrester JV. Fundal white dots: the spectrum of a similar pathological process. *Br J Ophthalmol* 1995;79:856–860.

Brown J, Folk JC, Reddy CV, et al. Visual prognosis of multifocal choroiditis, punctate inner choroidopathy, and diffuse subretinal fibrosis syndrome. *Ophthalmology* 1996;103:1100–1105.

Cantrill HL, Folk JC. Multifocal choroiditis associated with progressive subretinal fibrosis. *Am J Ophthalmol* 1986;101:170–180.

Dreyer RF, Gass JDM. Multifocal choroiditis and panuveitis: a syndrome that mimics ocular histoplasmosis. *Arch Ophthalmol* 1984;102:1776–1784.

Dunlop AAS, Cree IA, Hague S, et al. Multifocal choroiditis. Clinicopathologic correlation. *Arch Ophthalmol* 1998;116:801–803.

Lardenoye CWTA, Van der Lelij A, de Loos WS, et al. Peripheral multifocal choroiditis. A distinct clinical entity? *Ophthalmology* 1997;104:1820–1826.

Morgan CM, Schatz H. Recurrent multifocal choroiditis. *Ophthalmology* 1986;93:1138–1147.

Nozik RA, Dorsch W. A new chorioretinopathy associated with anterior uveitis. *Am J Ophthalmol* 1973;76:758–762.

Punctate inner choroidopathy

Diagnosis

Punctate inner choroidopathy (PIC) is an uncommon, idiopathic disease which typically affects young myopic women. Both eyes are frequently involved, but not simultaneosly.

1. **Presentation** is with blurring of central vision or paracentral scotomas which may be associated with photopsia.

2. **Signs**

- Multiple, small, yellow, indistinct spots at the level of the inner choroid. The lesions are all of the same age, range in diameter from 100–300 μm, and principally involve the posterior pole (Figure 4.90a).

- Plentiful lesions occasionally may be associated with a serous sensory retinal detachment.

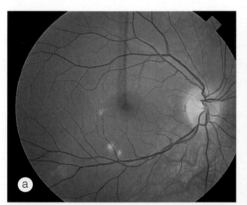
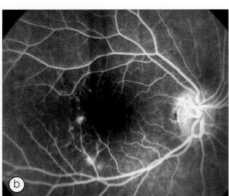
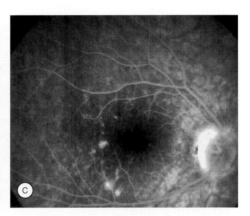

Figure 4.90 Punctate inner choroidopathy (see the text)

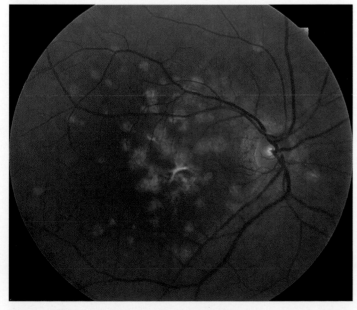

Figure 4.91 Inactive punctate inner choroidopathy

- Absence of intraocular inflammation.

3. **Course**

- After a few weeks the acute lesions resolve to leave behind sharply demarcated atrophic scars.

- With time, the scars may enlarge and become pigmented (Figure 4.91).

- After a variable period of time the fellow eye frequently becomes similarly involved.

4. **FA** shows hyperfluorescence of the lesions due to RPE window defects (see Figure 4.90b and 4.90c).

5. **ERG** is normal.

Prognosis

The prognosis is guarded, because central vision may become compromised by either foveal involvement by a lesion (Figure 4.92) or the development of CNV from one of the scars

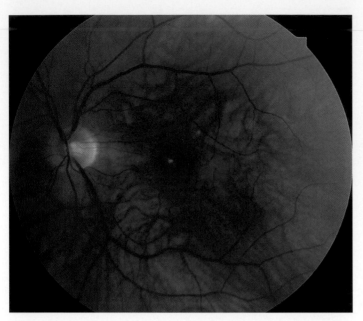

Figure 4.92 Fresh punctate inner choroidopathy involving the fovea

which usually occurs within the first year of presentation (see below).

Treatment

There is no medical treatment for PIC. Eyes with extrafoveal CNV may benefit from laser photocoagulation. It has also been suggested that systemic steroid therapy in patients with subfoveal CNV may reduce subretinal vascular leakage and stabilize vision. Surgical excision of subfoveal CNV may be appropriate in selected cases.

Differential diagnosis

1. Multifocal choroiditis and panuveitis

- *Similarities* – similar lesions when they affect the posterior pole and CNV.

- *Differences* – presence of intraocular inflammation and involvement of the peripheral fundus.

2. Ocular histoplasmosis

- *Similarities* – punched-out chorioretinal scars, presence of CNV and absence of intraocular inflammation.

- *Differences* – peripapillary atrophy, linear peripheral streaks and peripheral lesions.

3. Myopic maculopathy

- *Similarities* – maculopathy, CNV and absence of intraocular inflammation.

- *Differences* – degree of myopia is greater and other degenerative changes are present.

FURTHER READING

Eldlam B, Sener C. Punctate inner choriodopathy and its differential diagnosis. *Ann Ophthalmol* 1991;23:153–158.

Olsen TW, Capone A Jr, Sternberg P Jr, et al. Subfoveal choroidal neovascularization in punctate inner choroidopathy. Surgical management and pathologic findings. *Ophthalmology* 1996;103:2061–2069.

Watzke RC, Packer AJ, Folk JC, et al. Punctate inner choroidopathy. *Am J Ophthalmol* 1984;98:572–584.

Case study

1. History

A 35-year-old woman presented with a four-week history of photopsia followed by distortion of the central vision of her left eye.

2. Examination: left eye

- Visual acuity was 6/36.

- Slitlamp examination showed absence of intra-ocular inflammation.

- Fundus examination showed multiple, deep, yellow spots of variable diameter involving the posterior pole. One large spot, just superonasal to the fovea, was associated with slight retinal edema and was surrounded by small hard exudates (Figure 4.93a).

3. FA

- *Arteriovenous phase* showed hyperfluorescence of the small spots due to RPE window defects. Also present is a larger hyperfluorescent spot supero-nasal to the fovea (Figure 4.93b).

- *Early venous phase* showed increased hyper-fluorescence of the large spot (Figure 4.93c).

- *Late phase* showed an increase in size of the large hyperfluorescent spot due to leakage (Figure 4.93d).

4. Diagnosis

- Juxtafoveal CNV associated with PIC.

5. Treatment

- Laser photocoagulation to CNV.

6. Outcome

- Three months later visual acuity was 6/12 and there was no evidence of recurrence of CNV.

7. Comment

This patient had a favorable result of laser photocoagulation to CNV associated with PIC. Unlike CNV associated with age-related macular degeneration, the long-term prognosis is good as the risk of recurrence is small.

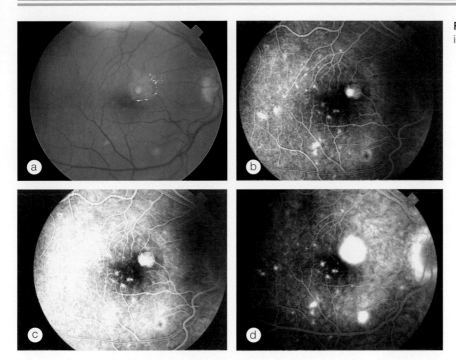

Figure 4.93 CNV associated with punctate inner choriodopathy (see the text)

Multiple evanescent white dot syndrome

Multiple evanescent white dot syndrome (MEWDS) is an uncommon, idiopathic, self-limiting, multifocal inflammatory disease which typically affects healthy young individuals. Females are more commonly affected than males by a 4:1 ratio. The condition is usually unilateral and may be anteceded by a viral-like illness. Although uncommon, it is important to be aware of MEWDS because the subtle signs may be overlooked and a misdiagnosis made of a more serious disorder such as retrobulbar neuritis with its possible implications.

1. **Presentation** is with sudden onset decreased vision or paracentral scotomas which may be associated with photopsia which typically affects the temporal visual field.

2. **Signs**

- Numerous, very small, white dots at the level of the deep retina and RPE involving the posterior pole but sparing the fovea (Figure 4.94a).

Figure 4.94 Active multiple evanescent white dot syndrome (see the text)

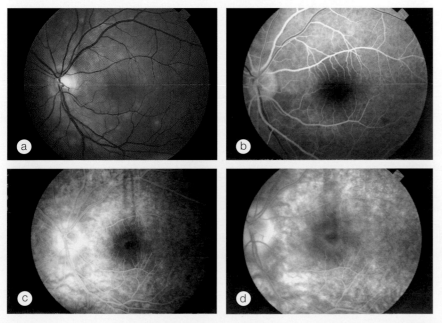

- The fovea has a granular appearance which renders the foveal reflex abnormal or absent.

- Mild vitritis and vasculitis.

- Optic disc edema and enlargement of the physiological blind spot.

3. **Course** lasts a few weeks during which visual acuity recovers, the white dots fade and the disc edema resolves, but the fovea retains its abnormal appearance (Figure 4.95). Recurrences occur in about 10% of cases and a very small minority of patients develop CNV.

4. **FA** of active lesions shows a normal early phase (see Figure 4.94b). The late phases shows hyperfluorescence which may have a 'wreath-like' appearance (see Figure 4.94c and 4.94d).

5. **ERG** shows a decrease in a-wave amplitude.

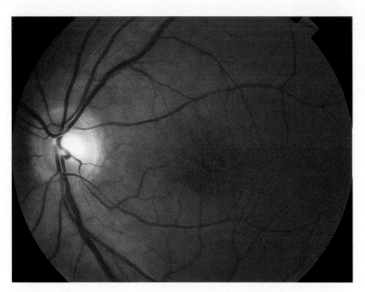

Figure 4.95 Residual foveal granularity in multiple evanescent white dot syndrome

FURTHER READING

Barile GR, Reppucci VS, Schiff WM, et al. Circumpapillary chorioretinopathy in multiple evanescent white dot syndrome. *Retina* 1997;17:75–77.

Borruat FX, Auer CA, Piguet B. Choroidopathy in multiple evanescent white dot syndrome. *Arch Ophthalmol* 1995;113:1569–1570.

Ie D, Glaser BM, Murphy RP, et al. Indocyanine green angiography in multiple evanescent white dot syndrome. *Am J Ophthalmol* 1994;117:7–12.

Jampol LM, Sieving PA, Pugh D, et al. Multiple evanescent white dot syndropme. I. Clinical findings. *Arch Ophthalmol* 1984;102:671–674.

Mamalis N, Daily MJ. Multiple evanescent white dot syndrome. A report of eight cases. *Ophthalmology* 1987;94:1209–1212.

Singh K, de Frank MP, Shults WT, et al. Acute idiopathic blind spot enlargement – a spectrum of disease. *Ophthalmology* 1991;98:497–502.

Acute retinal pigment epitheliitis

Acute retinal pigment epitheliitis is a rare, idiopathic, self-limiting inflammatory condition of the macular RPE. It typically affects otherwise healthy young adults and although there is no treatment the visual prognosis is excellent. The condition is unilateral in 75% of cases.

1. **Presentation** is with sudden onset impairment of central vision which may be associated with metamorphopsia.

2. **Signs**

- The fovea shows a blunted reflex with discrete clusters, of a few, subtle, small, brown or grey spots at the level of the RPE which may be surrounded by hypopigmented yellow halos (Figure 4.96).

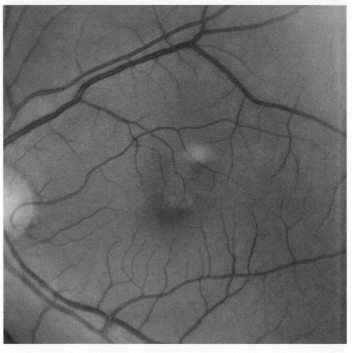

Figure 4.96 Acute retinal pigment epitheliitis

- Absence of intraocular inflammation.

3. **FA** shows small hyperfluorescent dots with hypofluorescent centres ('honeycomb' appearance) without leakage (Figure 4.97).

4. **EOG** is decreased.

5. **Course** is 6–12 weeks, during which the acute fundus lesions resolve and visual acuity returns to normal. Innocuous residual pigment clumping at the fovea may remain. Recurrences may occur but are uncommon.

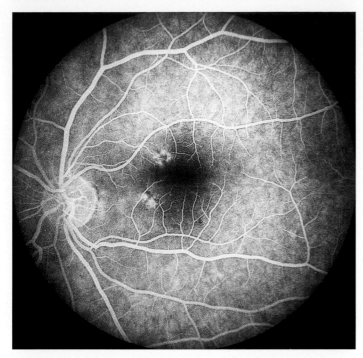

Figure 4.97 FA of acute retinal pigment epitheliitis showing small hyperfluorescent dots with hypofluorescent centres

FURTHER READING

Deutman AF. Acute retinal pigment epitheliitis. *Am J Ophthalmol* 1974;78:571–578.

Eifrig DE, Knobloch WH, Moran JA. Retinal pigment epitheliitis. *Ann Ophthalmol* 1977;9:639–642.

Friedman MW. Bilateral recurrent acute retinal pigment epitheliitis. *Am J Ophthalmol* 1975;79:567–570.

Krill AE, Deutman AF. Acute retinal pigment epitheliitis. *Am J Ophthalmol* 1972;74:193–205.

Luttrull JK. Acute retinal pigment epitheliitis. *Am J Ophthalmol* 1997;123:127–129.

Prost M. Long-term observations of patients with acute retinal pigment epitheliitis. *Ophthalmologica* 1989;199:84–89.

Unilateral acute idiopathic maculopathy

Acute idiopathic maculopathy is a very rare inflammatory condition which typically affects young adults. It is most frequently unilateral and may be preceded by a flu-like illness.

1. **Presentation** is with a unilateral sudden and severe loss of vision.

2. **Signs**

- Wedge-shaped detachment of the sensory retina at the macula with an irregular outline (Figure 4.98a).

- Smaller, grayish subretinal thickening at the level of the RPE beneath the sensory detachment is frequently present.

- Associated features include cells in the posterior vitreous and papillitis.

3. **FA** in the early phase shows minimal subretinal hypofluorescence and hyperfluorescence beneath the sensory retinal detachment (Figure 4.98b). The late phase shows complete staining of the overlying sensory retinal detachment (Figure 4.98d).

4. **Course** is short with complete resolution of the exudative changes and nearly complete recovery of vision. Innocuous residual RPE atrophic changes which may have a 'bulls eye' pattern remain. A few patients may subsequently develop CNV.

FURTHER READING

Freund KB, Yannuzzi LA, Barile GR, et al. The expanding clinical spectrum of unilateral acute idiopathic maculopathy. *Arch Ophthalmol* 1996;114:555–559.

Yannuzzi LA, Jampol LM, Rabb, et al. Unilateral acute idiopathic maculopathy. *Arch Ophthalmol* 1991;109:1411–1416.

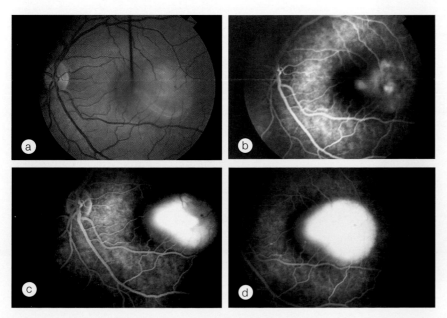

Figure 4.98 Unilateral acute idiopathic maculopathy (see the text)

Neuroretinitis

Neuroretinitis, which is also referred to as Leber is idiopathic stellate neuroretinitis, is an uncommon type of optic neuritis which affects both the optic nerve and retina. Although many cases are idiopathic, neuroretinitis may be associated with a variety of systemic disorders such as viral infections, Lyme disease, cat-scratch disease and syphilis. It is, however, never associated with multiple sclerosis.

1. **Presentation** is with unilateral visual impairment which starts gradually and then becomes most marked after about a week.

2. **Signs**

- Visual acuity is impaired to a variable degree.

- Afferent pupillary conduction defect.

- Impaired colour vision.

- Impaired light brightness appreciation.

- Optic disc swelling (papillitis), which may be associated with splinter-shaped hemorrhages in severe cases, and a macular star figure composed of hard exudates (Figure 4.99) which may not be present initially.

- Peripapillary retinal edema and serous elevation of the macula may be present in some cases.

3. **Course** in most cases lasts between 6–12 months, with return to normal or near-normal visual acuity in the majority of patients with resolution of the papillitis and then of the macular hard exudates. Initially, however, the hard exudates tend to become more prominent as the optic disc swelling is resolving. Recurrences in the same eye are very unusual although some patients may subsequently develop involvement of the other eye.

4. **FA** shows diffuse leakage from superficial disc vessels.

5. **Treatment** depends on the underlying cause. Presumed idiopathic or viral neuroretinitis does not require treatment because there is no evidence that systemic steroid therapy alters either the speed of recovery or the final visual outcome. Systemic antibiotics may be beneficial in patients with associated Lyme disease, cat-scratch disease or syphilis.

FURTHER READING

Bar S, Segal M, Shapiro R, et al. Neuroretinitis associated with cat scratch disease. *Am J Ophthalmol* 1990;110:703–705.

Carroll DM, Franklin RM. Leber's idiopathic stellate retinopathy. *Am J Ophthalmol* 1982;93:96–101.

Dreyer RF, Hopen G, Gass DM, et al. Leber's idiopathic stellate neuroretinitis. *Arch Ophthalmol* 1984;102:1140–1145.

Foster RE, Lowder CY, Meisler DM, et al. Mumps neuroretinitis in an adolescent. *Am J Ophthalmol* 1990;110:91–93.

Maitland CG, Miller NR. Neuroretinitis. *Arch Ophthalmol* 1984;102:1146–1150.

Acute macular neuroretinopathy

Acute macular neuroretinopathy is a rare idiopathic condition that typically affects healthy females between the second and fourth decades of life. The disease may affect one or both eyes and may be preceded by a flu-like illness. Although there is no treatment the condition is self-limited.

1. **Presentation** is with sudden visual impairment which may be associated with paracentral scotomas.

2. **Signs**

- Several, small, circular or oval, dark red or brown parafoveal lesions within the deep retina or RPE.

- Absence of intraocular inflammation.

3. **FA** is normal.

4. **ERG** is normal.

5. **Course** lasts several months with gradual improvement in visual symptoms and fading but not complete resolution of the fundus lesions. Recurrences are uncommon.

FURTHER READING

Bos PJM, Deutman AF. Acute macular neuroretinopathy. *Am J Ophthalmol* 1975;80:573–584.

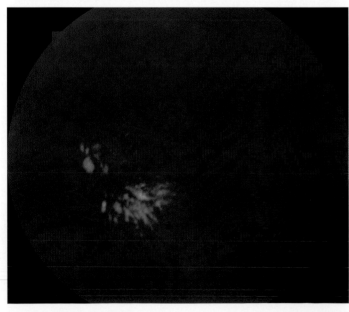

Figure 4.99 Neuroretinitis

Acute multifocal retinitis

Acute multifocal retinitis is a very rare idiopathic condition that typically affects healthy, young to middle aged adults. It may be preceded by a flu-like illness. The condition is frequently bilateral.

1. **Presentation** is with sudden onset of mild visual loss.

2. **Signs**

- Several, white, retinal infiltrates of variable size (Figure 4.100).

- Mild vitritis and disc edema are frequent.

- A macular star is present in a few cases.

3. **FA** shows early hypofluorescence due to blockage with late staining of the lesions.

4. **Course** lasts two to four months with resolution of the fundus lesions and return of visual acuity to normal with little or no residual fundus changes. Small retinal branch artery occlusions may occur in a minority of cases.

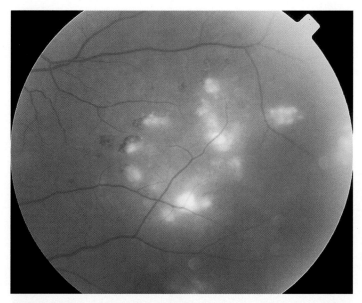

Figure 4.100 Acute multifocal retinitis

Progressive subretinal fibrosis and uveitis syndrome

The progressive subretinal fibrosis and uveitis syndrome is a rare, idiopathic, bilateral condition which typically affects healthy young adult females.

1. **Presentation** is with gradual unilateral blurring of vision although both eyes are usually eventually involved.

2. **Signs**

- Yellow, indistinct subretinal lesions which coalesce into dirty-yellow mounds.

- Vitritis.

3. **Course** is gradual with expansion of the lesions to involve most of the fundus. The prognosis is poor because of subretinal opaque bands and RPE changes at the macula (Figure 4.101).

4. **ERG** is decreased.

5. **Treatment** with systemic steroids is usually not effective, although there are anecdotal reports that it may protect the fellow eye. Other immunosuppresive agents may, however, have some benefit.

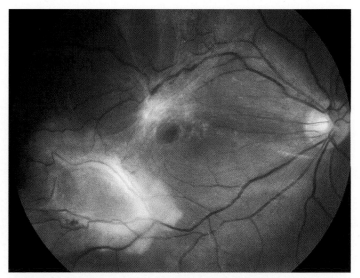

Figure 4.101 Progressive subretinal fibrosis and uveitis syndrome

FURTHER READING

Cunningham ET Jr, Schatz H, McDonald HR, et al. Acute multifocal retinitis. *Am J Ophthalmol* 1997;123:347–357.
Foster RE, Gutman FA, Myers SM, et al. Acute multifocal inner retinitis. *Am J Ophthalmol* 1991;111:673–681.
Golstein BG, Pavan PR. Retinal infiltrates in six patients with an associated viral syndrome. *Retina* 1985;5:144–150.

FURTHER READING

Palestine AG, Nussenblatt RB, Parver LM, et al. Progressive subretinal fibriosis and uveitis. *Br J Ophthalmol* 1984;68:667–673.
Palestine AG, Nussenblatt RB, Chan CC, et al. Histopathology of the subretinal fibrosis and uveitis syndrome. *Ophthalmology* 1985;92:838–844.

Acute zonal outer retinopathies

The acute zonal outer retinopathies (AZOR) are a group of very rare, idiopathic syndromes characterized by acute onset of loss of one or more zones of visual field caused by damage to the retinal receptor elements. During the acute stage these syndromes can be subclassified on the basis of ophthalmoscopic and FA characteristics into two types: (a) those with primary retinal receptor damage, and (b) those with combined retinal receptor and RPE involvement (see below). Although AZOR is a rare condition, it is important to be aware of its existence to save the patient inappropriate and unrewarding medical and neurological investigations.

Classification

1. Primary retinal receptor involvement

- *Absence of fundus and FA changes*
  - a. Acute zonal occult outer retinopathy.
  - b. AZOR, occult + multifocal chorioretinal lesions.
  - c. AZOR, occult annular type: white ring.

- *Fundus changes corresponding to zones of visual field loss*
  - a. AZOR, overt retinal type: white retina without FA changes.

2. Combined retinal receptor and RPE involvement

- *Presence of fundus and FA changes*
  - a. AZOR, overt combined retinal and RPE
  - b. AZOR, overt annular type: white or yellow orange ring.

Acute zonal occult outer retinopathy

Because acute zonal occult outer retinopathy is the most common of the AZOR syndromes, it will be discussed in more detail. The condition typically affects healthy, young, frequently myopic women some of whom have an antecedant viral-like illness and is bilateral in 50% of cases.

1. Presentation

- Acute visual loss affecting one or more zones which is frequently associated with photopsia.

- The temporal field is frequently involved but the central field is usually spared.

2. Signs in chronological order are as follows:

- Initially the fundus is normal.

- Several weeks later there may be mild vitritis, attenuation of retinal vessels in the affected zone and occasionally periphlebitis.

- The zones may enlarge, or less frequently they remain the same or improve.

- In 50% of cases visual field loss stabilizes within 4–6 months.

- Late findings include mild RPE mottling and bone-spicule pigmentary changes (Figure 4.102) in 50% of cases, in the remainder the fundus appearance remains normal.

3. ERG amplitudes in the affected area are abnormal.

4. Prognosis is relatively good with a final visual acuity of 6/12 in at least one eye in 85% of cases.

FURTHER READING

Arai M, Nao-I N, Sawada A, et al. Multifocal electroretinogram indicates visual field loss in acute zonal occult outer retinopathy. *Am J Ophthalmol* 1998;126:446–449.

Fekrat S, Wilkinson CP, Chang B, et al. Acute annular outer retinopathy: report of four cases. *Am J Ophthalmol* 2000;130:636–644.

Gass JDM. Acute zonal occult outer retinopathy. Donders lecture. The Netherlands Ophthalmological Society, Maastricht, Holland, June 19, 1992. *J Clin Neuro Ophthalmol* 1993;13:79–97.

Gass JDM. The acute zonal outer retinopathies. Editorial. *Am J Ophthalmol* 2000;130:655–657.

Gass JDM, Stern C. Acute annular outer retinopathy as a variant of acute zonular occult outer retinopathy. *Am J Ophthalmol* 1995;119:330–334.

Holz FG, Kim RY, Schwartz SD, et al. Acute zonal occult outer retinopathy (AZOOR) associated with multifocal choroidopathy. *Eye* 1994;8:77–83.

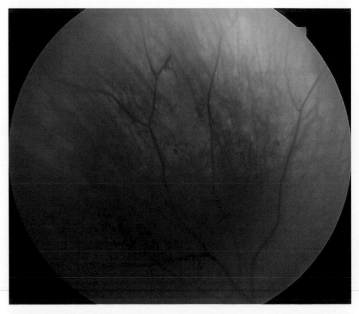

Figure 4.102 Subtle, residual bone-spicule pigmentary changes in acute zonal occult outer retinopathy

Chapter **5**

Hereditary fundus dystrophies

Retinitis pigmentosa

Typical retinitis pigmentosa

Retinitis pigmentosa (RP) is a generic name for a group of hereditary disorders characterized by progressive loss of photoreceptor and RPE function. The prevalence is approximately 1:4000. The clinical features of RP vary among patients and even among family members with the disease. Typical RP is a diffuse, usually bilaterally symmetrical, retinal dystrophy. Although both cones and rods are involved, damage to the rod system is predominant. In some cases the causative gene has been identified.

Inheritance

The age of onset, rate of progression, amount of eventual visual loss and the presence or absence of associated ocular features are frequently related to the mode of inheritance. Retinitis pigmentosa may occur as an isolated disorder, or be inherited as autosomal dominant, autosomal recessive or X-linked. It may occur in association with certain systemic disorders (see below) which are usually autosomal recessive in inheritance. The frequency of the various modes of inheritance differs in various countries.

1. **Isolated**, without any family history, is common and may either represent autosomal recessive inheritance or a fresh autosomal dominant or X-linked mutation.

2. **Autosomal dominant** is also common and has the best prognosis.

3. **Autosomal recessive** is less common than the dominant form and has an intermediate prognosis.

4. **X-linked** is the least common but is the most severe. Female carriers may have normal fundi or show a 'golden-metallic' tapetal reflex temporal to the macula which is virtually pathognomonic. In other cases, carriers may show peripheral retinal atrophy and pigmentary irregularities involving one sector of the fundus.

Diagnosis

The diagnosis of RP is established when the following criteria are present: bilateral involvement, loss of peripheral vision, rod dysfunction and progressive loss of photoreceptor function. The classic clinical triad of RP is: (a) *arteriolar attenuation*; (b) *retinal bone-spicule pigmentation*; and (c) *waxy disc pallor*.

1. **Presentation** is usually with defective dark adaptation (night blindness – nyctalopia). By age 30 years over 75% of patients are symptomatic.

2. **Signs** in chronological order are as follows:

- Arteriolar narrowing, fine dust-like intraretinal pigmentation and loss of pigment from the RPE with a normal optic disc (Figure 5.1). In the past this appearance was referred to as RP *sine pigmento*. A minority of

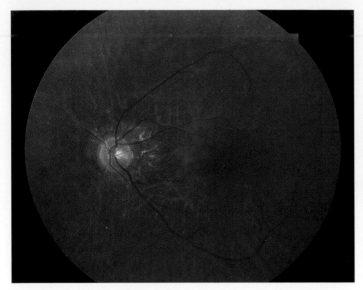

Figure 5.1 Retinitis pigmentosa with minimal pigmentary changes

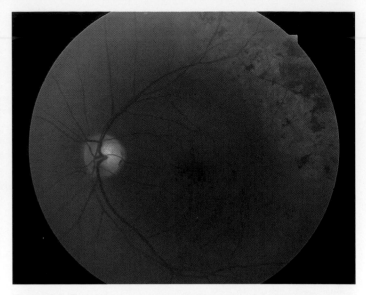

Figure 5.2 Retinitis pigmentosa with 'bone-spicule' pigmentary changes

patients also have scattered white dots which are most numerous at the equator. This appearance is referred to as *retinitis punctata albescens*.

- Coarser pigmentary changes with a perivascular 'bone-spicule' configuration, which are initially observed in the mid-retinal periphery and becomes denser with time (Figure 5.2).

- Gradually, the pigmentation spreads both anteriorly (Figure 5.3) and posteriorly (Figure 5.4).

- The three types of maculopathy which may be seen are: atrophic, cellophane and CME. The latter may respond to systemic acetazolamide.

3. **Perimetry** is useful in monitoring the progression of the disease and will show peripheral field loss and a ring-like scotoma.

4. **Dark adaptation testing** may be useful in early cases where the diagnosis is uncertain.

5. **FA**, which is not required to make the diagnosis, shows diffuse hyperfluorescence due to window defects and small areas of hypofluorescence corresponding to masking by pigment (Figure 5.5c and 5.5d).

6. **ERG** is abnormal even during the early stages of the disease, in which the fundus changes are minimal. There is reduced amplitude initially of scotopic and later of the photopic b-wave. There is also delay in time between the flash of light and the peak of the b-wave (delayed implicit time).

7. **EOG** shows an absence of the light rise.

8. **Course** is characterized by gradual but progressive contraction of the visual fields which ultimately leaves only a tiny island of central vision which may eventually be extinguished. At this stage the optic nerve begins to assume a waxy pallor which is the least

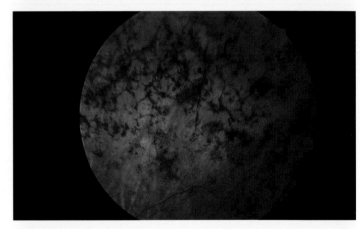

Figure 5.3 Advanced retinitis pigmentosa with anterior involvement

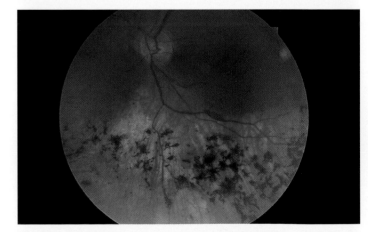

Figure 5.4 Advanced retinitis pigmentosa with posterior involvement

reliable sign of the RP triad. Advanced features are characterized by unmasking of the larger choroidal blood vessels giving the fundus a tessellated appearance, severe arteriolar attenuation and marked optic disc pallor (Figure 5.6).

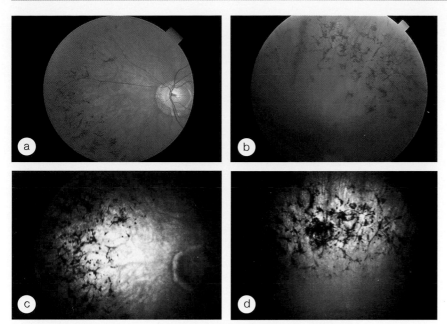

Figure 5.5 Retinitis pigmentosa (see the text)

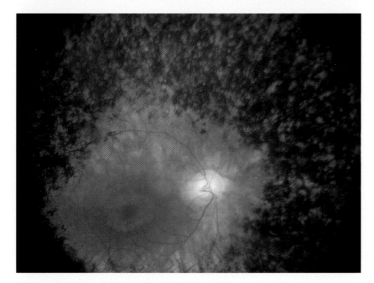

Figure 5.6 Very advanced retinitis pigmentosa

Associated ocular conditions

It is important to follow up patients with RP because they may develop other vision-threatening complications, some of which may be amenable to treatment.

1. **Posterior subcapsular cataracts** are common in all forms of RP. Extraction often leads to visual improvement, particularly in milder forms of RP.

2. **Open-angle glaucoma** occurs in 3% of patients.

3. **Myopia** is frequent.

4. **Keratoconus** is uncommon.

5. **Vitreous changes**, which are common, consist of posterior vitreous detachment and occasionally intermediate uveitis.

6. **Optic disc drusen** are more frequently seen in patients with RP than in normals.

Prognosis

The prognosis in the long-term is poor, with eventual loss of central vision resulting from direct involvement of the fovea by RP itself or maculopathy. It has been suggested that daily administration of supplemental vitamin A, if instituted early, may retard the progression of RP. The overall prognosis is as follows:

- About 25% of patients maintain good visual acuity and are able to read throughout their working life, despite unrecordable ERG and 2–3° central field.

- Under the age of 20 years, only a few patients will have a visual acuity of 6/60 or worse.

- By the age of 50 years an appreciable number will have very poor visual acuity.

Differential diagnosis

The following conditions should be considered in the differential diagnosis of advanced RP.

1. **End-stage chloroquine retinopathy**

- *Similarities* – bilateral loss of the RPE with unmasking of choroidal vessels and arteriolar attenuation.

- *Differences* – pigmentary changes do not have a paravascular 'bone corpuscle' configuration; optic atrophy is not waxy.

2. **End-stage thioridazine retinopathy**

- *Similarities* – bilateral diffuse loss of RPE.

- *Differences* – the pigmentary changes are plaque-like and there is no nyctalopia.

3. End-stage syphilic neuroretinitis

- *Similarities* – gross restriction of visual fields, vascular attenuation and pigmentary changes.

- *Differences* – nyctalopia is not severe, asymmetrical involvement and mild or absent choroidal unmasking.

4. Cancer-related retinopathy

- *Similarities* – nyctalopia, restriction of peripheral visual field, arteriolar attenuation and extinguished ERG.

- *Differences* – more rapid course and mild or absent pigmentary changes.

Atypical retinitis pigmentosa

1. Sector RP is characterized by involvement of only one quadrant (usually nasal) (Figure 5.7) or one half (usually inferior) of the fundus. Progression is slow and many cases remain stationary.

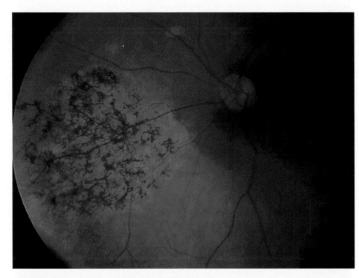

Figure 5.7 Sector retinitis pigmentosa

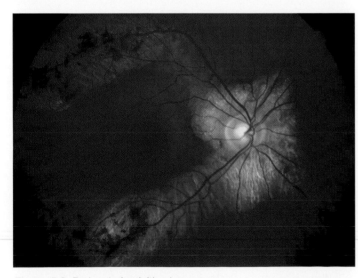

Figure 5.8 Pericentral retinitis pigmentosa

2. Pericentral RP in which the pigmentary abnormalities eminate from the disc and extend along the temporal arcades and nasal to the disc (Figure 5.8).

Systemic associations

Retinitis pigmentosa, often of the atypical type, may be associated with a wide variety of systemic disorders. Only the more important associations are described.

Bassen-Kornzweig syndrome

Bassen-Kornzweig syndrome is a rare disease characterized by deficiency in beta-lipoprotein resulting in malabsorption and secondary vitamin A deficiency. Jejunal biopsy is diagnostic.

1. Inheritance is autosomal recessive.

2. Presentation is in adolescence with steatorrhea due to fat malabsorption.

3. Signs

- Spinocerebellar ataxia.

- Acanthocytosis in the peripheral blood.

4. Retinopathy develops towards the end of the first decade. The pigment clumps are often larger than in classic RP and are not confined to the equatorial regions. Peripheral white dots are also common.

5. Other ocular features are ophthalmoplegia and ptosis.

6. Treatment with vitamin E, if instituted early, may be beneficial for neurological lesions.

Refsum disease

Refsum disease (heredopathia atactica polyneuritiformis) is a rare inborn error of metabolism due to a deficiency in the enzyme phytanic acid 2-hydroxylase resulting in the accumulation of phytanic acid in the blood and body tissues.

1. Inheritance is autosomal recessive.

2. Presentation is in the second decade with nyctalopia followed by neurological problems.

3. Signs

- Mixed motor and sensory polyneuropathy.

- Cerebellar ataxia.

- Deafness and anosmia.

- Cardiomyopathy.

- Ichthyosis.

- Epiphyseal dysplasia.

- Elevated CSF protein in the absence of pleocytosis (cytoalbuminous inversion).

4. **Retinopathy**, which is not typical RP, is characterized by generalized 'salt-and-pepper' changes.

5. **Other ocular features** are cataract, miotic pupils and prominent corneal nerves.

6. **Treatment**, initially with plasmaphoresis and later with a phytanic-acid-free diet, may prevent progression of both systemic and retinal involvement.

Usher syndrome

Usher syndrome accounts for about 5% of all cases of profound deafness in children, and is responsible for about half of all cases of combined deafness and blindness.

1. **Inheritance** is autosomal recessive.

2. **Subtypes**

- *Usher 1* is characterized by severe congenital deafness with absent vestibular function.

- *Usher 2* is characterized by less severe congenital deafness with normal vestibular function.

- *Usher 3* is characterized by progressive deafness.

3. **RP** develops before puberty in all three subtypes.

Kearns-Sayre syndrome

Kearns-Sayre syndrome is a rare mitochondrial cytopathy associated with mitochondrial DNA deletions.

1. **Presentation** is in childhood or adolescence with an insidious onset of ptosis and progressive external ophthalmoplegia (ocular myopathy).

2. **Signs**

- Heart block which may cause sudden death.

- Ataxia.

- Proximal muscle wasting.

- Short stature.

3. **Retinopathy**, which is not typical RP, is characterized by coarse pigment clumping which principally affects the central fundus.

Bardet-Biedl syndrome

1. **Inheritance** is autosomal recessive.

2. **Signs**

- Mental handicap which is mild to moderate.

- Polydactyly.

- Obesity.

- Hypogenitalism.

- Renal disease.

3. **RP** is serious and almost 75% of patients are blind by the age of 20 years. Some patients develop a bull's eye maculopathy.

FURTHER READING

Berson EL, Sandberg MA, Rosner B, et al. Natural history of retinitis pigmentosa over a three-year period. *Am J Ophthalmol* 1985;99:240–251.

Berson EL, Rosner B, Sandberg MA, et al. Ocular findings in patients with autosomal dominant retinitis pigmentosa and a rhodopsin gene defect (Pro-23-His). *Arch Ophthalmol* 1991;109:92–101.

Berson EL, Rosner B, Sandberg MA, et al. A randomised trial of vitamin-A and vitamin-E supplementation for retinitis pigmentosa. *Arch Ophthalmol* 1993;111:761–772.

Dryja TP. Rhodopsin and autosomal dominant retinitis pigmentosa. *Eye* 1992;6:1–10.

Heckenliveley JR, Rodriguez JA, Daiger SP, et al. Autosomal dominant sectoral retinitis pigmentosa: Two families with transversion mutation in codon 23 of rhodopsin. *Arch Ophthalmol* 1991;109:84–91.

Inglehearn CF. Molecular genetics of human retinal dystrophies. *Eye* 1998;12:571–579.

Jacobson SG, Kemp CM, Sung C-H, et al. Retinal function and rhodopsin levels in autosomal dominant retinitis pigmentosa with rhodopsin mutations. *Am J Ophthalmol* 1991;112:256–271.

Massof RW, Finkelstein D, Starr SJ. Bilateral symmetry of vision disorders in typical retinitis pigmentosa. *Br J Ophthalmol* 1979;63:90–96.

Moore AT, Fitzke FW, Kemp CM, et al. Abnormal dark adaptation kinetics in autosomal dominant sector retinitis pigmentosa due to rhodopsin mutation. *Br J Ophthalmol* 1992;76:465–469.

Skalka W. Asymmetric retinitis pigmentosa, luetic retinopathy and the question of unilateral retinitis pigmentosa. *Acta Ophthalmol* 1979;57:351–357.

Progressive cone dystrophies

The progressive cone dystrophies comprise a heterogenous group of rare disorders. Patients with pure cone dystrophy have initially only cone dysfunction. Those with cone-rod dystrophy have an associated but less severe rod dysfunction. However, in many patients with initially pure cone dysfunction the rod system also becomes subsequently affected. For this reason the description cone-rod dystrophies would be more appropriate. Although inheritance may be autosomal dominant, autosomal recessive or X-linked recessive, most cases are sporadic. The most common established inheritance pattern is autosomal dominant.

1. **Presentation** is usually between the first and third decades with gradual bilateral impairment of central and color vision which may later be associated with photophobia.

2. Signs

- Initially the fundus may be virtually normal although the patient is symptomatic.

- 'Bull's eye' macular lesion is classically described but is not universal (Figure 5.9).

- Mild 'bone-spicule' pigmentary changes may subsequently develop (Figure 5.10).

3. ERG typically shows severely reduced cone responses with preserved rod function, at least in the early stages.

4. FA shows a round hyperfluorescent window defect with a hypofluorescent centre.

5. Color vision defects are varied and can be used in early cases to distinguish between the various subtypes of the disease.

6. Course is characterized by slowly progressive RPE atrophy at the macula (Figure 5.11) and the eventual development of geographic atrophy.

7. Prognosis is dependent on the severity of rod involvement. Patients with the least rod involvement having a better prognosis, at least in the intermediate term, but the long term prognosis is usually poor.

Differential diagnosis

Other hereditary fundus dystrophies that may be associated with a bull's eye maculopathy include the following:

1. Advanced Stargardt disease.

3. Fenestrated sheen dystrophy is a rare dominantly inherited condition which presents in young adult life. Bull's eye maculopathy is a late feature.

3. Benign concentric annular macular dystrophy is a very rare dominantly inherited condition which may cause a mild impairment of central vision.

4. Batten disease.

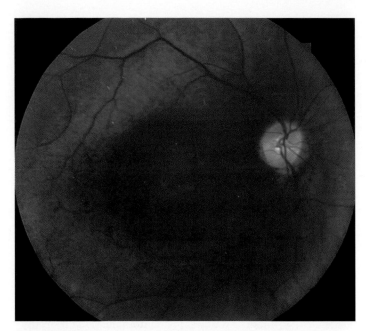

Figure 5.9 Progressive cone dystrophy with bull's eye macular lesions

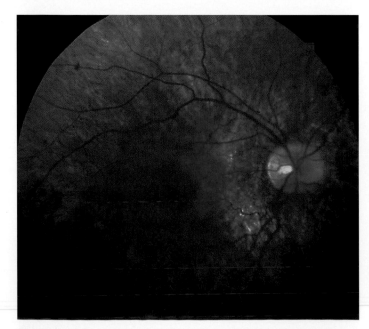

Figure 5.10 Progressive cone dystrophy with mild 'bone-spicule' pigmentary changes

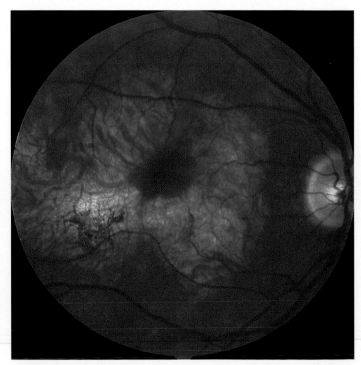

Figure 5.11 Progressive cone dystrophy with RPE atrophy at the macula

FURTHER READING

Fujii N, Shiono T, Wada Y, et al. Autosomal dominant cone-rod dystrophy with negative electroretinogram. *Br J Ophthalmol* 1995;79:916–921.

Jacobson DM, Thompson HS, Bartley JA. X-linked progressive cone dystrophy: clinical characteristics of affected males and female carriers. *Ophthalmology* 1989;96:885–895.

Krauss HR, Heckenlively JR. Visual field changes in cone-rod dystrophy. *Arch Ophthalmol* 1982;100:1784–1790.

Meire F, Bergan AA, de Rouck A, et al. X-linked progressive cone dystrophy: localisation of the gene locus to Xp21–p11.1 by linkage analysis. *Br J Ophthalmol* 1994;78:103–108.

Ripps H, Noble KG, Greenstein VC, et al. Progressive cone dystrophy. *Ophthalmology* 1987;94:1401–1409.

Simunovic MP, Moore AT. The cone dytrophies. *Eye* 1998;12:553–565.

Szlyk J, Fishman GA, Alexander KR, et al. Clinical subtypes of cone-rod dystrophy. *Arch Ophthalmol* 1993;111:781–788.

van Schooneveld MJ, Went LN, Oosterhuis JA, et al. Dominant cone dystrophy starting with blue cone involvement. *Br J Ophthalmol* 1991;75:332–336.

Yagasaki K, Jacobson SG. Cone-rod dystrophy phenotypic diversity by retinal function testing. *Arch Ophthalmol* 1989;107:701–708.

Albinism

Albinism is a genetically determined heterogeneous group of disorders involving deficiency in the enzyme tyrosinase, which mediates the conversion of tyrosine to melanin. The two main types are: (a) *oculocutaneous* and (b) *ocular*. Oculocutaneous albinism may be either tyrosinase-negative or tyrosinase-positive.

Tyrosinase-negative oculocutaneous albinism

Tyrosinase-negative oculocutaneous albinos are incapable of synthesizing melanin. They have blond hair and a very pale skin (Figure 5.12). Inheritance is autosomal recessive. The ocular features are as follows:

1. **Diaphanous blue iris** with complete iris translucency (Figure 5.13) which gives rise to a 'pink-eyed' appearance (Figure 5.14).

2. **Ophthalmoscopy**

- Lack of pigment with conspicuously large choroidal vessels (Figure 5.15).

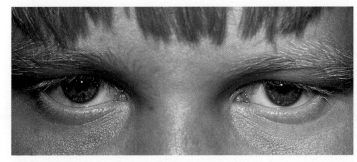

Figure 5.12 Oculocutaneous albinism

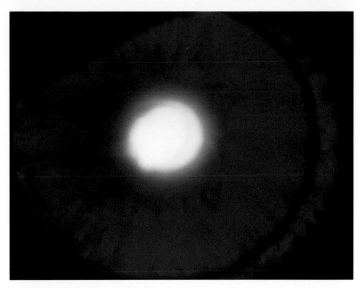

Figure 5.13 Marked iris translucency in albinism

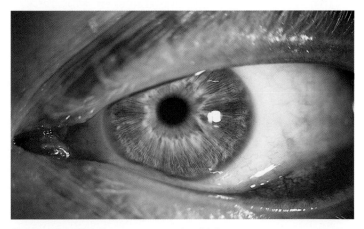

Figure 5.14 Pink eye appearance in albinism

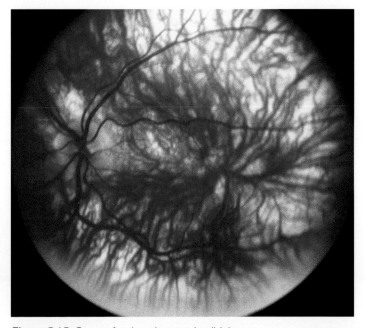

Figure 5.15 Severe fundus changes in albinism

- There may be a marked reduction of vessels forming the perimacular arcades.

- The fovea may not be formed and the optic disc may be hypoplastic.

3. **Refractive errors**, both myopic and hypermetropic, are common and visual acuity is usually less than 6/60.

4. **Nystagmus** is usually pendular and horizontal, and increases on bright illumination. Its severity may lessen with age.

5. **Chiasm** has a decreased number of uncrossed nerve fibers and there are abnormal visual pathways from the lateral geniculate body to the occipital cortex.

Tyrosinase-positive oculocutaneous albinism

Tyrosinase-positive albinos can synthesize variable amounts of melanin and vary in complexion from very fair to normal.

1. **Iris color** may be blue or dark-brown with variable degrees of iris translucency.

2. **Fundus hypopigmentation** is variable (Figure 5.16).

3. **Visual acuity** is usually impaired from lack of differentiation of the fovea.

Associated syndromes

1. **Chediak-Higashi syndrome** is a very rare dominantly inherited life-threatening disorder. It presents in childhood with recurrent pyogenic infections resulting from a leucocyte killing defect. Systemic manifestations include lymphadenopathy and hepatomegaly with an early demise as a result of overwhelming infection or lymphoma.

2. **Hermansky-Pudlak syndrome** is a very rare recessively inherited lysosomal storage disease of the reticuloendothelial syndrome. It is characterized by easy bruising, especially after aspirin ingestion as a result of platelet dysfunction.

Ocular albinism

Clinically, the eyes are predominantly affected and there may be less evident dilution of skin and hair. Inheritance is X-linked or, less commonly, autosomal recessive. Females with X-linked ocular albinism are asymptomatic and have normal vision, although they may show partial iris translucency (Figure 5.17), macular stippling and scattered areas of depigmentation and granularity in the mid-periphery (Figure 5.18).

FURTHER READING

Bergsma DR, Kaiser-Kupfer M. A new form of albinism. *Am J Ophthalmol* 1979;77:837–844.

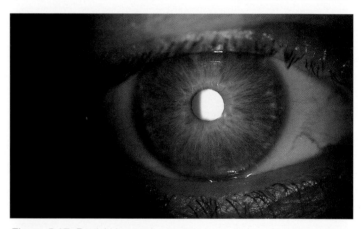

Figure 5.17 Partial iris translucency

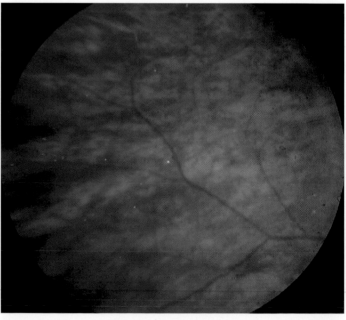

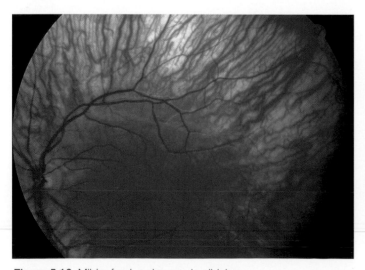

Figure 5.16 Milder fundus changes in albinism

Figure 5.18 Peripheral retinal changes in a carrier of ocular albinism

Castronuovo S, Simon JW, Kandel GL, et al. Variable expression of albinism within a single kindren. *Am J Ophthalmol* 1991;111:419–426.

Charles SJ, Green JS, Grant JW, et al. Clinical features of affected males with X-linked ocular albinism. *Br J Ophthalmol* 1993;77:222–227.

Creel D. Problems of ocular miswiring in albinism, Duane's syndrome and Marcus Gunn phenomenon. *Int Ophthalmol Clin* 1984;24:165–176.

Kriss A, Russell-Eggitt I, Harris CM, et al. Aspects of albinism. *Ophthal Paediatr Genet* 1992;13:89–100.

O'Donnell FE, Green WR, Fleischman JA, et al. X-linked ocular albinism in blacks. *Arch Ophthalmol* 1978;96:1189–1192.

Russell-Eggitt I, Kriss A, Taylor DSI. Albinism in childhood – a flash VEP and ERG study. *Br J Ophthalmol* 1990;74:136–140.

Congenital retinoschisis

Congenital retinoschisis, also called juvenile X-linked retinoschisis, is an uncommon, bilateral, vitreoretinal degeneration which develops early in life. The gene responsible for the disease is designated *XLRS1*. The disease is bilateral but may be asymmetrical with variable severity. The basic defect is present in the Müller cell layer, causing splitting of the retinal nerve fiber layer from the rest of the sensory retina. This differs from acquired (senile) retinoschisis in which there is splitting of the middle retinal layers.

1. **Presentation** is usually between the age of 5 and 10 years with reading difficulties as a result of maculopathy. Less frequently the disease presents in infancy with squint or nystagmus associated with advanced peripheral retinoschisis often with vitreous hemorrhage.

2. **Maculopathy**, which is almost universal, is characterized by the following:

- Foveal schisis is characterized by tiny cystoid spaces with a 'bicycle-wheel' pattern of radial striae (Figure 5.19) which are more apparent when examined with red-free light.

- With time the radial folds become less evident leaving a somewhat blunted foveal reflex (Figure 5.20).

3. **Retinoschisis**, which is present in about 50% of patients, predominantly involves the inferotemporal quadrant.

- The inner wall of the schisis is extremely thin because it consists only of the internal limiting membrane and the retinal nerve fiber layer.

- In older patients, a breakdown of the inner layer breaks may lead to formation of varying degrees of round or oval defects (Figure 5.21).

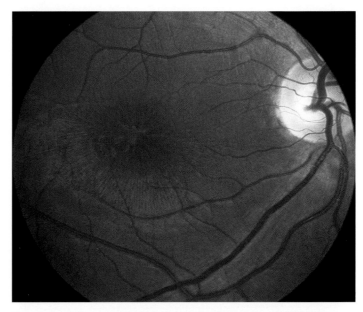

Figure 5.19 Maculopathy in congenital retinoschisis showing the typical 'bicycle-wheel' appearance

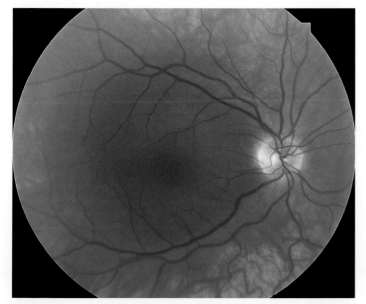

Figure 5.20 Late maculopathy in congenital retinoschisis showing a less evident 'bicycle-wheel' appearance

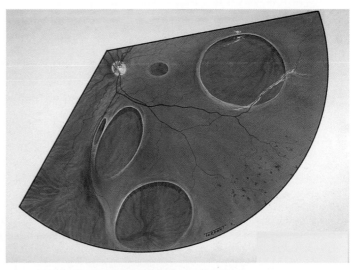

Figure 5.21 Large defects in peripheral congenital retinoschisis

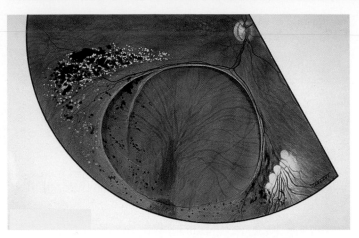

Figure 5.22 Coalescent defects in peripheral congenital retinoschisis

- In extreme cases, these defects may coalesce (Figure 5.22), leaving only retinal blood vessels floating in the vitreous ('vitreous veils').

- The peripheral retina may have a 'golden-glistening' appearance.

4. **Other signs** include perivascular sheathing, nasal dragging of the retinal vessels, retinal flecks, subretinal exudates and neovascularization.

5. **ERG** is characteristic and diagnostic by showing a disproportional decrease in the b-wave as compared with that of the a-wave.

6. **FA** does not show fluorescence of the macular lesions.

7. **Course** is one of progressive visual deterioration during the first two decades of life. After puberty the disease may be stationary or slightly progressive until the fifth or sixth decades when further deterioration occurs.

8. **Prognosis** is poor because of progressive maculopathy. Serious complications of peripheral retinoschisis are vitreous hemorrhage, intraschisis hemorrhage and retinal detachment, which occur in up to 40% of cases. In some cases vitreoretinal surgery for complications may improve the prognosis.

FURTHER READING

Condon GP, Brownstein S, Wang N-S, et al. Congenital hereditary (juvenile X-linked) retinoschisis: histopathologic and ultrastructural findings in three eyes. *Arch Ophthalmol* 1986;104:576–583.

Eksandh LC, Ponjavic V, Ayyagari R, et al. Phenotypic expressions of juvenile X-linked retinoschisis in Swedish families with different mutations in the *XLRS1* gene. *Arch Ophthalmol* 2000;118:1098–1104.

Ferrone PJ, Trese MT, Lewis H. Vitreoretinal surgery of congenital retinoschisis. *Am J Ophthalmol* 1997;123:742–747.

George NDL, Yates JRW, Moore AT. Perspectives. X-linked retinoschisis. *Br J Ophthalmol* 1995;79:697–702.

George NDL, Yates JRW, Moore AT. Clinical features in affected males with X-linked retinoschisis. *Arch Ophthalmol* 1996;114:278–280.

Inoue Y, Yamamoto S, Okada M, et al. X-linked retinoschisis with point mutations in the *XLRS1* gene. *Arch Ophthalmol* 2000;118:93–96.

Regillo CD, Tasman WS, Brown GC. Surgical management of complications associated with X-linked retinoschisis. *Arch Ophthalmol* 1993;111:1080–1086.

Tanna AP, Asrani S, Zeimer R, et al. Optical cross-sectional imaging of the macula with the retinal thickness analyzer in X-linked retinoschisis. *Arch Ophthalmol* 1998;116:1036–1041.

Yamaguchi K, Hara S. Autosomal juvenile retinoschisis without foveal involvement. *Br J Ophthalmol* 1989;73:470–473.

Stargardt disease and fundus flavimaculatus

Stargardt disease and fundus flavimaculatus are regarded as being variants of the same disease despite the fact that they present at different times and have a different prognosis.

Stargardt disease

Stargardt disease is the most common of the hereditary macular dystrophies. Inheritance is usually autosomal recessive and occasionally autosomal dominant.

1. **Presentation** is during childhood with bilateral, gradual impairment of central vision.

2. **Signs** in chronological order are as follows:

- Non-specific mottling at the fovea may be the only finding and malingering may be suspected.

- Oval macular lesion about 1.5 disc diameters in size which has a 'snail-slime' or 'beaten-bronze' appearance (Figure 5.23), which may or may not be surrounded by yellow-white spots or flecks.

- Atrophic maculopathy (Figure 5.24a) which may sometimes assume a bull's-eye configuration.

3. **ERG** and **EOG** are abnormal only in advanced cases when the changes have progressed to diffusely involve the RPE, choroid and sensory retina.

4. **FA**

- Eyes with atrophic maculopathy show hyperfluorescence at the macula and of the surrounding flecks due to RPE window defects (Figure 5.24b–5.24d).

- A 'dark choroid' is seen in about 75% of cases and is caused by blockage of background choroidal fluorescence by lipofuscin deposits within the RPE. It is characterized by absence of normal background fluorescence during dye

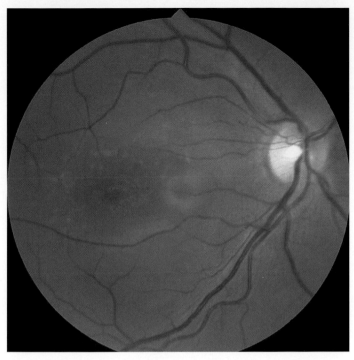

Figure 5.23 Maculopathy in Stargardt disease without flecks

transit resulting in enhanced prominence of the retinal circulation (Figure 5.25).

5. **Course** is slowly progressive with increasing atrophy of the RPE and choriocapillaris at the macula.

6. **Prognosis** is poor. Once visual acuity drops below 6/12 it tends to decrease rapidly and then stabilize at about 6/60 or less due to severe atrophic macular degeneration (Figure 5.26).

Fundus flavimaculatus

1. **Presentation** is in adult life, although in the absence of macular involvement the condition may be asymptomatic and discovered by chance.

2. **Signs** in chronological order, are as follows:

- Bilateral, ill-defined, yellow-white spots or flecks, at the level of the RPE scattered throughout the posterior pole and mid-periphery (Figure 5.27). The lesions may be round, oval, linear, semilunar or pisciform (fish-tail-like).

- The fundus has a vermilion color in about 50% of cases.

3. **FA** shows hypofluorescence of new flecks and hyperfluorescence of old flecks due to associated atrophy of the RPE.

4. **ERG** may be reduced in advanced cases.

5. **Course** is slow with the development of new lesions as older lesions resorb. Fresh lesions are usually dense with distinct borders, whereas older lesions are ill-defined and softer.

6. **Prognosis** is relatively good and patients may remain asymptomatic for many years unless one of the spots or flecks involves the foveola. However, some patients develop significant visual loss due to atrophic maculopathy (Figure 5.28).

Disease patterns

In patients with Stargardt-flavimaculatus four patterns of lesions are seen at a given stage of the disease:

- Maculopathy without flecks (see Figure 5.23).

- Maculopathy with perifoveal flecks (see Figure 5.24).

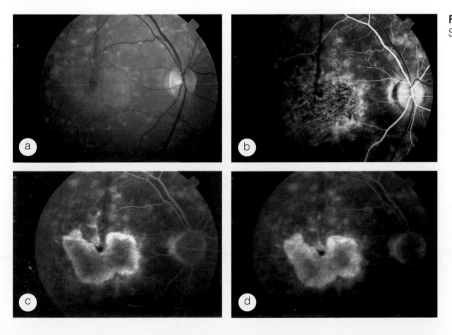

Figure 5.24 Atrophic maculopathy in Stargardt disease (see the text)

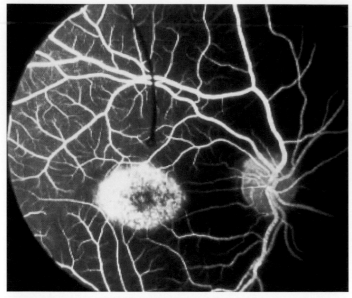

Figure 5.25 FA of Stargardt disease showing a generalized dark choroid

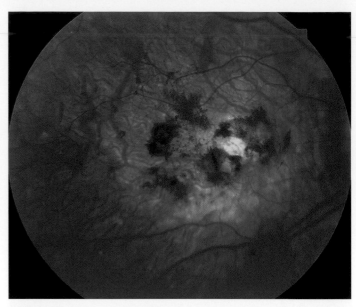

Figure 5.26 End-stage Stargardt disease

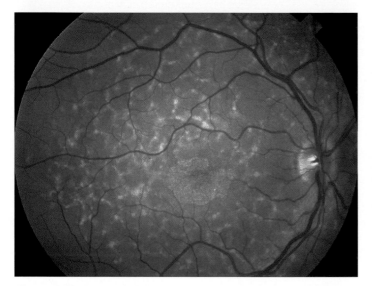

Figure 5.27 Fundus flavimaculatus with mild atrophic maculopathy

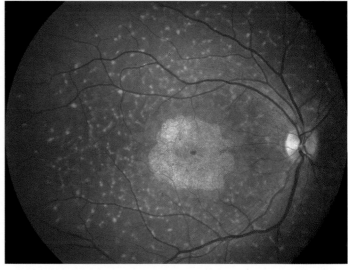

Figure 5.28 Fundus flavimaculatus with severe atrophic maculopathy

- Diffuse flecks without maculopathy (see Figure 5.27).
- Diffuse flecks with maculopathy (see Figure 5.28).

Differential diagnosis of fundus flecks

1. **Benign familial fleck retina**

- *Differences* – shape of flecks is highly variable: many are larger and spare the macula.

2. **Alport syndrome**

- *Differences* – macular flecks are pale and punctate; periphery flecks are confluent.

3. **Early North Carolina macular dystrophy**

- *Differences* – flecks at the macula are smaller and tightly packed together.

4. **Fundus albipunctatus**

- *Differences* – flecks are punctate and spare the macula.

5. **Basal lamina drusen**

- *Differences* – flecks are more numerous, smaller and more subtle.

FURTHER READING

Armstrong JD, Meyer D, Xu S, et al. Long-term follow-up of Stargardt's disease and fundus flavimaculatus. *Ophthalmology* 1998;105:448–458.

Fishman GA, Farber M, Patel BS, et al. Visual acuity loss in patients with Stargardt's macular dystrophy. *Ophthalmology* 1987;94:809–814.

Fishman GA, Farbman JS, Alexander KR. Delayed rod dark adaptation in patients with Stargardt's disease. *Ophthalmology* 1991;98:957–962.

Krill AE, Klein BA. Flecked retina syndrome. *Arch Ophthalmol* 1965;74:496–508.

Lopez PF, Maumenee IH, Cruz Z, et al. Autosomal-dominant fundus flavimaculatus: clinicopathologic correlation. *Ophthalmology* 1988;59:798–809.

Stone EM, Nichols BE, Kimura AE, et al. Clinical features of a Stargardt-like dominant progressive macular dystrophy with genomic linkage to chromosome 6q. *Arch Ophthalmol* 1994;112:765–772.

Weleber RG. Stargardt's macular dystrophy. *Arch Ophthalmol* 1994;112:752–754.

Zhang K, Garibaldi DC, Kniazeva M, et al. A novel mutation in the *ABCR* gene in four patients with autosomal recessive Stargardt's disease. *Am J Ophthalmol* 1999;128:720–724.

Vitelliform macular dystrophies

Juvenile Best disease

Juvenile Best disease is a very rare autosomal dominant condition dominant with variable penetrance and expressively. The EOG is severely subnormal during all stages of the disease as well as in carriers with normal fundi. The macular lesion gradually evolves through five stages as follows:

1. **Stage 0** (pre-vitelliform) is characterized by a subnormal EOG in an asymptomatic child with a normal fundus appearance.

2. **Stage 1** is characterized by pigment mottling at the macula.

3. **Stage 2** (vitelliform) is characterized by the classic 'egg-yolk' or 'sunny-side-up' macular lesion which varies in diameter from 1–5 mm (Figure 5.29). It consist of subretinal deposition of lipofuscin. This stage of the disease is usually detected during the first and second decades of life. Visual acuity may be normal or slightly decreased. FA shows a corresponding area of blocked background choroidal fluorescence (Figure 5.30).

4. **Stage 3** (pseudohypopyon) may occur when part of the lesion becomes absorbed (Figure 5.31). Occasionally, the whole lesion becomes absorbed with little effect on vision.

5. **Stage 4** (vitelliruptive) during which the 'egg-yolk' begins to break up and assumes a 'scrambled egg' appearance (Figure 5.32). At this point the patient usually develops visual impairment.

6. **Prognosis** is reasonably good until the fifth decade, after which visual acuity declines and some patients become legally blind as a result of one of the following macular degenerative changes:

- Hypertrophic scar (Figure 5.33).

- Fibrovascular scar associated with CNV.

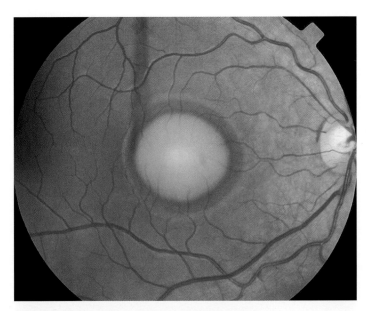

Figure 5.29 Vitelliform stage of juvenile Best disease

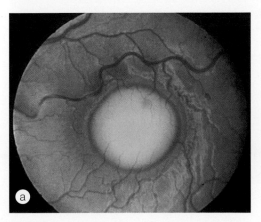

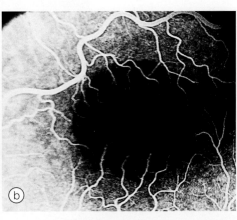

Figure 5.30 Vitelliform stage of juvenile Best disease (see the text)

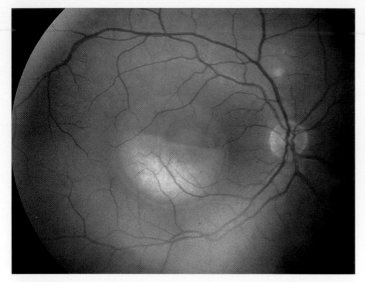

Figure 5.31 Pseudohypopyon stage of juvenile Best disease

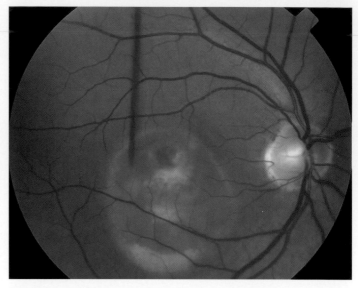

Figure 5.32 Vitelliruptive stage of juvenile Best disease

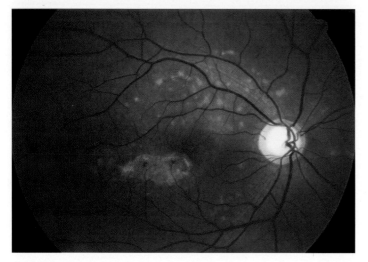

Figure 5.33 End-stage of juvenile Best disease

2. Signs

- Bilateral, symmetrical, round or oval, slightly elevated, yellow, subfoveal deposits which are approximately one-third or one-half disc diameters in size (Figure 5.34).

- The surface of the lesions may contain one or more pigmented spots.

3. ERG is normal.

4. Course – the yellow material tends to fade with time.

5. Prognosis is good in the majority of cases, although some patients develop secondary degenerative changes.

- Geographic atrophy.

- Macular hole formation which may lead to retinal detachment.

Adult vitelliform macular dystrophy

Adult vitelliform macular dystrophy is an uncommon condition which may be inherited as an autosomal dominant trait. In contrast to juvenile Best disease, the foveal lesions are smaller, present later and do not demonstrate the evolutionary changes. It is considered by some authorities to belong to the category of 'pattern dystrophies'.

1. Presentation is usually during the fourth or sixth decades with mild metamorphopsia. However, in many patients the condition may be asymptomatic and discovered by chance.

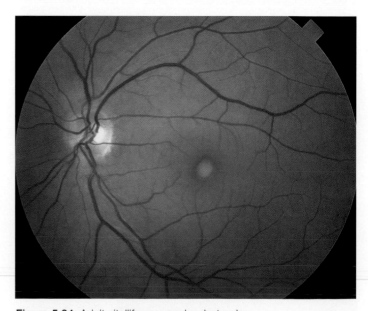

Figure 5.34 Adult vitelliform macular dystrophy

Multifocal Best disease

Multifocal Best disease (Figure 5.35) is a very unusual form of the disease that can occur in patients without a family history. It may develop acutely in adult life and give rise to diagnostic difficulties.

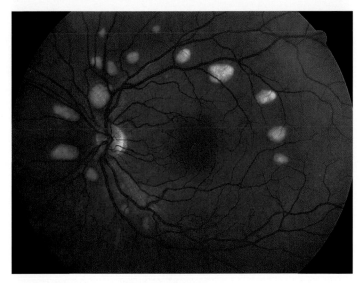

Figure 5.35 Multifocal Best disease

FURTHER READING

Cuilla TA, Frederick AR. Acute progressive multifocal Best's disease. *Am J Ophthalmol* 1997;123:129–131.

Feist RM, White MF Jr, Skalka H, et al. Choroidal neovascularization in a patient with adult foveomacular dystrophy and a mutation in the retinal degeneration slow gene. *Am J Ophthalmol* 1994;118:259–260.

Fishman GA, Baca W, Alexander KR, et al. Visual acuity in patients with Best's vitelliform macular dystrophy. *Ophthalmology* 1990;100:1665–1670.

Miller S. Multifocal Best vitelliform dystrophy. *Arch Ophthalmol* 1977;95:984–990.

Mohler CW, Fine SL. Long-term evaluation of patients with Best's vitelliform dystrophy. *Ophthalmology* 1981;688–692.

O'Gorman S, Flaherty WA, Fishman GA, et al. Histopathologic findings in Best's vitelliform macular dystrophy. *Arch Ophthalmol* 1988;106:1261–1268.

Patrinely JR, Lewis RA, Foni RL. Foveomacular vitelliform dystrophy, adult type. A clinicopathologic study, including electron microscopic observation. *Ophthalmology* 1985;92:1712–1718.

Choroideremia

Choroideremia is a very rare but serious choroidal dystrophy. Inheritance is X-linked recessive so that only males are affected. This has the following implications:

- All daughters of affected fathers will be carriers.

- Half of the sons of female carriers will develop the disease.

- Half of the daughters of female carriers will also be carriers.

1. **Female carriers** show mild, usually innocuous, fundus changes in the form of patchy atrophy and mottling of the RPE and brown granular pigment dispersion in the fundus periphery (Figure 5.36).

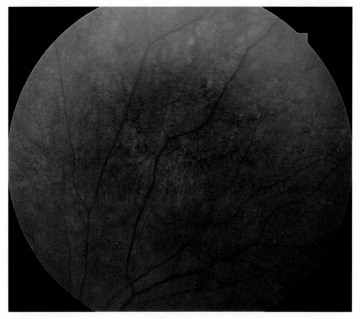

Figure 5.36 Peripheral fundus changes in a carrier of choroideremia

2. **Presentation** is usually in the first decade with nyctalopia.

3. **Signs** in chronological order are as follows:

- Patches of RPE atrophy and clumping involving the mid and far periphery of the fundus.

- Fibrillary vitreous degeneration.

- Patches of choroidal atrophy in the mid periphery (Figure 5.37).

- Diffuse atrophy of the RPE and choriocapillaris making the intermediate and larger choroidal vessels more prominent (Figure 5.38).

- Atrophy of intermediate and larger choroidal vessels with exposure of the underlying sclera (Figure 5.39).

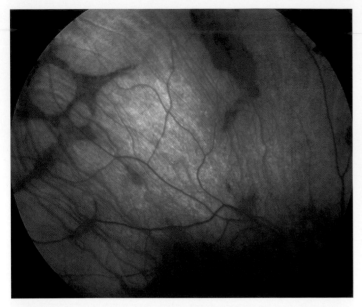

Figure 5.37 Mid-peripheral changes in choroideremia

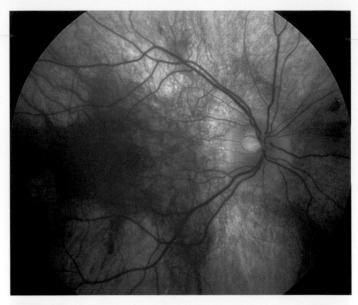

Figure 5.38 Moderately advanced choroideremia

4. **ERG** during the early stages may be normal, but by the end of the first decade the scotopic ERG usually becomes non-recordable and the photopic ERG is severely reduced.

5. **FA** of advanced cases shows the following: the early phase shows normal filling of the retinal and large choroidal vessels but not of the choriocapillaris, hypofluorescence corresponding to the intact fovea and a surrounding area of hyperfluorescence (Figure 5.40b). The late phases show fading of the previously hyperfluorescent areas and new increasing diffuse hyperfluorescence due to staining of the sclera (Figures 5.40c and 5.40d).

6. **Course** is very gradual, with central spread of the atrophic changes with sparing of the macula until very late (Figure 5.40a). In contrast to primary retinal dystrophies, the optic disc and retinal blood vessels remain relatively normal.

7. **Prognosis** is eventually very poor. Although most patients retain useful vision until the sixth decade, there is very severe visual loss thereafter.

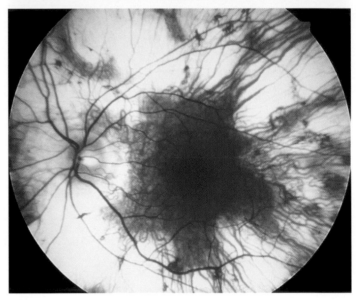

Figure 5.39 Advanced choroideremia

FURTHER READING

Cameron DJ, Fine BS, Shapiro I. Histopathologic observations in choroideremia with emphasis of vascular changes of the uveal tract. *Ophthalmology* 1987;94:187–196.

Flannery JG, Bird AC, Farber DB, et al. A histopathologic study of choroideremia. *Invest Ophthalmol Vis Sci.* 1990;31:229–236.

Ghosh M, McCulloch C, Parker JA. Pathological study in a female carrier of choroideremia. *Can J Ophthalmol* 1988;23:181–186.

Krill AE, Archer D. Classification of the choroidal atrophies. *Am J Ophthalmol* 1971;72:562–585.

Sieving PA, Niffenegger JH, Berson EL. Electroretinographic findings in selected pedigrees with choroideremia. *Am J Ophthalmol* 1986;101:361–367.

Rodrigues MM, Ballintine EJ, Wiggert BN, et al. Choroideremia: a clinical, electron micropscopic, and biochemical report. *Ophthalmology* 1984;91:873–883.

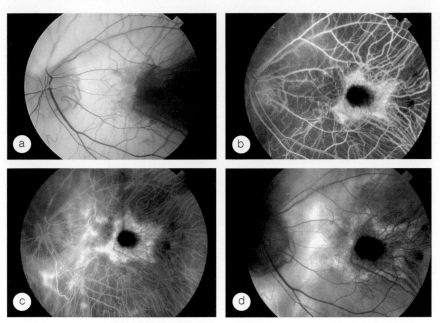

Figure 5.40 End-stage choroideremia (see the text)

Gyrate atrophy

Gyrate atrophy of the choroid and retina is a rare autosomal recessive disease caused by a deficiency of the mitochondrial matrix enzyme ornithine keto-acid aminotransferase. It is associated with increased levels of ornithine in the plasma, urine, CSF and aqueous humor.

1. **Presentation** is in early childhood with the development of axial myopia. Most patients have nyctalopia and reduced peripheral visual fields by the age of ten years.

2. **Signs** in chronological order are as follows:

   • Circular patches of chorioretinal atrophy in the far and mid-periphery (Figure 5.41) associated with vitreous degeneration.

   • Increase in number and size of the lesions which become confluent and form a scalloped border (Figure 5.42).

   • Extreme attenuation of the retinal vasculature, in contrast to choroideremia.

3. **ERG** is either markedly depressed or flat.

4. **Course** is very gradual with central and peripheral spread (Figure 5.43) with sparing of the fovea (Figure 5.44) until very late.

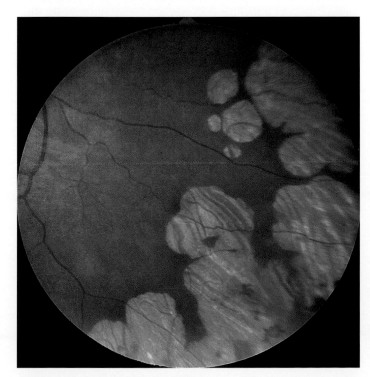

Figure 5.41 Patches of gyrate atrophy

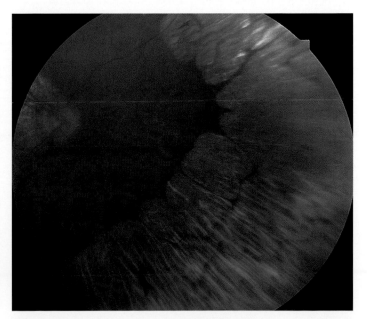

Figure 5.42 Confluent lesions of gyrate atrophy

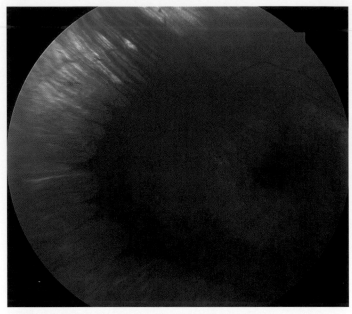

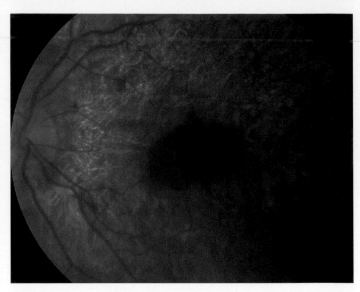

Figure 5.44 Advanced gyrate atrophy

Figure 5.43 Macular involvement with foveal sparing in gyrate atrophy

5. **Prognosis** is poor, with legal blindness occurring by the fourth to seventh decade from macular involvement by the atrophic process, although central vision may fail earlier as a result of CME, epiretinal membrane formation or the development of posterior subcapsular cataract.

6. **Treatment**. There are two clinically different subtypes of gyrate atrophy based on response to pyridoxine (vitamin B6), which may normalize plasma and urinary ornithine levels. Patients responsive to vitamin B6 generally have a less severe and more slowly progressive clinical course than patients who are not responsive. Reduction in ornithine levels with an arginine-restricted diet is also beneficial in slowing progression of gyrate atrophy.

FURTHER READING

Feldman RB, Mayo SS, Robertson DM, et al. Epiretinal membrane and cystoid macular edema in gyrate atrophy of the choroid and retina. *Retina* 1989;9:139–142.

McCulloch JC, Arshinoff SA, Marliss EB, et al. Hyperornithinemia and gyrate atrophy of the choroid and retina. *Ophthalmology* 1978;85:918–228.

Kaiser-Kupfer MI, Kuwabara T, Askansas V, et al. Systemic manifestations of gyrate atrophy of the choroid and retina. *Ophthalmology* 1981;88:302–306.

Kaiser-Kupfer MI, Caruso RC, Valle D. Gyrate atrophy of the retina and choroid – long-term reduction of ornithine slows retinal degeneration. *Arch Ophthalmol* 1991;109:1539–1548.

Takki KK, Milton RC. The natural history of gyrate atrophy of the choroid and retina. *Ophthalmology* 1981;88:292–301.

Wilson DJ, Weleber RG, Green WR. Ocular clinicopathologic study of gyrate atrophy. *Am J Ophthalmol* 1991;111:24–33.

Cherry-red spot at macula syndromes

The cherry-red spot is the most striking retinal lesion in a rare group of inherited metabolic diseases which comprise the sphingolipidoses. These diseases are characterized by the progressive intracellular storage of excessive quantities of certain glycolipids and phospholipids in various tissues of the body, including the retina. The lipids are stored in the ganglion cell layer of the retina, giving the retina a white appearance. As ganglion cells are absent at the foveola, this area contrasts with the surrounding opaque retina (Figure 5.45). With the passage of time the ganglion cells die and the spot becomes less evident. The late stage of the disease is characterized by atrophy of the retinal nerve fibre layer and consecutive optic atrophy.

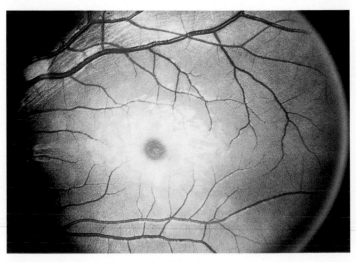

Figure 5.45 Cherry-red spot at the macula

Systemic associations

1. **Tay-Sachs disease** (Gm2 gangliosidosis type 1), also called infantile amaurotic familial idiocy, is an autosomal recessive disease with an onset during the first year of life, usually ending in death before the age of two years. It typically affects the European Jewish population and is characterized by progressive neurological involvement and eventual blindness. A cherry-red spot is present in about 90% of cases.

2. **Niemann-Pick disease** is divided on a clinical and chemical basis into the following four groups:

   * *Group A* with severe early CNS deterioration.

   * *Group B* with normal CNS function.

   * *Group C* with moderate CNS involvement and a slow course.

   * *Group D* with a late onset and eventual severe CNS involvement.
     The incidence of the cherry-red spot is lower than in Tay-Sachs disease.

3. **Sandhoff disease** (Gm2 gangliosidosis type 2) is almost identical with Tay-Sachs disease.

4. **Generalized gangliosidosis** (Gm1 gangliosidosis type 1) is characterized by hypoactivity, edema of the face and extremities, and skeletal anomalies from birth.

5. **Sialidosis types 1 and 2** (cherry-red spot myoclonus syndrome) are characterized by myoclonic jerks, pain in the limbs and unsteadiness. A cherry-red spot may be the initial finding.

Familial dominant drusen

Familial dominant drusen (Doyne honeycomb retinal dystrophy) is an uncommon autosomal dominant condition mapped to chromosome 2p16. The disorder is fully penetrant, although there is great variation in severity of involvement.

1. **Presentation** is during the third to fourth decades of life with the development of asymptomatic and symmetrical fundus lesions.

2. **Signs**, according to disease severity are as follows:

   * *Mild disease* is characterized by a few small, discrete, hard drusen confined to the macula (Figure 5.46). The lesions typically appear during the third decade of life, do not affect visual acuity and carry a good long-term visual prognosis.

   * *Moderate disease* is characterized by large, soft drusen at the posterior pole and peripapillary region (Figure 5.47). It is usually seen after the third decade of life and is associated with normal or mild impairment of visual acuity. The long-term prognosis is guarded, particularly in patients with confluent lesions.

   * *Advanced disease*, which is uncommon, is seen after the fifth decade of life and is associated with profound impairment of visual acuity. One of the following fundus appearances are seen:

   a. Macular drusen associated with subretinal scarring (Figure 5.48) secondary to exudative maculopathy associated with submacular choroidal neovascularization (CNV).

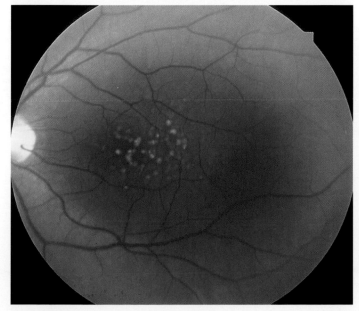

Figure 5.46 Mild familial dominant drusen

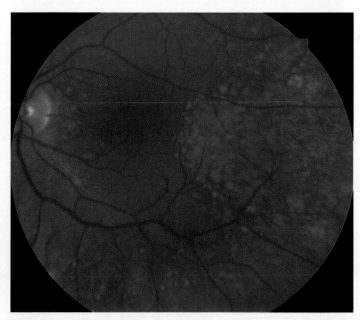

Figure 5.47 Severe familial dominant drusen

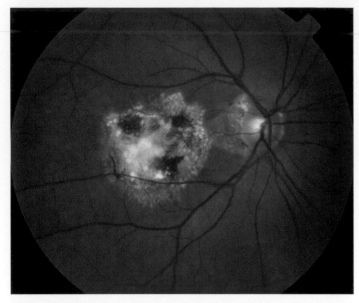

Figure 5.48 Maculopathy in familial dominant drusen

b. Atrophic maculopathy, usually not associated with drusen which had presumably resolved with the onset of retinal atrophy.

3. **ERG** is abnormal only patients with advanced disease.

4. **FA** shows well-defined hyperfluorescent spots due to window defects beginning in the arterial phase. The lesions appear more extensive on FA than seen clinically (Figure 5.49)

FURTHER READING

Deutman AF, Hansen LMAA. Dominantly inherited drusen of Bruch's membrane. *Br J Ophthalmol* 1970;34:373–382.

Evans K, Gregory CY, Wijesuriya SD, et al. Assessment of the phenotype range seen in Doyne honeycomb retinal dystrophy. *Arch Ophthalmol* 1997;115:904–910.

Heon E, Piquet B, Munier F, et al. Linkage of autosomal dominant radial drusen (malattia levantinese) to chromosome 2p16–21. *Arch Ophthalmol* 1996;114:193–198.

Jay M, Plant C, Evans K, et al. Doyne's revisited. *Eye* 1996;10:469–472.

Piquet B, Haimovici R, Bird AC. Dominantly inherited drusen represent more than one disorder. *Eye* 1995;9:34–41.

Sorsby pseudo-inflammatory macular dystrophy

Sorsby pseudo-inflammatory macular dystrophy, which is also referred to as hereditary hemorrhagic macular dystrophy, is a very rare but serious condition. Inheritance is autosomal dominant.

1. **Presentation** is during the second and fourth decades with initially unilateral impairment of central vision and metamorphopsia.

2. **Signs**. Yellow-white, confluent spots located along the arcades and nasal to the optic disc (Figure 5.50).

3. **ERG** is normal.

4. **Prognosis** is poor due to the development, during the fifth decade of life, of exudative maculopathy (Figure 5.51) and subsequent subretinal scarring (Figure 5.52); similar to that seen in age-related macular degeneration.

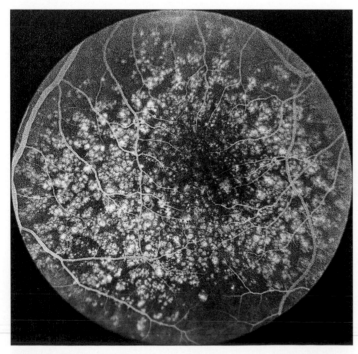

Figure 5.49 FA in familial dominant drusen showing well-defined hyperfluorescent spots due to window defects

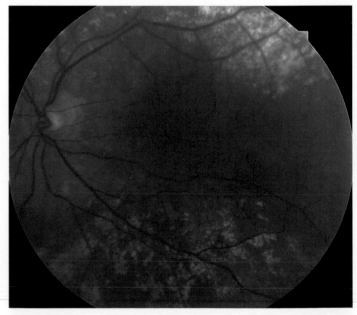

Figure 5.50 Early Sorsby pseudo-inflammatory macular dystrophy showing confluent spots along the arcades

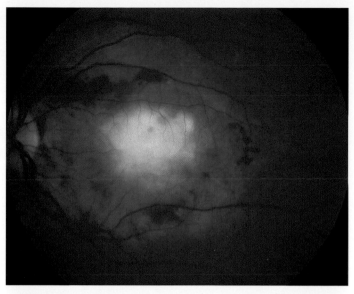

Figure 5.51 Exudative maculopathy in Sorsby pseudo-inflammatory macular dystrophy

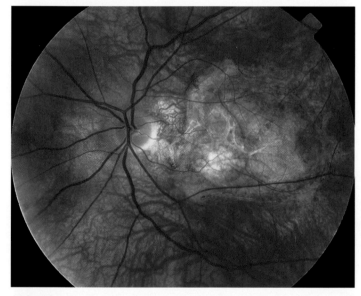

Figure 5.52 End-stage Sorsby pseudo-inflammatory macular dystrophy

FURTHER READING

Capon MR, Marshall J, Kraff JI, et al. Sorsby's fundus dystrophy. A light and electron microscopic study. *Ophthalmology* 1989;96:1769–1777.

Carr RE, Noble KG, Nasaduke I. Hereditary hemorrhagic macular dystrophy. *Am J Ophthalmol* 1978;85:318–328.

Forsius HR, Eriksson AW, Suvanta EA, et al. Pseudoinflammatory fundus dystrophy with autosomal recessive inheritance. *Am J Ophthalmol* 1982;94:634–639.

Hamilton WK, Ewing CC, Ives EJ, et al. Sorsby's fundus dystrophy. *Ophthalmology* 1989;96:1755–1762.

Polkinghorne PJ, Capon MRC, Berninger T, et al. Sorsby's fundus dystrophy. *Ophthalmology* 1989;96:1763–1768.

North Carolina macular dystrophy

North Carolina macular dystrophy is a very rare but serious condition. Inheritance is autosomal dominant with complete penetrance but highly variable expressivity.

1. **Presentation** is during the second decade with the development of asymptomatic fundus lesions.

2. **Signs** can be grades as follows:

- *Grade 1* is characterized by yellow-white, drusen-like deposits at the periphery (Figure 5.53) and the macula with normal visual acuity. The long-term visual prognosis is excellent and most patients remain asymptomatic.

- *Grade 2* is characterized by deep, confluent macular deposits (Figure 5.54). The long-term visual prognosis is less favorable because some patients exudative maculopathy (Figure 5.55) and subretinal scarring (Figure 5.56).

- *Grade 3* is characterized by bilateral coloboma-like atrophic macular lesions (Figure 5.57) which are associated with variable impairment of visual acuity (6/12 to 3/60).

3 **ERG** is normal.

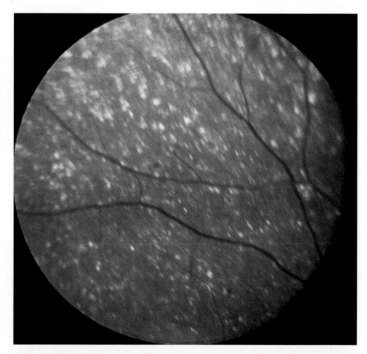

Figure 5.53 Grade 1 of North Carolina macular dystrophy

FURTHER READING

Small KW, Hermson V, Gurney N, et al. North Carolina macular dystrophy and central areolar choroidal pigment epithelial dystrophy: one family, one disease. *Arch Ophthalmol* 1992;110:515–518.

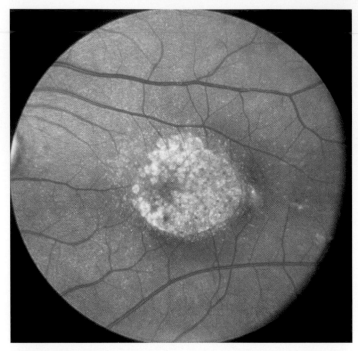

Figure 5.54 Grade 2 of North Carolina macular dystrophy

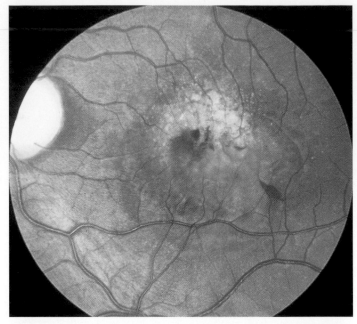

Figure 5.55 Exudative maculopathy in grade 2 North Carolina macular dystrophy

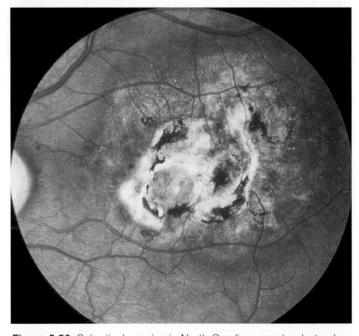

Figure 5.56 Subretinal scarring in North Carolina macular dystrophy

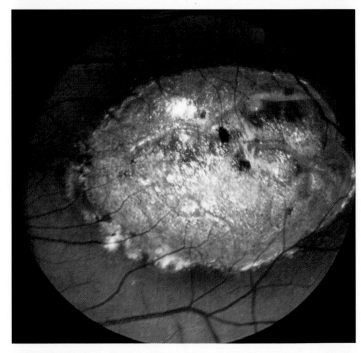

Figure 5.57 Grade 3 of North Carolina macular dystrophy

Butterfly dystrophy

Butterfly dystrophy is a rare and relatively innocuous condition. Inheritance is usually autosomal dominant.

1. **Presentation** is at any time between the early teens and middle-age, which may be asymptomatic or associated with mild disturbance of central vision.

2. **Signs** include yellow pigment at the center of the macula arranged in a triradiate manner (Figure 5.58).

3. **ERG** is normal.

4. **Prognosis** is generally good, although a minority of patients may develop visual impairment.

FURTHER READING

Deutman AF, van Blommestein JDA, Henkes HE, et al. Butterfly-shaped pigment dystrophy of the fovea. *Arch Ophthalmol* 1970;83:558–569.

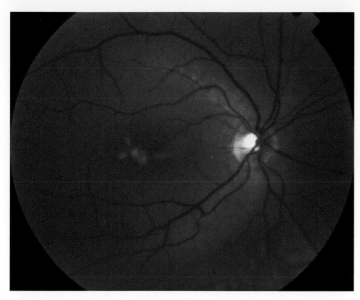

Figure 5.58 Butterfly dystrophy

Dominant cystoid macular edema

Dominant cystoid macular oedema (CME) is an extremely rare but serious condition. Inheritance is autosomal dominant.

1. Presentation is during the first decade with gradual bilateral blurring of central vision.

2. Signs

- Bilateral CME (Figure 5.59) secondary to parafoveal capillary leakage which does not respond to treatment with systemic acetazolamide.

3. FA shows the typical flower-petal pattern of leakage at the fovea (see Figure 2.48).

4. ERG is normal

5. Prognosis is poor because the disease is progressive with the eventual development of pericentric pigmentaty changes and a decline of visual acuity to counting fingers.

FURTHER READING

Loeffler KU, Li Z-L, Fishman GA, et al. Dominantly inherited cystoid macular edema. A histopathologic study. *Ophthalmology* 1992;99:1385–1392.

Central areolar choroidal dystrophy

Central areolar choroidal dystrophy is a very rare but serious condition. Inheritance is autosomal dominant.

1 Presentation is in the fourth decade with gradual, bilateral impairment of central vision.

2. Signs in chronological order are as follows:

- Non-specific RPE changes at the macula.

- Areas of RPE atrophy and loss of the choriocapillaris at the macula (Figure 5.60).

- Geographic atrophy characterized by circumscribed macular lesions between 1–3 disc diameters in size within which the larger choroidal vessels are prominent (Figure 5.61).

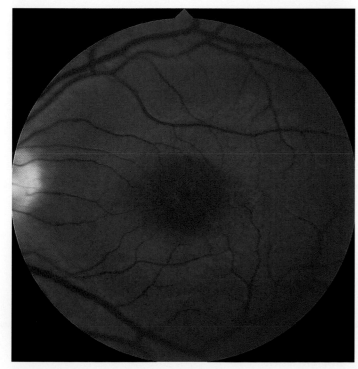

Figure 5.59 Dominant cystoid macular edema

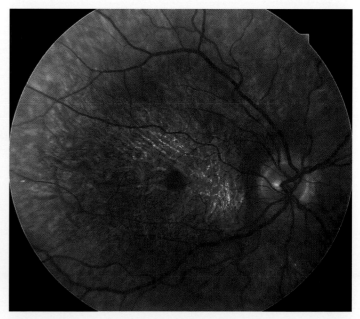

Figure 5.60 Early central areolar choroidal dystrophy

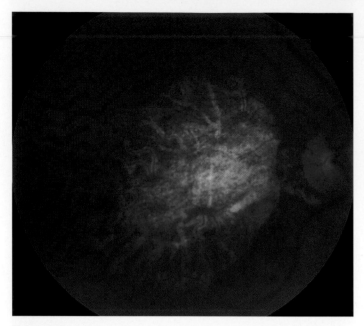

Figure 5.61 Advanced central areolar choroidal dystrophy

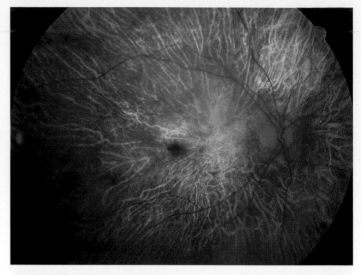

Figure 5.62 Diffuse choroidal atrophy

3. ERG is normal.

4. Prognosis is poor with severe visual loss occurring by the sixth or seventh decades of life.

Diffuse choroidal atrophy

Diffuse choroidal atrophy is a very rare but serious condition. Inheritance is autosomal dominant.

1. Presentation is during the fourth or fifth decades with either impairment of central vision or nyctalopia.

2. Signs in chronological order are as follows:

* Peripapillary and pericentral atrophy of the RPE and choriocapillaris rendering visibility of the larger choroidal vessels.

* Gradual enlargement of the atrophic areas until the entire fundus is affected (Figure 5.62).

* Atrophy of most of the larger choroidal vessels rendering visibility of the sclera (Figure 5.63).

* The retinal vessels may be normal or slightly constricted.

3. ERG is subnormal.

4. Prognosis is very poor because of early macular involvement.

Progressive bifocal chorioretinal atrophy

Progressive bifocal chorioretinal atrophy is an extremely rare but serious condition. Inheritance is autosomal dominant.

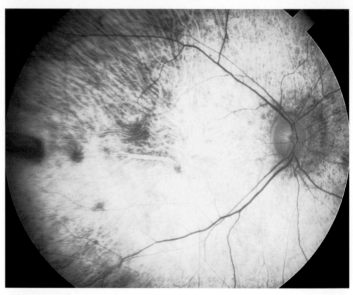

Figure 5.63 End-stage of diffuse choroidal atrophy

1. Presentation is at birth.

2. Signs in chronological order are as follows:

* Focus of chorioretinal atrophy temporal to the disc which enlarges in all directions.

* Later a similar lesion develops nasally.

* The end result are two separate areas of chorioretinal atrophy separated by a normal segment (Figure 5.64).

3. Prognosis is poor because macular involvement is inevitable.

FURTHER READING

Godley BF, Tiffin PA, Evans K, et al. Clinical features of progressive bifocal chorioretinal atrophy: a retinal dystrophy linked to chromosome 6q. *Ophthalmology* 1996;103:893–898.

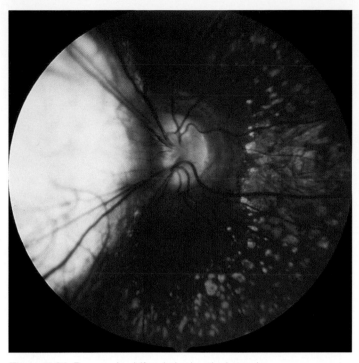

Figure 5.64 Progressive bifocal chorioretinal atrophy

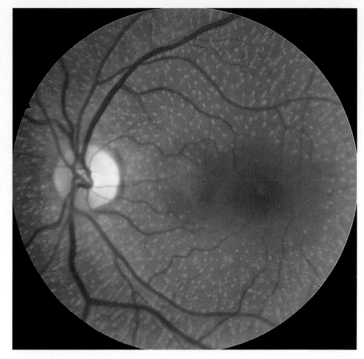

Figure 5.65 Fundus albipunctatus

Fundus albipunctatus

Fundus albipunctatus is a very rare but innocuous condition which is characterized by congenital stationary night blindness. Inheritance is autosomal recessive.

1. Signs

- Normal visual acuity and peripheral visual fields.

- A multitude of tiny yellow-white spots which extend from the posterior pole, where they are most dense, to the midperiphery (Figure 5.65).

- The fovea itself is spared and the retinal vasculature is normal.

2. ERG and **EOG** may be abnormal when tested routinely, but revert to normal on prolonged dark adaptation.

3. Dark adaptation shows marked delay.

4. Prognosis is excellent.

Bietti crystalline dystrophy

Bietti crystalline dystrophy is a very rare condition which predominantly affects males. Inheritance may be either X-linked or autosomal recessive. It is characterized by the deposition of crystals in the peripheral cornea and retina.

1. Presentation is in the third decade of life with progressive visual loss.

2. Signs in chronological order:

- Yellow-white crystals scattered throughout the posterior fundus (Figure 5.66).

- Localized atrophy of the RPE and choriocapillaris at the posterior pole.

- Diffuse atrophy of the choriocapillaris.

- Gradual confluence and expansion of the atrophic areas into the retinal periphery.

3. ERG and **EOG** are subnormal.

4. Prognosis is variable, because the rate of disease progression differs in individual cases.

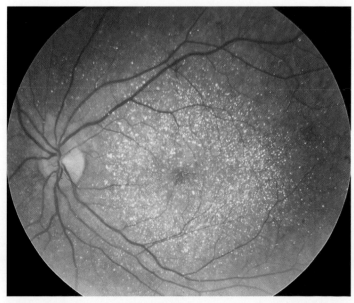

Figure 5.66 Bietti crystalline dystrophy

FURTHER READING

Wilson DJ, Weleber RG, Klein ML, et al. Bietti's crystalline dystrophy. *Arch Ophthalmol* 1989;107:213–221.

Kaiser-Kupfer MI, Chan C, Markello T, et al. Clinical, biochemical and pathologic correlations in Bietti's crystalline dystrophy. *Am J Ophthalmol* 1994;118:567–582.

Alport syndrome

Alport syndrome is a rare abnormality of glomerular basement membrane which is characterized by chronic renal failure and sensorineural deafness. Inheritance is X-linked dominant.

1. **Signs**

* Scattered, pale, yellow, punctate flecks at the macula (Figure 5.67) with normal visual acuity.

* Larger flecks, some of which may be confuent, in the periphery (Figure 5.68).

* Anterior lenticonus (Figure 5.69).

2. **ERG** is usually normal.

3. **Prognosis** is excellent because the retinal changes are innocuous.

FURTHER READING

Gelisken O, Hendrikse F, Schroeder CH, et al. Retinal abnormalities in Alport's syndrome. *Acta Ophthalmol* 1988;66:713–717.

Govan JA. Ocular manifestations of Alport's syndrome. *Br J Ophthalmol* 1983;67:493–503.

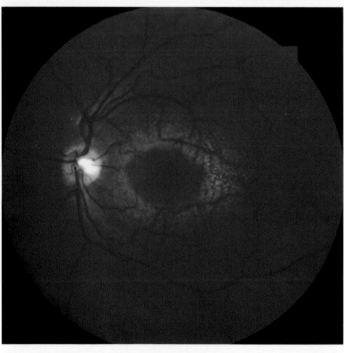

Figure 5.67 Macular flecks in Alport syndrome

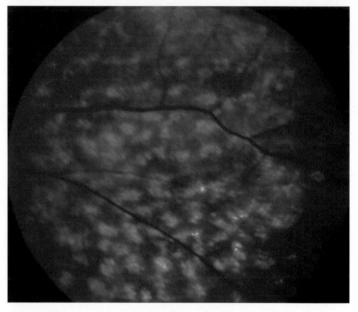

Figure 5.68 Larger peripheral flecks in Alport syndrome

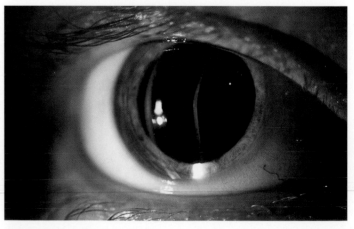

Figure 5.69 Anterior lenticonus